Mother Nature's
HERBAL

Mother Nature's
HERBAL

JUDY GRIFFIN, PH.D.

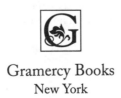

Gramercy Books
New York

This book is dedicated to Mother Nature.

ᴖ

May she always grow and bloom on our land and in our hearts.

This 2000 edition is published by Gramercy Books™, an imprint of Random House Value Publishing, Inc. 280 Park Avenue, New York, N.Y. 10017, by arrangement with Llewellyn Publications, St. Paul, MN

Gramercy Books™ and design are trademarks of Random House Value Publishing, Inc.

Illustrations, unless otherwise noted, are used courtesy of Dover Publications.
Illustrations of aphid, carrot weevil, cutworm, and scale in Chapter 11 by Carrie Westfall
Illustrations of kiva in Chapter 2 and rosemary in Chapter 5 by Fran Gorham
Landscape drawings in Chapter 11 by Pat Cowan
Landscape designs by Judy Griffin and Pat Cowan
Permission to quote from *The Story of Corn* by Betty Fussell (1992) granted by Alfred A. Knopf, Inc., New York

Note: The old-fashioned remedies in this book are historical references used for teaching purposes only. The recipes are not for commercial use or profit. The contents are not meant to diagnose, treat, prescribe, or substitute consultation with a licensed healthcare professional. New herbal recipes should be taken in small amounts to allow the body to adjust.

Random House
New York • Toronto • London • Sydney • Auckland
http://www.randomhouse.com/

Printed and bound in the United States of America.

Library of Congress Cataloging–in–Publication Data

Griffin, Judy.
  Mother nature's herbal / Judy Griffin.
       p. cm.
  Includes bibliographical references and index.
  Previously published: St. Paul, Minn. : Llewellyn Publications, c1997.
  ISBN 0-517-16228-8
    1. Materia medica, Vegetable. 2. Herbals. I. Title.

RS164 .G678 2000
615'.321–dc21

                                                00-037144

9 8 7 6 5 4 3 2 1

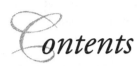

Contents

Section II: *Grow and Use Your Own Herbs*

Section III: *Appendices*

Introduction

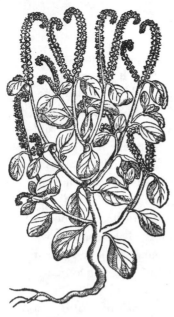

HELIOTROPE

Of herbs, and other country messes,
Which the neat-handed Phyllis dresses.
—Milton

Have we forgotten how simple it is to enhance our own well-being? Have we become too dependent on a quick fix and neglected to really care for our bodies? Have we exchanged the joys of gardening for the drive-through at a fast-food restaurant?

Mother Nature's Herbal is written for those who are ready to learn and experience the beauty, knowledge, and synergy of everything that grows. The focus is on familiar herbs we all know and love. I emphasize companion planting, kitchen gardens, and herbal repellents the way American colonists gardened. The pioneers combined their methods with the knowledge of the Native Americans to develop a unique herbal lore.

America is blessed with herbs from many cultures. Over the past three hundred years, America has experienced a cultural expansion. With each culture, new herbs and foods are introduced to us. My interest in herbs, spices, and foods led me to research these ancient secrets of herbal folk remedies and plants. I learned to appreciate new, and sometimes unusual, herbs by studying the history, cuisine, and medicine of various cultures.

America is blessed with herbs from many cultures.

~

My interest in herbs began in childhood as I learned to grow and use Mediterranean herbs from my parents and great aunt. It greatly intensified after having twins with immune deficiencies, asthma, eczema, anaphylactic shock, and multiple allergic reactions. I had to find new foods the twins could eat in a variety of ethnic grocery stores and remedies and tonics to build their immune system. As I searched for new foods, I began to research each culture's ancient secrets of herbal folk remedies. I attracted many teachers over a period of twenty years, from curanderos to cooks. During this time span, I traveled to several countries and areas in the United States to learn first-hand knowledge of herbal remedies and gain a better understanding of health and disease. I also had my own health to regain after having my last child; my youngest son and I went through several years of health problems that had me searching for remedies for chronic disease.

Each cultural experience expanded my knowledge of health to a greater level of awareness. From the Asians, I learned a system of harmony and balance that leads to radiant health. The Native Americans of many tribes taught me how to reduce acute symptoms with bitter tonics, while the Mediterraneans infused a passion for health that is celebrated in the preparation of every nutritious meal. Africans and African Americans taught me to utilize every part of Nature for remedies. The Far Eastern cultures expanded my knowledge of the immune system by using aromatic essential oils for stress reduction. Mexican and Latin American travels amplified my culinary and horticultural skills with the same skills used by their ancestors thousands of years ago.

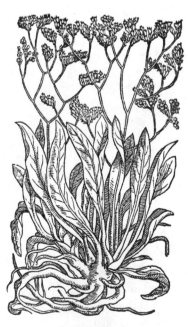

SEA LAVENDER

Every culture has an innate understanding of Nature I named "the path of least resistance." Their knowledge is very deep and experiential, flavored with a great respect for Mother Nature. Foods are a part of their medicine and their medicine is in harmony with Nature, not a separate entity. Healers are accomplished gardeners and cooks. Their understanding of Nature enhances the nurturing qualities of each herb as they plant, nurture, and harvest in rhythm with the cycles of Mother Nature.

Disease is believed by the indigenous natives of many cultures to be caused by an imbalance in the mental, emotional, and physical harmonics of the personality. Their healers teach us how to maintain health and cultivate wellness by treating the person and the condition. The ultimate treatment is to change the lifestyle of the individual to enhance the attitude and conditions that allow the personality to thrive and express unique creativity. Since the body knows no age or order of difficulty, the person often looks younger as health improves.

Herbs are given not only to prevent imbalance, but also to bring out the potential of each individual. Herbs are organically grown or located nearby in the wild. They are utilized in foods, massage, acupuncture, sweats (saunas), aromatherapy, and baths to enhance vital energy, clear the mind, and open the heart, as only the heart can perceive reality without illusion and experience real joy. Besides herbal usage, prevention is encouraged through the practice of moderation, silent contemplation, and ever-expanding goals that will benefit humanity.

Herbs bring out the potential of each individual.

~

These simple folk express passion for life in everything they do. Their food is prepared with precision and care. Herbs and spices are fresh, chosen to enhance each individual's well-being, and served with great pride. Each participates in family time and comments on how the food makes them feel. These statements are generally meant to complement the cook. No one hooks their mouth to their plate and watches television. Rather, an atmosphere of comfort initiates a warm feeling of relaxation. Once again, life is safe to experience and the healing begins.

Folk remedies exude the same innocence and expectation. Suffering is not required to achieve healthiness. Healers see the goodness in each person and help them to express this through better health. The body easily responds to the love that goes into the preparation of every simple tea or compress. Each culture believes in the individual's ability to heal simply by stepping into Mother Nature's herbal.

The last three hundred years have brought us a variety of new cultures with enthusiastic herbalists who want to share their knowledge and expertise. Each chapter of *Mother Nature's Herbal* helps us explore the cuisine, beauty secrets, and folk remedies of selected cultures. The recipes will ignite your curiosity for more new experiences. My teaching is limited to the space available in this book, but not my enthusiasm or experience. There is much more knowledge I want to share with you.

I encourage you to step into *Mother Nature's Herbal* daily and continue to grow and learn from her gentle guidance. My intention is to encourage an understanding of herbs as a part of our cultural heritage. I have no desire to coerce those who doubt the beneficial experience of growing and using herbs. A humble teacher once told me, "It is a great sin to awaken one who is fast asleep." Over the years, I have come to understand that herbs are not for people who "believe," but for people who "know." These are the people Mother Nature awaits with open arms to unveil the ancient secrets of times too long forgotten. When you hear her calling, allow her wisdom to permeate your awareness and attract only those who will inspire, aid, and assist you in attaining your highest goals. Only then will you "walk your own path" and "make your own medicine."

Judy Griffin

SECTION I

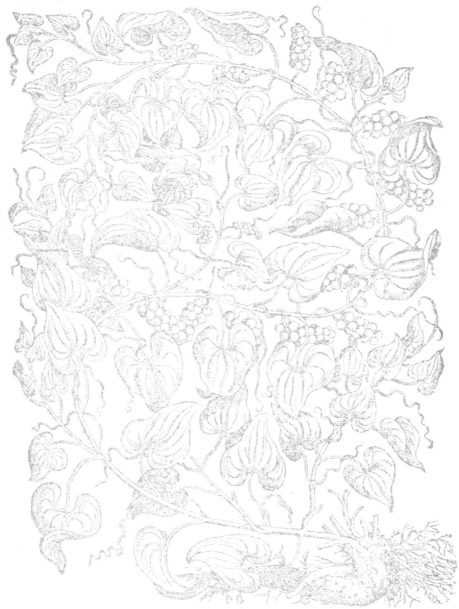

A Cultural Herbal

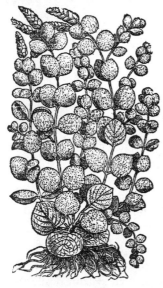

1

A Gardener's Almanac

A Walk in Moontime

Though I am an old man, I am but a young gardener.
—Thomas Jefferson

Traditional folklore has become more popular as our world rapidly advances through a technological revolution. The key to our imagination and development of psyche lies in the customs and beliefs of centuries past. Many gardeners continue to follow the traditions of their ancestors. An example is planting by the moon or hanging sea squill at the entrance of a vineyard to protect the grapes from harm. The following ideas come from the common knowledge once shared by ancient gardeners. I refer to this knowledge as "moontime." It is ageless and timeless, part of a deeper knowledge we inherited. Our true nature is rooted in the soil, making something from nothing and bringing it into full bloom.

Step into moontime and take a walk into a garden of transformed beauty. Ancient gardeners were guided by instinct and imagination. They lived in a world of wonder, populated by fairies, nymphs, elves, trees that talked, and flowers who became guardian spirits. Their world was one of good and evil, with only plants to protect them on the earth level. They planted by the waxing of the moon. The soil was prepared and tested for warmth before sowing by resting one's elbow on the earth. Seeds were germinated overnight in manure tea. Manure was steeped in

Step into moontime and take a walk into a garden of transformed beauty.

~

3

an equal amount of water twenty-four hours, strained and diluted again until a clear amber color appeared. Hard-coated seeds were exposed to frost or buried in the cold to enhance germination. Fine seed was mixed with sand and sprinkled to evenly coat the soil. After sowing, the ground was immediately firmed by walking over it. Another covering of loose soil was applied and the ground firmed again. Seeds were then watered with warm water.

Gardeners followed special traditions for planting food crops and flowers. Beans were sown next to sunflowers in soil laden with hair. Unscented flower seeds were soaked overnight in floral water to produce a perfumed scent. Leeks were planted in open air to protect houses from fire and electrical storms.

Like people, plants had friends. They were planted synergistically to complement each other. Lavender planted near crocus kept the birds away. Black currants planted in a bed of nettles would produce exceptionally fine fruit. Strawberries were mulched with pine needles to produce the juiciest flavor. Garlic cloves were bruised before planting to produce a hardy crop. Roses dressed with tea leaves and banana skins dug into the soil produced the best aromas. Seeds and starts were always planted before sunset to assure a good night's rest before sprouting the next day.

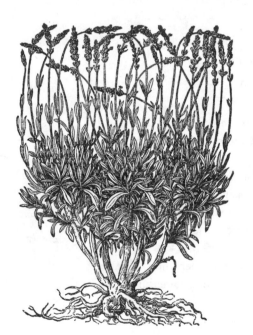

LAVENDER

Gardeners from the past worked diligently to outsmart pests. They accepted bugs as part of Nature and worked to create a balance in their favor. The best deterrents were aromatic herbs, which snails and slugs particularly dislike. In the event of infestation, damaged leaves were removed and tobacco was dusted on the plants. An observant gardener would watch for snails climbing the blades of grass, for wet weather was soon to follow. If birds became a nuisance in newly sown beds, they were deterred by placing potatoes with feathers stuck into them on sticks. Gardeners knew the birds would later be allies, eating unwanted insects and cutworms.

To early farmers, moles represented the power of darkness. Settlers planted milk spurge, *Euphorbia lathyrus,* and herbs high in camphor (such as basil) to deter them. If the moles still posed a problem, long-necked wine bottles were sunk a few inches below ground so wind would produce a high singing sound, driving them to a neighbor's pasture.

Field mice were deterred by watering the plants with a cat's bath water. If there were no cats to be cleaned, prickly holly leaves were scattered amongst the garden with spearmint leaves and chamomile flowers. Mice were also repelled by elder leaves and poisonous oleanders.

Rats were poisoned by the sea squill onion still used commercially today. The smelly valerian was planted as a deterrent and drunk as a sleep-inducing tea by tired farmers.

Wild rabbits were deterred by a liberal planting of onion and foxglove. Since dill is a favorite of rabbits, compassionate gardeners would plant a patch for the rabbits far away from their gardens.

Ants were considered beneficial in areas with clay or rocky soil. However, gardeners discouraged the ants from climbing the trunks of their elm and fruit trees by crushing lupine blooms and rubbing the juicy gel on the base of the trees. Herbs were also used with some success as deterrents. Tansy roots, pennyroyal, garlic chives, and marigolds were very

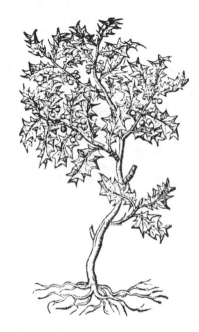

HOLLY

popular. Other deterrents included hyssop, sage, lavender, and thyme. Today, gardeners mix baker's yeast with sugar for a lethal effect. They lay the mixture on leaves and bark to protect the soil of any imbalance from the yeast. Remember that ants control the flea population, so allow Nature to find its balance.

Aphids were deterred by companion planting silvery-leaved plants. Nasturtiums were planted at the bases of apple trees and chervil between rows of lettuce to repel aphids. An aphid never landed on roses skirted with garlic. For a preventative measure, a soap was made from soapwort and lathered on the leaves. Rhubarb or nettle leaves were boiled in the sudsy mixture, which was used to wash the leaves of vegetables.

Southernwood and other varieties of artemisia were used to keep flies away. Tansy was planted in the garden as a deterrent and hung at the entrance of doorways for the same purpose. Walnut leaves were spread to keep flies from laying eggs. Wasps were easier. Containers of sugar water were hung, attracting the wasps to their death by drowning.

Did you ever wonder what Empress Josephine sprayed on her roses if blackspot occurred? A decoction of horsetail was used effectively to reduce fungal diseases. An ounce was boiled in a pint of water for thirty minutes and hand-painted on each rose leaf in Josephine's garden. Laurel leaves were allowed to ferment and used as a deadly fumigant for insects. Potato water was used to wash the stone pathways. Salt and wood ashes were sprinkled on moss to remove the fungus from pathways.

We can learn much from these moontime gardeners.

~

We can learn much from these moontime gardeners. Their simple solutions sound ingenious to us today. It should be no surprise to learn that gardeners of every culture talked to their plants, a common practice still. Flowers were dug and taken for cart rides around the garden to encourage them to bloom. Luther Burbank, a renowned horticulturist of the early twentieth century, believed with all his heart that love was the food that attuned plants. He lived in San Francisco during the disastrous 1906 earthquake. Every one of his plants in the greenhouses survived.

Historical Uses of Herbs

You will find the following terms used often in herbal lore as a common language of herbal properties. They refer to the energetic pathway of how a herb affects the body.

ALTERATIVES are blood cleansers. They help assimilate nutrients and eliminate metabolic waste products. Examples: Alfalfa, echinacea, dandelion root, sarsaparilla.

ANALGESICS relieve pain. Examples: Chamomile, catnip, cramp bark, lobelia, valerian.

ANTACIDS neutralize excess stomach acid. Examples: Fennel, Irish moss, kelp, slippery elm.

ANTIABORTIVES inhibit simultaneous abortion and bleeding. Examples: False unicorn root, red raspberry, skullcap, cramp bark.

ANTIASTHMATICS relieve wheezing. Examples: Lobelia, mullein, wild cherry bark.

ANTIBIOTICS inhibit or destroy bacteria and viruses while stimulating the body's immune response. Examples: Chaparral, echinacea, goldenseal, thyme, juniper berries.

ANTICATARRHALS eliminate and help prevent excess mucus formation. Examples: Cayenne, ginger, cinnamon, anise, mullein, yerba santa.

ANTIPYRETICS reduce fever by neutralizing acidic blood and cooling the body. Examples: Elder flowers, peppermint, basil, skullcap.

ANTISEPTICS inhibit bacteria growth both internally and externally. Examples: Myrrh, thyme, sage.

ANTISPASMODICS relax muscle spasms and cramps. Examples: Lobelia, tang kuei, black cohosh, blue cohosh, valerian, skullcap. **Note:** Blue cohosh and lobelia should not be used by people with hypertension.

APHRODISIACS rejuvenate sexual organs and their functions. Examples: Tang kuei, ginseng, angelica, garlic.

ASTRINGENTS dry up discharges, swollen tonsils, and hemorrhoids. They are symptomatic, not preventative. Examples: Aloe juice, shepherd's purse, white oak bark, blackberry leaves, self-heal, turmeric.

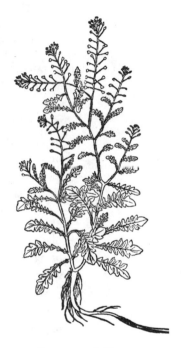

SHEPHERD'S PURSE

CARMINATIVES relieve gas and intestinal stagnation, while increasing circulation. These aromatic spices can be used daily to promote better digestion, assimilation, and elimination.

Warming carminatives work best for people who have weak digestion. Examples: Anise, basil, bay leaves, ginger, cinnamon, cloves.

Cooling carminatives work well for people who get toxic headaches from the foods they eat or overeat. Examples: Mints, chrysanthemum, coriander, cumin, dill, fennel.

CHOLAGOGUES promote bile flow and stimulate peristalsis. Examples: Aloe vera, barberry, Oregon grape root, Culver's root, wild yam root.

DEMULCENTS soothe inflamed tissue. Examples: Comfrey leaves and root, marshmallow root, slippery elm, flaxseed tea, fenugreek.

DIAPHORETICS promote sweating as a warm tea and act as diuretics when served cold. Primary action is on the respiratory system and sinuses. Examples: Ginger, flaxseed, sage.

Stimulating diaphoretics are hot and pungent. They drain the lymphatics. Examples: Angelica, camphor, basil, bayberry, cardamom, cinnamon, cloves, ephedra, eucalyptus, ginger, sage, thyme. **Note:** Ephedra should not be used by people with hypertension.

Relaxing (cooling) diaphoretics reduce fevers and remove toxins from the skin. They perform well at the onset of acute symptoms or hysteria. Examples: Catnip, chamomile, chrysanthemum, peppermint, elder flowers, yarrow flowers, boneset.

DIGESTANTS increase circulation, organic function, digestion, and appetite. Their hot, spicy nature aids in the elimination of accumulated mucous and toxins. For best results, use small amounts as a seasoning. Examples: Asafoetida, cayenne, black pepper, dry ginger, horseradish, mustard, garlic, prickly ash. **Note:** Digestants are not to be taken during pregnancy, lactation, or when inflammation or ulceration is possible. They can increase hypertension and produce insomnia.

DIURETICS increase urination and elimination through the kidneys and bladder. Their cooling nature alleviates toxins in the blood and brings energy downward to reduce edema and swelling from the waist down. They are used in weight reduction. Examples: Buchu leaves, cleavers, corn silk, dandelion, parsley, chickweed, gravel root, horsetail, uva ursi, juniper berries, plantain. **Note:** A small amount of a demulcent herb, like marshmallow root, should be added as a buffer.

EMMENAGOGUES promote menses and may increase the flow.

Warming emmenagogues alleviate dysmenorrhea, amenorrhea, anxiety, cramps, and pain. Examples: Tang kuei, angelica, ginger, cinnamon, valerian, red raspberry.

Cooling emmenagogues calm excited, emotional conditions and irritability. Examples: Blessed thistle, chamomile flowers, chrysanthemum flowers, rose petals, squawvine. **Note:** Not to be taken in excess of two cups daily during pregnancy.

Tonic emmenagogues build blood and promote sexual function. They counteract aging and organ weakness. Examples: Licorice, false unicorn, wild yam root, jasmine, peony root. **Note:** Do not use licorice if hypertension exists.

EMOLLIENTS protect the skin by soothing and softening. Examples: Marshmallow root, comfrey root, slippery elm, oils of almond, apricot kernel, sesame, olive, flaxseed (externally).

EXPECTORANTS expel mucous from the sinuses, lungs, and stomach. Coughs can be relieved by their antispasmodic action. Examples: Anise, wild cherry bark, lobelia, mullein, yerba santa, horehound, slippery elm, comfrey root, lungwort, flaxseed tea.

GALACTOGOGUES increase milk production and flow. Examples: Anise, blessed thistle, fennel, vervain.

HEMOSTATICS stop hemorrhaging. They are astringent. Examples: Blackberry leaves, cayenne, cranesbill, mullein, goldenseal, white oak bark, yellow dock, yarrow (externally).

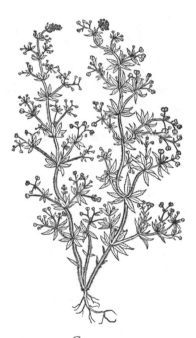

LAXATIVES promote peristalsis. They combine well with stimulants like fennel, anise, or ginger to dispel gas and enhance digestion. Many blood cleansers also have laxative properties. The three types of laxatives are given below.

Stimulant laxatives promote bile flow and increase digestive enzymes. Examples: Cascara sagrada, rhubarb, gentian.

Lithotriptics dissolve and eliminate kidney or gallstones. Examples: Gravel root, parsley, dandelion, uva ursi, nettles, cleavers.

Lubricants moisten and add bulk. They contain many nutrients. Examples: Flaxseed tea, slippery elm bark, psyllium seed, whole wheat bran.

CLEAVERS

NERVINES calm and nourish neuronal function. They can promote mental clarity and relieve spasms, pain, and congestion. The two types of nervines are given below.

Warming nervines aid people with chronic disorders. Examples: Valerian, basil, lady's slipper.

Cooling nervines alleviate anger, hypertension, and migraines. Examples: Gotu kola, hops, wood betony, skullcap.

OXYTOXICS induce labor by stimulating uterine contractions. These herbs may also tone uterine muscles. Examples: Black cohosh, blue cohosh, raspberry leaves, wild ginger. **Note:** Do not use blue cohosh if hypertension exists. Consult your physician before hastening childbirth.

PARASITICIDES kill parasites in the intestines and on the scalp and skin. Examples: Garlic, thyme, black walnut leaves, cinnamon oil, thyme oil (externally).

PURGATIVES are irritants and weaken digestion and bowel tone with prolonged use. They are useful upon occasion to remove accumulated toxins in the large and small bowel. Examples: Aloe vera, senna leaves, castor oil, epsom salts.

Use aloe vera as a compress to promote cell growth and repair.

~

REJUVENATIVES renew the optimal function of the body and mind. They are anti-aging, increasing sensitivity and awareness. Examples: Gotu kola, ginseng, oatstraw, ginko biloba.

RUBEFACIENTS increase surface blood flow and produce redness. They alleviate arthritis, rheumatism, aches, and pains. Examples: Mustard seed oil, ginger, thyme oil, eucalyptus, cayenne (as a compress). External use only.

SIALAGOGUES increase saliva to improve digestion of starches. Examples: Echinacea, cayenne, ginger, licorice, yerba santa. **Note:** Do not use licorice if hypertension exists.

TONICS are nutritive and building. They harmonize body function and build the blood and lymphatic system. Examples: Tang kuei, angelica, comfrey root, Irish moss, marshmallow root, slippery elm.

VULNERARIES promote cell growth and repair. Examples: Aloe vera, comfrey, fenugreek, marshmallow root, slippery elm. Use as a compress.

The Language of Herbal Folklore

*L*overs have long used the beauty of flowers and herbs to express true feelings from their hearts. The individual meaning of each herb, spice, and flower began in the Orient and was introduced to the West in 1716 by Lady Montague while her husband served as the English ambassador to the Turkish government in Constantinople. The language of herbs and flowers soon spread to France and reached its height of popularity in the nineteenth century. Flowers and herbs added spontaneity to romance and made flirting great fun. I believe each herb and plant still has a silent message for each of us. As we learn to harmonize with Mother Nature, we will gain more understanding of the nonverbal communication that speaks from our hearts.

The following is adapted from *The Language of Flowers* (Dover, 1965) and *The Folklore of Plants* (Dyer, 1889).

ALOE is for patience. The Native Americans know it as "the burn plant." I learn more patience every time I burn myself cooking!

ANGELICA is for protection and blooms at the feast day of Michael the Archangel.

ARTEMISIA is believed to have grown in the path left by the serpent in the Garden of Eden. It is also known as wormwood.

BASIL is the herb of romance, placed outside a maiden's window when she is ready to receive her lover. In India, "holy basil" is used at funerals to assure safe passage into heaven.

BAY LAUREL is a sign of greatness and honor for those who wear it in a garland.

BEE BALM, also known as Oswego tea, was drunk by American colonists following the Boston Tea Party.

ATROPA BELLADONNA is named after the goddess of fate. (It's also toxic!)

BETONY LAMB'S EARS were grown to ward off evil spirits. They take on an ethereal quality in the moonlight.

BORAGE is for courage. Roman soldiers drank a wine made from borage flowers before going off to battle.

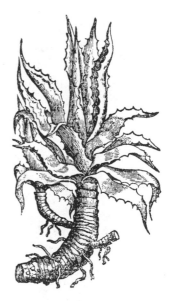

ALOE

BURNET protects the blood. The leaves were used by the Greeks to arrest bleeding.

CHAMOMILE is for relaxation. It is revered in Ayurvedic East Indian medicine for its ability to calm the body, mind, and spirit.

CARROT is for night vision and for increasing fertility.

CATNIP protects the throat. It was used in ancient European cultures to soothe a crying baby and to reduce colic.

CHIVES were hung in homes to drive away evil. In medieval times an "evil" could mean a virus or plague.

COMFREY is known as "bone-knit," closing fractures and wounds. It was brought to America by early colonists, who cultivated comfrey for external compresses.

COSTMARY is known as "Bible leaf" and used as a bookmark.

CRESS is the herb of stability. It is known and loved as "peppergrass" in England, eaten at lunch to give people fuel to finish their day.

CRETE DITTANY represents passion. The strong flavor was believed to excite Mediterraneans who used this herb in their cuisine.

CURRY often represents hidden worth. Those who grow curry soon learn to admire her stamina and modest qualities.

DANDELION is French for "lion's tooth," alluding to the stamina gained by using the herb. The Mohegan Native Americans drank dandelion tea for an energy tonic.

DILL garlands crowned war heroes and protected commoners from the "evil eye" of "witches."

ECHINACEA was used by Native Americans to counteract snakebites.

EPAZOTE, known as "wormseed" in Mexico, has long been used as a vermifuge for parasites.

FENNEL is the herb of sight. Ancient Roman physicians used an extract of fennel root to clear the cloudy vision of cataracts.

GARLIC is the herb of endurance, having magical powers against evil. I believe it has something to do with the smell!

SCENTED GERANIUMS are the herbs of true friendship. They can mimic any flavor (such as lemon rose, peach, lime, peppermint, coconut, and cinnamon) and were used in Victorian nosegays to welcome guests. Their origin is African.

GERMANDER was the herb most used for rheumatism and pain. It was a favorite in George Washington's knot gardens.

GROUND IVY is the herb of humility. We literally walk on it.

HOREHOUND was used to break spells and is one of the bitter herbs of Passover.

HYSSOP is the holy herb of cleanliness, a Biblical herb known for its antiseptic qualities.

LAVENDER is the herb of chastity. In Latin, *lavare* means "to wash."

LEMON BALM is the herb of sympathy, known to the Greeks as the bee plant.

LEMON GRASS is the herb of concentration. It is used as a tea, in culinary dishes, and as an essential oil to "awaken" the mind.

LEMON VERBENA is the herb of marital fidelity. It is native to South America.

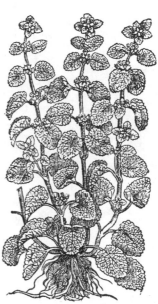

HOREHOUND

POT MARIGOLD (Calendula) is the herb of joy, enabling one to see fairies.

MARIGOLD is the herb for indecision about a lover(s)!

MARJORAM enhances marital bliss.

MINT is the herb of virtue, believed to relieve mental and emotional tension. "When the heart is right, for and against is forgotten" (Lao Tzu).

MULLEIN is the candle plant. American settlers dipped the bloom stalk in tallow and used it as a candle.

OREGANO is a wild Greek herb. Its name means "joy of the mountain."

PARSLEY is an herb of festivity. It is chewed to sweeten the breath.

PERIWINKLE is the herb for pleasant memories. Slip one into your pillowcase or add it to an herbal pillow.

ROSEMARY is the herb of remembrance. It was given to lovers so they would think of each other when they were apart.

RUE is the herb of grace. It is dipped in holy water in Eastern Orthodox rituals.

SAGE is the herb of salvation and virtue. It was used to calm excess desires and passions and became a cure-all in medieval folklore.

Join us in moontime!

~

SANTOLINA LAVENDER COTTON is the herb of trust and was planted in every medieval knot garden.

SAVORY is the herb of sexual enticement—evidenced by the fact that it is a favorite bee plant!

SPEEDWELL is for feminine fidelity.

SORREL is for maternal tenderness. The seed pods are used in dried arrangements and given to mothers who have just delivered a newborn.

TANSY is the herb of immortality. It was used in medieval Europe to clean the blood of "ill humors." (It is highly toxic!)

TARRAGON was given to travelers to prevent fatigue. It was rubbed, chewed, or sniffed to promote endurance.

THYME houses fairies. It was used as a strewing herb because of its antiseptic and aromatic qualities. Encased in a pillow, thyme promotes safe dreams.

VIOLET: Blue is for faithfulness; white is for modesty. Violets are used for spring bouquets and weddings.

YARROW is the herb of cavepeople; yarrow fossils date back 60,000 years. Today, yarrow may be known as the oldest weed. It is a relative of the ancient ferns and is believed to grow wherever people have traveled.

Join us in moontime!

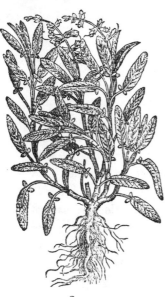

SAGE

2

The Roots of Mother Nature

One land with many features, one people with many faces,

and one harvest to provide all our needs.

The secrets of Mother Nature unfold by studying the land, the various people who have tilled it, and the indigenous plants that sustained them. Let us step into the adventures of myth and time to experience how Mother Nature nurtures us in North America. We will learn what is valuable about our past and how we can grow together in the future.

Native American Ancestry

From the womb of Mother Earth emerged the Anasazi, "the Ancient Ones," the Basketmakers of the four corners of New Mexico, Colorado, Utah, and Arizona. The four corners include an arid plateau stretching diagonally from northeast to southwest across Arizona and New Mexico. The squared edges of New Mexico and Arizona meet Utah and Colorado to create the four corners, where the Anasazi culture grew into what is now known as the Pueblos. They lived in harmony with the sagebrush, grasslands, red canyons, and pine-covered mountains. For over one thousand years the Pueblos lived as cliff dwellers, in open mound pueblos and caves, as a mother clan (matriarchal) society. For generations the natives

How can we grow together in the future?

~

sang for the corn, drummed for the rain, danced for the cotton, and called for the spirit of Mother Nature to fire their pottery.

The religious centers that developed in the community were known as kivas. Kivas were circular, subterranean chambers representing the underworld birthing center of all creation—the womb of time. It is here, where the ancestral and cosmic forces erupt from the belly of the earth, the men gathered for ceremonial and religious practices. Benches lined the circular walls, adorned with paintings of their gods. In the center of the room is the mystical hole, called the sipapu, representing the place of emergence from the womb of Mother Nature. The sipapu was an altar symbolizing the power of the feminine, where a fire blazed in honor of all the hearth fires of civilization.

The kivas were governed by a clan of priests and their initiates. Since the women governed the homes and fields, the kiva was a sanctuary for the men where no women were allowed. The kiva was placed to the Southeast, where the earliest light of Father Sun initiates life. The central location of the kiva, between the communal house and the cemetery, represented migration between the spirits of the living and the dead. The young men learned to perform rituals and communicate with the dead ancestors' spirits. These initiates learned to renew their ties with spirit by journeying into the center of Mother Earth, symbolized by how they entered the kiva through a hole in the roof. They learned how spirit sustains all creation, not by measurement of time, but by listening to their hearts.

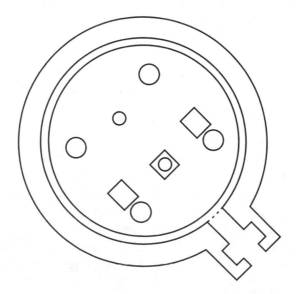

ILLUSTRATION OF A KIVA, A NATIVE AMERICAN RELIGIOUS CENTER.

The Rhythm of the Corn Dance

Adapted from the Zuni story of creation from *The Story of Corn* by Betty Fussell (New York: Alfred Knopf, Inc., 1992).

In the beginning there was watery darkness from which the Sun Father rose to give light and life from his skin. He rolled balls of flesh that became Earth Mother and Sky Father. The Earth and Sky embraced each other. Earth Mother then conceived in her four cavernous wombs the first men and creatures. Sky Father spread out his hand and of his palm were yellow grains to guide his children. From a bowl of foam, Earth Mother created the boundaries of the Earth, but their parents were afraid to let them go; from foam, Sun Father created twin warriors with rainbows and thunderbolts for bows and arrows. They split the womb of Earth Mother and gave the children of darkness a tall ladder to climb into the kiva of twilight and into the light of the Sun.

Spirit sustains all creation by listening to our hearts.

Their chiefs taught them sacred words and rituals and divided them into clans, each with a magical medicine. They wandered for generations until they reached the Middle of the World. When they came upon The Place of Misty Waters, they discovered the Seed People, who challenged them to show their powers. They planted prayer sticks and it rained for eight days. For eight days following, the Seed People danced and sang until the prayer sticks turned into seven corn plants.

These are the flesh of seven maidens, our own sisters. The eldest sister was yellow, the next blue, then red, white, speckled, and black. The youngest was to remain sweet corn, in honor of innocence.

Each color of corn gave an element and direction: yellow originated in the North from winter; blue came out of the waters from the West; red erupted from the South during the summer; white was born of daylight in the East; the speckled rained from the clouds, and the black came from the Womb of Earth Mother.

The Seed Clan and Cave Clan then drummed and danced. Their union gave birth to the Corn Clan and their corn maidens created the dance of the Corn Wands. The Corn Clan then traveled together until they heard the beautiful music of flutes rising from the Cave of the Rainbow. Two brave warriors followed the sound of the music to be greeted by the Father of Dew and the Father of Medicine, Pai' a tu ma, who taught them new dances.

That night, as the lovely corn maidens danced, the flute players filed out of their cave and became immediately love-struck at the first sight of the corn maidens. Sensing the flute players' desires, the corn maidens simultaneously pressed their hands to their bodies and vanished. Only their seed was left behind to nurture the Corn Clan.

The people missed their lovely sisters and called the eagle to find them. The eagle soared from the highest clouds where the Great Sky Father dwelled. Then the people called on the tiniest sparrow to look for the corn maidens in crevices of the highest mountains. The hawk was then called to receive any omens or messages from the Spirit that unites all life. No detail evaded the hawk's keen perception, for he flies close to the light of Sun Father. Crow was called to search the supernatural, for he was the master of illusion. But the corn maidens were not to be found, and the people mourned their sisters.

Only the God of Dew could find them. He could follow the origin of the flute to the dwellers of time, singing in eternity. He was guided to the Land of Everlasting Summer. Here he found the lovely maidens singing to the children of the Earth:

> The Sun, who is the Father of all.
> The Earth, who is the Mother of men.
> The Water, who is the Grandfather.
> The Fire, who is the Grandmother.
> Our brothers and sisters, the corn, and seeds of growing things.
> So we have given our flesh to you . . .
> The milk of mankind.

The Native American Path

Everything is alive, sacred, and connected to the Oneness of the Life Force—the Center is everywhere and within each of us.

We belong to the Earth and it is our sacred path to protect and honor it. Life is our gift. We share with those in need. Peace is not only an absence of conflict, but also a nurturing life force joining the earth and sky, the physical and the metaphysical.

The Native Americans call us to seek a personal truth and become a clear channel for us to express spirit through our souls.

Native Americans of all cultures represent our responsibility of shared humanity for all races, conditions, and cultures. By honoring the Earth, we respect all she bears forth. Herbs and herbal traditions represent our commitment to our culture and to Mother Nature.

The Path of the Healer

To the Native Americans, all healing is supernatural. They believed all disease originated from the soul disassociating from the body. The most ancient form of native healing in the Eastern and Western Old World was through the medium of a hollow bone called a soul catcher. Medicine men, endowed with the power of animal spirits, would use a bone, a soul catcher, to suck or blow the illness from the diseased. The healer would shake the tent with animal energy flowing through him and remove the evil spirit through fasting and entering a trance state.

The ability to endow animal spirits for healing came to a healer through a conscious-altering illness and subsequent vision. Healers could also be chosen through a dream state; for example, dreams of a bear in an inner journey indicated the calling of a medicine man. Healers could mend a broken ego or a broken bone by invoking the greater power of *nunwati,* or health. Nunwati was a personal experience enhanced by all of Nature. The healer could receive a cure for an illness in a dream or trance. The cure could be derived from a local plant, animal, or mineral. The healers found a use for everything in their environment to encourage systemic harmony.

When using plants, the roots were most often used for healing. Prayers were said as the roots were dug. The location and time of day for the dig were usually given to the healer in a dream. Most of the roots they dug were bitters to relieve acute disease.

Ancient civilizations died more from injury and childbirth than nutritional deficiencies. The average life span was twenty-eight to thirty-seven years. Only one hundred diseases plagued early humans, compared to over thirty thousand today. As the average life span increased, so did the opportunity to contract disease. Native Americans believed their food would provide great health. The food was grown or provided locally and organically before erosion and industry depleted the land. Most of their herbal treatments were rejuvenative tonics, vapors, and compresses. The Native Americans recuperated from illness as effortlessly as animals and trees. They acknowledged their Creator in every part of Nature and believed in their innate right to celebrate life through good health. Their unique relationship with Nature ensured good health. They understood all their needs to have been provided through Nature.

Believe in your innate right to celebrate life through good health.

~

Being in harmony with Nature enabled medicine men to utilize what is now called the Doctrine of Signatures to identify medicinal plants by their shape, color, and texture. For every illness, Native Americans found a cure in a plant's similarity to a disease or symptom; for example, a juicy leaf would decrease thirst and reduce a fever, a milky stem would promote lactation, and a kidney bean would benefit the kidney. The color, shape, and size of every plant would reveal its secrets.

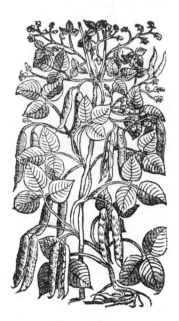

Kidney Bean

The Native Americans also learned about herbal cures from observing animals' instinctive intelligence to find what they needed in their environment. From observation, they learned when to gather a plant and when it was most potent. Plants were always taken from an abundant source in the appropriate season. Roots were dug during autumn, when their nutrition content was highest. Leaves were gathered during spring and dried in the shade. Bark was stripped during early spring or winter months.

Medicinal teas were prepared from dried roots and leaves by a Native American healer. A decoction was prepared by boiling and steeping an herb for ten to twenty minutes. Native Americans often used just one herb for healing, which they prepared and drank only once during an illness, as opposed to our repeated intake of medications.

The application of medicine would vary according to the symptom and preference of the healer. When fresh roots were used, they were macerated and applied locally. Some roots were chewed. For example, dental cavities were a problem for Native Americans, who consumed a high amount of cereal. Echinacea root (the purple coneflower) has a numbing effect and was used to abate toothaches. It was also chewed by the Native Americans of the Plains as an antidote for snakebites and insect stings.

External applications of herbal poultices were prepared from fresh or powdered dried roots boiled in animal grease. These were applied to the skin as emollients to set fractures. Herbal poultices were pricked into the skin with a sharp flint. Herbal compresses were applied to induce blood-letting, removing toxins from an infected area. An appropriate poultice was then applied to heal the wound. Steam and herbal vapors for bronchial or rheumatic complaints were also used. Since all healing was considered supernatural, Native Americans also returned to Nature to achieve greater health.

The Midewiwin and the Grand Medicine Society

𝒯he Midewiwin Grand Medicine Society first appeared among the Ojibwas, known as the Chippewa, and spread to other Great Lakes tribes, such as the Winnebego and Omaha. The Midewiwin Grand Medicine Society replaced shamanistic medicine men as a path of healers. The Midewiwin organized the use of herbal medicine into tonics affecting major organs, lungs and chest, liver and intestines. Their elders initiated healers into each tribe, initiating women as well as men. This new order of healers inspired confidence in their people and taught them the responsibility of self-healing, called "right living." Every person was encouraged to eat a balanced diet of grains and vegetables, improve personal hygiene with baths and skincare, and avoid alcohol. The Midewiwins believed the body to be self-healing, similar to holistic healers today.

The Midewiwin, known as Mide, looked to the power of Mother Nature for cures. Every tree, herb, and flower held potential. Their lives were in tune with nature, allowing the secrets of local herbs to call them as medicine. Each Midewiwin found their cures after individually identifying and using many local plants as initiates. They advanced through many degrees with special instruction and time-honored remedies from the elders of the secret society. These herbal cures have been handed down to many generations who followed "the path of the bear." The strongest medicine became known as bear medicine.

The Midewiwins believe that the body is self-healing.

The Mide searched for bitter roots to heal the most stubborn diseases. Bitters are very cleansing and detoxifying, a natural remedy for acute illness. After locating the herb, the Mide dug a hole beside the plant to fill it with tobacco as an offering. Silent reverence or a spoken prayer of thanksgiving honored the herb.

Midewiwins paid for the knowledge of a time-honored remedy with tobacco to an elder Midewiwin. In recent times, cures were handed down through the families of the Midewiwins. The tradition of payment assured the remedy would be respected and given proper treatment.

Midewiwin Tonics

Family remedies developed into a combination of several synergistic herbs. These formulas were originated by the Chippewa, also known as the Ojibwa of the Great Lakes region, and later given the name of "tonics." **Note:** Always contact your physician for proper evaluation.

∾ *Decongestant Tonic* ∾

Midewiwins of the Rocky Mountains treated bronchitis, congestion, and chronic upper respiratory problems with osha root, a sacred herb of the Midwest. It is a spicy, odorous root stimulating the flow of mucus. Even smoke of the burning leaves can stimulate mucus. The following combination is effective as a expectorant cough syrup. Expectorants should not be used for a dry, hacking cough.

  ⅓ cup dried osha root *(Ligusticum porteri)*, chopped
  ¼ cup each dried elecampane root and flowers *(Inula helinium)*
  2 (1-inch) pieces of dried licorice root *(Glycyrrhiza glabra)*, optional
  ¼ cup dried wild cherry bark *(Prunus serotina)*
  1 tablespoon dried mullein leaves *(Verbascum thaspus)*
  1 pound sugar, raw is best

Simmer the roots and bark in 4 cups of water for 30 minutes, uncovered (do not use licorice if hypertension exists). Reduce the liquid to 2 cups. Turn off the heat, add the mullein leaves and elecampane flowers, and cover. In another pan, boil the sugar in 2 cups of water to form a syrup. Remove from heat. Strain herbs; add the liquid to the syrup. Take 1 tablespoon 3–4 times daily. Bottle and refrigerate the tonic. The Native Americans kept it covered in a cool, dark place. This syrup keeps 3 months refrigerated.

∾ *Tonic for Craziness* ∾

Mental and emotional affliction was treated with inhalants such as this one. The Winnebego Mides gathered blueberry flowers from the *Vaccinium* family, dried them for twenty-four hours in the shade, and placed them on hot stones to produce a vapor. The affected person inhaled the fumes to restore balance. The Native Americans used other inhalants to cleanse the aura and home of an affected person. After the person inhaled fumes of the blueberry flowers, the room and aura of the individual would be cleansed by burning dried mugwort, *Artemisia frigida,* or wormwood.

✌ *Bitter Tonic* ✌

Drink this cleansing liver tonic to increase longevity. The southwestern Mides prepared a bitter tea, cleansing the liver and blood in acute diseases. Today, it may be used for a spring tonic and for chronic biliary disorders. Use fresh leaves and root when possible, although dried may also be used.

- 1 tablespoon dandelion root *(Taraxacum officinale)* [2-year-old roots are best]
- 1 tablespoon dried and ground goldenseal root *(Hydrastis canadensis),* optional
- 1 tablespoon aerial portions of thistle *(Sylibum marianum)*
- 1 tablespoon dandelion leaves

In a covered glass pot, simmer the roots in 4 cups of water for 20 minutes. Add the thistle and dandelion leaves. Remove from heat and cover. Steep 15 minutes. Strain; drink 1–2 cups daily for three days. Reduce if diarrhea occurs. Refrigerate leftover tea. This tea is bitter and should not be sweetened. Lemon may be added to soften the bitterness. It is safe to drink 1 cup weekly for maintenance. **Note:** Do not use goldenseal if hypoglycemia exists.

✌ *Kidney Tonic* ✌

This tonic promotes the free flow of urine. Cherokee Mides made it to alleviate cystitis, urinary spasms, and stone formation. It can also be used for prostatitis.

- 1 tablespoon marshmallow root *(Althea officinalis)*
- 2 teaspoons hydrangea root *(Hydrangea arborescens)*
- 2 teaspoons uva ursi leaves *(Arctostaphylos,* also known as bearberry), soaked overnight in ½ cup cold water
- 2 teaspoons cramp bark *(Viburnum opulus)*

Simmer the roots and bark in 4 cups of water for 30 minutes. Remove the boiled roots. Strain uva ursi leaves and retain the water to add to the root and bark tea. Drink half a cup four times daily.

Midewiwin Skincare and Personal Hygiene

The Midewiwins taught "right living," which included personal hygiene as well as skincare to enhance well-being. The following chart entails a few examples of the tonics and skin preparations taught by the Midewiwins to their fellow Native Americans.

Therapeutic Baths

HERB	PREPARATION	RESULT
Anemone root *(Anemone canadensis)*	The root was pounded and boiled.	An antiseptic wash was applied to sores and wounds.
Joe Pye weed *(Eupatorium maculatum)*	Infusion of whole plant added to bathwater.	Induce a crying child to sleep.
White Trillium root *(Trillium grandiflorum)*	The pulverized root was steeped in water and applied to sore nipples.	Reduces sore nipples during lactation.
Wild Plum root *(Prunus americana)*	Infusion of the powdered or macerated root was used as a skin wash.	Topical disinfectant as a wash.
Wormwood *(Artemisia absinthium)*	Infusion of tops added to bathwater or applied warm as a compress.	Reduces muscle strain.
Yarrow *(Achillea millefolium)*	The whole plant was steeped in hot water.	Used to bathe bruises to reduce internal bleeding and bruising.

Hair Tonics

HERB	PREPARATION	RESULTS
Chokecherry bark *(Prunus virginiana)*	A decoction was made from boiling the bark in water.	Hairwash to strengthen the hair and encourage growth.

Columbine flowers *(Aquilegia columbine)*	The flowers were steeped in hot water.	Hair rinse.
Mugwort flowers *(Artemisia vulgaris)*	Flowers were dried and steeped.	Hair rinse.
Scouring rush *(Equisetum hymale)*	The fern stalks were boiled in water.	Hairwash to eliminate fleas and mites.
Soapwort root *(Saponaria officinalis)*	The powdered root was pounded and mixed with hot water.	Hairwash for dandruff and itchy scalp.

Skincare

HERB	PREPARATION	RESULTS
Yellow Dock root *(Rumex crispus)*	Moisten dried powdered root and apply as a poultice.	Reduces itching and skin eruptions.
Wild Lettuce *(Lactuca canadensis)*	Squeeze the white juice from the stalk and apply locally.	Removes warts.
Peppermint *(Mentha piperita)*	The fresh leaves were chewed to freshen the breath.	Antiseptic mouthwash.
Wild Geranium *(Geranium maculatum)*	The autumn roots were steeped in hot water.	Mouthwash to reduce pyorrhea.
Juniper berries *(Juniperus species)*	The berries were crushed to extract the oil to apply externally.	Insect repellent.
Sage leaves *(Salvia species)*	Sage leaves were bruised and used to clean teeth.	Tooth whitener.
Sumac root *(Rhus glabra)*	The fresh root was chewed.	Heal mouth sores.
Bloodroot, also called pyccoon *(Sanguinaria canadensis)*	The root was dried, ground, and mixed with water.	Face paint.

A Native American Herbal

*H*ere is a sampling of herbs we may find in a Native American's medicine pouch. Remember that Native Americans ingested their remedy only once as necessary to abate symptoms.

*P*luck not

where you

never planted.

—Native American
proverb

∾

AMERICAN GINSENG *(Panax quinquefolius)*. Woodland Native Americans dug and boiled ginseng roots to relieve cold symptoms and nausea. The Pawnee of the Caddoan tribes made a love potion using ginseng, wild parsley, columbine, and cardinal flowers to attract a spouse.

AMERICAN IPECAC *(Gillenia stipulata)*. Native Americans from many tribes gathered this root in September and ate one or two grams (about 1 teaspoon) raw to purge their system as an emetic. Native Americans traditionally purged before fasting.

BLOODROOT *(Sanguinaria canadensis)*. Woodland Native Americans east of the Mississippi River collected the rhizome in the late fall and prepared a tea for rheumatic pain. The red juice was also applied to their skin as an insect repellent. Since it is a toxic relative of the opium poppy, some Native Americans used it to induce vomiting. **Note:** Only external use is recommended.

BLUE COHOSH ROOT *(Caulophyllum thalictroides)*. Omaha and Allegheny Mountain Native Americans gathered this root in the fall and boiled it with water to make a tea to reduce fever. Other tribes, such as the Menominees, Ojibwas, and Potawatomis, made a tea to induce and expedite labor. The tea was taken daily one to two weeks before delivery. Early white settlers borrowed this practice for female and labor complications, naming it "squawroot." **Note:** Blue Cohosh root is not recommended for those who suffer from hypertension.

BONESET *(Eupatorium perfoliatum)*. The Iroquois and Mohegans gathered and dried the leaves and flowers of this wetland weed in August. They prepared a tea for colds, fevers, and body aches. An infusion of leaves and flowers produces copious sweating and the taste produces nausea.

CATNIP *(Nepeta cataria)*. The Mohegans used catnip extensively for colicky babies, colds, and as a sedative. They harvested the leaves and white flowers in early autumn and dried them in the shade before brewing a tea over hot coals.

CHAPARRAL *(Larrea tridentata)*. Southwestern and desert Native Americans used dried chaparral leaves, stems, and gum for wounds, female problems, diuresis, colds, and stomachaches. They sprinkled the dried leaves in their shoes to prevent rheumatism and foot problems. Western herbalists later used chaparral tea for upper respiratory diseases. An infusion of one-half ounce chaparral infused in two cups of water was used locally to prevent dental cavities, eczema, and dandruff.

CHESTNUT *(Castanea dentata)*. Northeastern tribes steeped fresh leaves in boiled water for whooping cough. The Native Americans roasted the nuts and ate them or pounded them into a nutritious flour.

CLOVER *(Trifolium species)*. Many tribes on the West coast enjoyed clover as food, combining it with peppernuts dipped in saltwater. The Pomo celebrated the emergence of the clover in early spring with dance and celebration. As medicine, clover was infused as a tea to relieve spasmodic coughing and applied with grease to soothe topical ulcers, sores, and burns. Clover has recently been found to thicken the blood and may be preventive of certain heart diseases.

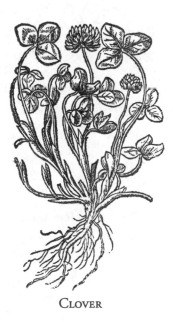

CLOVER

COMFREY *(Symphytum officinale)*. Comfrey was introduced to the Northeast Native Americans by early colonists, who would not leave home without it. Comfrey leaves and roots were infused and applied to burns, broken bones, sores, and insect stings. A tea was drunk upon occasion for bronchial complaints, gastritis, and intestinal distress. **Note:** Comfrey may cause liver damage if taken internally often or in large doses.

CORN *(Zea mays)*. Ancient Aztec and Inca tribes cultivated wild corn and utilized it as food and medicine. The corn silk was steeped in boiled water to treat urinary complaints. Corn smut, a predecessor to penicillin, was used to abate headaches. Cornstarch was dampened and applied locally to relieve itchy skin. The Iroquois of the Northeastern Atlantic coast prepared a coffee by parching dried ears on hot embers. The Chickasaw east of the Mississippi River used corn oil to abate dandruff by rubbing it into their scalp.

DANDELION *(Taraxacum officinale)*. Dandelions were introduced by early colonists to the Native Americans as greens. The Iroquois boiled dandelion leaves with fatty meats. The bitter taste made the meats more digestible. The Ojibwas of the Great Lake region made a tea of boiled roots to relieve heartburn and indigestion. The Mohegans of Connecticut drank a tea from fresh leaves as a spring tonic.

ELDERBERRY *(Sambucus canadensis)*. The Iroquois tribes of the Atlantic coast enjoyed many parts of the American elderberry. The inner bark was stripped before winter and boiled to produce an analgesic. The leaves were dried and crushed into animal grease for an insect repellent. The flowers are diaphoretic and induce sweating to reduce fever. Mohegans used the flowers in a tea for colicky babies, probably as a compress. The berries were eaten to regulate the bowels and fermented by many Eastern tribes for a delicious wine.

The Zuni chewed and swallowed the juice of goldenrod flowers to relieve sore throats.

GOLDENROD *(Solidago species)*. The Zuni of New Mexico chewed and swallowed the juice of goldenrod flowers to relieve sore throats. The Meskwaki of Minnesota ground the flowers and applied them to insect stings.

HOPS *(Humulus lupulus)*. The Mohegans used the strobiles, cone-like flowers, in a sedative tea, while the Meskwaki found hops a cure for insomnia. Hops belong to the hemp family and were utilized by many Native Americans as a tonic for nervous complaints.

ICELAND MOSS *(Cetraria islandica)*. Northern tribes boiled Iceland moss into a gelatinous tea and drank a cup daily to break up mucous congestion.

JEWELWEED *(Impatiens capensis)*. The Potawatomi of the Great Lakes region found jewelweed growing next to poison ivy and used the juice as an antidote for poison ivy and eczema.

JUNIPER *(Juniper communis)*. Many Native American groups crushed the blueberries of the juniper and applied the oil as an insect repellent. The fragrant wax is first removed by boiling. The bark and branches were burned to produce a healing antiseptic inhalant.

LICORICE *(Glycyrrhiza glabra)*. Northwest Native Americans roasted and ate nutritious licorice roots as a survival food. The roots are mildly laxative. The leaves were brewed, strained, and applied externally to relieve earaches.

LOBELIA *(Lobelia inflata)*. Central and Eastern Native American tribes smoked dried lobelia leaves to relieve asthma. Lobeline alkaloid removes mucous from the bronchial passages. This remedy was not used until the late eighteenth century. Lobeline is chemically similar to nicotine and is presently used in over-the-counter remedies to stop smoking. It is also known as "Indian tobacco." The red lobelia or cardinal flower was ground and added to an arguing couple's meal to promote harmony. **Note:** Lobelia is toxic in large doses, producing vomiting and heart palpitations. It is toxic when ingested, not inhaled.

MILKWEED *(Asclepias syriaca)*. Common milkweed was used by the Navajo women as a contraceptive following childbirth. They prepared a tea from boiling the entire plant and only drank it once. Native Americans of the Northeast seacoast used the juice topically to remove warts and treat ringworm. **Note:** Topical use only.

MULLEIN *(Verbascum thapsus)*. The Mohegans steeped fresh mullein leaves in water and molasses for a cough syrup. Other tribes smoked dried leaves to relieve asthma. The golden yellow flowers produce an oil used to treat hemorrhoids and earaches.

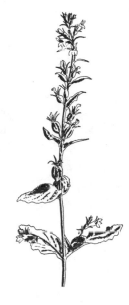

LOBELIA

NETTLE *(Urtica urens)*. The tops of stinging nettles were brewed as a tea to reduce rheumatic pain. It is comforting to know that stinging nettles are useful, but puzzling to think how the Native Americans picked the nettles safely! (Handle with gloves.)

PIPSISSEWA *(Chimaphilla umbellata)*. Northeastern tribes steeped the entire plant in boiled water as a compress to draw out blisters and reduce swelling. Many tribes also drank a tea to reduce fever and rheumatic pain. Pipsissewa is a member of the wintergreen family.

PLANTAIN *(Plantago major* or *lanceolata)*. The semi-nomadic Shoshoni of the Northwestern plains applied heated plantain leaves to wounds and abrasions. They chewed the root to alleviate toothaches and swallowed the seeds to remove parasites. For insect stings, Native Americans applied the bruised and macerated whole plant as a compress.

SASSAFRAS *(Sassafras albidum).* Many Native American tribes from Northeastern America found this native shrub to be very useful. The Rappahannock tribe of Virginia drank a tea of boiled roots to lower fevers and promote the onset of measles. The rootbeer taste makes sassafras tea a favorite tonic for many occasions.

SELFHEAL *(Prunella vulgaris).* The Quileute of Washington State used selfheal as a poultice for boils and skin ulcers.

SKULLCAP *(Scutellaria lateriflora).* The Cherokee of the Northern Allegheny Mountain region drank an infusion of skullcap leaves to induce suppressed menstruation. Many Southeastern U.S. tribes drank the tea for nervous complaints and spasms. Skullcap was used for tetanus and rabies, but the effectiveness is unknown. Skullcap is a non-aromatic mint with a bitter taste.

SQUASH *(Lagenaria* species). Squash seeds and pumpkin seeds were dried and chewed to expel worms. Roasted seed provided a source of protein.

TANSY *(Tanacetum vulgare).* Algonkian tribes of the Great Lakes, known as the People of Calumet (or *peace pipe),* used tansy leaves and flowers to kill lice and fleas. They crushed them over their bodies, releasing camphor and borneol, as an insecticide.

TOBACCO *(Nicotiana* species). Native Americans of every nation used wet tobacco leaves to abate bee stings and rubbed the chewed juice on their bodies to repel insects. Native Americans consider tobacco a messenger to the Creator because the smoke curled upward to the heavens. Some tribes used tobacco smoke to alleviate earaches, blowing the smoke into the ear. Tobacco remains one of the oldest plants in Creation. The Native Americans knew to use tobacco in small amounts on special occasions for its narcotic properties.

WATERMELON SEEDS *(Citrullus vulgaris).* The Hopis made a tea of dried watermelon seeds to alleviate urinary complaints by simmering one teaspoon of seeds in one cup of water for fifteen minutes.

WHITE SPRUCE *(Picea alba).* Iroquois and Algonkian tribes of the Northeast Atlantic coast used several varieties of spruce and pine needles and the inner bark to prevent scurvy. The needles are rich in vitamins C and A, used by the Native Americans for a survival food. Spruce beer was made from early shoots, twigs, and cones by boiling them in maple syrup.

WILD GERANIUM *(Geranium maculatum)*. Lake Heron Native Americans used the dried, powdered root of this beautiful native flower to stop bleeding wounds. Roots dug in the autumn had the most medicinal value. The roots were boiled with wild grapes to treat pyorrhea and sore throats.

WILD GINGER *(Asarum canadensis)*. Canadian Native Americans infused wild ginger root to reduce heart palpitations and to relieve earaches. Native Americans of many tribes dug ginger roots to flavor their food.

WILD LETTUCE *(Lactuca canadensis)*. Wild lettuce sprouts were eaten as greens and rubbed on people's skin to stop poison ivy itch. It has narcotic properties. **Note:** Only external use is recommended.

WILLOW *(Salix* species). Native Americans of many nations simmered willow roots and twigs for an analgesic tea to reduce rheumatic pain and fever. Native Americans led us to the discovery of aspirin, salicylic acid.

WITCH HAZEL *(Haemelis virginiana)*. The Iroquois boiled the seeds with maple sugar for a nutritious winter drink. The Mohawk and Stockbridge along the northeast coast made a liniment from boiling the twigs. They took their remedy west to the Wisconsin Native Americans, who rubbed the liniment on their limbs before hunting and sports.

YARROW *(Achillea millefolium)*. The Zunis of New Mexico crushed the leaves to stop bleeding and clean wounds. For burns, the Zunis steeped the ground plant in cool water and applied a compress.

YUCCA *(Liliacea* species). The desert Native American tribes used yucca to alleviate rheumatic and arthritic pain. First, it was split in two and allowed to dry. Then approximately one tablespoon of ground yucca was boiled in two cups of water for fifteen minutes for a medicinal tea.

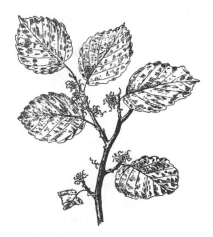

WITCH HAZEL

Origins of Native American Cuisine and Culture

The origins of American cuisine evolved from Native South Americans and Mesoamericans over eight thousand years ago. Wild botanicals, the most famous being the "three sisters" (squash, corn, and beans), were domesticated by the early Aztecs in Mexico, the Mayans of Central America, and the Incas of Peru. Through observation and experimentation, these early cultures domesticated and hybridized 150 varieties of corn and several species of beans and squash. Seventy-five percent of today's agricultural plants were introduced to Americans and Europeans by Native American tribes. Many herbs we grow today were enjoyed by our Native American forebearers as foods, beverages, skincare, medicines, and natural dyes.

Native Americans seasoned with herbs, enjoying a salt-free diet.

~

These early chefs also taught us how to cook. From them we have learned to make chowders, dumplings, stews, corn dishes, barbecue, breads, and even cranberry sauce. They seasoned with herbs, enjoying a salt-free diet.

Since early colonists failed miserably at farming, the natives equipped them with proper farming tools and knowledge of the land. Colonists were taught to store their bountiful harvest underground for the lean winter months.

The following stories exemplify how ceremony and cuisine are the basis for every agricultural society. Agricultural tribes renewed their spirits and health with group ceremonies culminating in seasonal feasts. This was a time for song and dance while enjoying the blessings of their labor. Both ceremonial and seasonal feasts promised a continuation of life, as each old and new generation looks forward to a new year.

The Mother Clan and Green Corn Ceremony

A matriarchal system, or Mother Clan, governed agricultural Native American tribes. Since the women worked the land, the women also governed the land and owned their homes. Even corn was given the name of "Mother." Property, including housing, was handed down to the women. The eldest matron, her daughters, sisters, and their husbands all lived together. Brothers and sons lived with the family members of their wives. This family of women worked and planned their lives together as one unit. A child's name was chosen from the mother's lineage and considered to belong to the family of women.

Marriage was arranged by women of two families. The new husband moved in with a whole clan of women, who not only ruled the household, but also presided over any quarreling couple. This was balanced by the mother-in-law avoidance rule. Both the mother-in-law and the son-in-law avoided speaking or even seeing each other, except on ceremonial occasions when gifts were exchanged between them in mutual respect (the only information located on a father-in-law taboo was with the Creek of the South). These "laws" were initiated to preserve the peace of the community.

The new couples were given a trial period until the new year started at the Green Corn Ceremony, which was held in July and marked a new year of fertility, growth, and renewal. At this time, all debts and grievances were forgiven, and trial marriages could be dissolved. Fasting and purification led to lighting a new fire, fueled with several ears of young, green corn. Dancing followed into the night to the rhythmic beat of hollow log drums, covered pottery, flutes, and bird-bone whistles.

Green corn leaf cakes were an integral part of the feast, and are still eaten in Mexico today. Green corn kernels were removed with pegs and scrapers and ground to a paste with stones. The paste was then wrapped in green corn leaves, covered with damp earth, and baked with hot coals in an earthen oven for one hour. The cakes were eaten with bear fat or sunflower seed oil. Leftovers were sun-dried and stored for winter meals.

The Great Iroquois Nation and the Dance of the Wild Strawberry Feast

The Great Iroquois Nation are renowned for their great contributions to horticulture. They were masters of the slash-and-burn method of agriculture used in forested areas. The men would slash trees, causing them to die and fall to the ground. They would then burn the trees, clearing a field for planting. The wood ash provided fertilization for three to four years, when new fields would again be prepared.

The Iroquois trusted women to plant their crops, believing women's magical childbearing ability was transferred to their crops. Women fertilized seeds as they planted corn, squash, and beans of many varieties and colors. Crops were guarded by the Spirit of the Three Sisters. The women talked and sang as they planted and tended the crops. First, rows of corn were planted and nurtured by the sun and rain. As the stalks grew tall, crops of beans and squash were sown. The beans wrapped around sister corn, while the squash grew as a ground cover, choking out weeds and mulching the soil to conserve moisture.

As the crops flourished, the women searched the forests for ripe, wild strawberries. *Fragaria vesca* species were native to forest lands and were enjoyed for their fragrant, sweet berries. Women filled their baskets in preparation for a feast. Native Americans understood the bounty of

Snowy winter,

a plentiful

harvest.

—Native American folk saying

Mother Nature as a gift for harmonious living and celebrated by sharing. Women danced in honor of the ripening berries as the men sang. The whole community joined in the celebration. War, politics, and differences were placed aside with tomahawks, as the great Nation gave precedence to the arrival of wild strawberries.

Berries were prepared in a variety of dishes. Any surplus were pressed and dried for the long winter months. But first the Native Americans feasted for days, as the fiercest warriors in North America waited like innocent children in great anticipation for their favorite wild strawberry bread. First, a Mohawk prayer in thanksgiving:

> Listen to her, my people, to the Earth, our Mother,
> and what she is saying. Listen!

∾ *Wild Strawberry Bread* ∾

An original Mohawk recipe.

- 1 cup cornmeal
- 1 cup oat or wheat flour
- 1 cup nut milk (see below)
- 2 tablespoons hazelnut acorn oil
- 1 cup wild strawberries

Combine the first four ingredients, stirring well. Fold in the wild strawberries and fry the batter in a well-oiled skillet, turning once.

∾ *Salt Substitute* ∾

A teaspoon of dried ground coltsfoot leaves *(tussilago farfara)* burned in a fire were often used as a salt substitute to flavor food.

∾ *Nut Milk or Oil* ∾

Nuts provided essential fatty acids, proteins, and carbohydrates to the Native American diet. Nut oils were made by pounding the nutmeats and boiling the meal in water. The oil rises to the top and is skimmed off. The nutmeats were removed and fried in hot animal fat coated with cornmeal and maple wood ash. Eastern woodland tribes pounded dried shelled nuts and boiled the nut meal in water. They strained off an oily cream-like milk and used it in cooking.

❧ *Nut and Seed Butters* ❧

Native Americans used nut and seed butters to enrich their breads.

  1 cup dried nuts or seeds (sunflower seeds, pecans, hazelnuts)
1–2 tablespoons maple syrup, honey, or water

Grind nuts or seeds in a blender. Add maple syrup, honey, or water to make a paste. Refrigerate for safekeeping. This butter is very rich. Sparingly serve with fresh fruit or vegetables, breads, muffins, and cakes, or use it as a butter substitute. Sunflower seeds yield up to fifty-five percent protein.

Variations: For variety and added flavor, combine 2 teaspoons of your favorite herb or spice while blending. For muffins, add cinnamon. For vegetables, add lemon thyme and tarragon. For legumes and lentils, add winter savory. For fresh fruit, add spearmint and/or lemon rose scented geranium leaves, finely chopped.

❧ *Dandelion Root Coffee* ❧

Here is a delicious caffeine-free coffee substitute you can grow in your own yard.

Dig dandelion taproots that are 2 years or older. Clean and pat dry. Slowly roast in a 250 degree oven 3 to 4 hours or longer until crisp and brown. Grind and store in an airtight container. Measure and brew like coffee. The finer grinds make the best coffee. Most people combine the dandelion grounds with chicory root grounds that have been roasted like dandelion roots. **Note:** Chop and grind roots in a coffee grinder for best results.

❧ *Toasted Pumpkin or Sunflower Seeds* ❧

Sprinkle any amount of cleaned seeds on a lightly oiled baking sheet. Flavor with herbs or spices as desired; for example, sprinkle cayenne over the roasted seeds and stir well before serving, or finely mince a garlic clove, stir well, and roast with the seeds. Roast 15–20 minutes at 325 degrees. Cool and store in airtight containers. Add vegetable no-salt herbal blend (page 287).

∾　*Sunflower Seed Coffee*　∾

This nutritious coffee can be used as a survival food or enjoyed on a campout.

Grind roasted sunflower seeds (unshelled) to make 1 tablespoon for each cup of "coffee" desired. Use as you would coffee grounds.

∾　*Sunflower Seed Oil*　∾

Sunflowers were one of the first plants domesticated by the southeastern Native Americans.

Bruise (lightly crush) 1 pound of shelled sunflower seeds, cover with distilled water, and boil. Skim off the oil. Use the ground paste as a butter. Any oil not used immediately should be covered in an airtight container and refrigerated.

∾　*Sunflower Seed Cakes*　∾

The Plains Native Americans enjoyed seed cakes similar to this recipe.

- 3 cups shelled sunflower seeds
- 3 cups water, soy milk, or nut milk (page 34)
- 6 tablespoons stoneground cornmeal, sifted
- 2 teaspoons vanilla
- ½ cup ground nutmeats or dried fruit (raisins, apricots, currants)

Simmer seeds in water, soy milk, or nut milk for 1 hour in a covered saucepan. Drain and grind. Combine with cornmeal, vanilla, and nutmeats or fruit to make a stiff dough. Shape into 3-inch flat cakes. Brown in hot oil. Drain and serve warm.

The Winter People and Native American Animal Guides

In the beginning, all spirits—Native Americans, ancestors, and animals—lived beneath the Earth. The Tewi Pueblos of the Anasazi called this sacred spot "the Sandy Place Lake to the North." Here cloud maidens dance on the lakeshore and the arc of a rainbow appears at twilight. There is no death; only the living reside peacefully here. Among the spirits dwell Blue Corn Woman Near Summer and the White Corn Maiden Near Winter. They call forth the Hunt Chief to find a safe passage for all Native Americans to emerge onto the land.

The Hunt Chief established two leaders for his people: the Blue Corn Chief of the Summer presided over the seven months of the growing season and the White Corn Chief of the Winter presided during the five months of the hunting season. The Summer Chief taught his people to live off the land; the Winter Chief taught his people how to hunt. Each leader kept their people in harmony with nature and the spirit world to assure abundant food and good health.

The people of the hunt looked to animals for guidance, just as the farmer looked to the sun and rain to provide abundant crops. They reconciled killing animals by believing they did not die, but took up form again to return to nature. If their flesh, skin, and skeleton were properly treated and prepared, the animals and fish could reform and return to serve humankind. Some tribes believed that animals were their ancestors who had died and returned to guide them and protect them.

Hunters honored their ancestors as animal guides, who symbolized oneness with nature. As the fire blazed, hunters journeyed in the direction of the Eastern sky, looking to their guides for direction. By drawing upon the strength of their animal guides, they developed new powers for the hunt.

After acknowledging their guides' strength, the Native Americans gazed to the South. Here they looked to animal guides with childlike innocence to root out fears or hidden insecurities.

Purged of fears, the Native Americans searched for an animal guide in the direction of the West. Here they visualized themselves as successful hunters aided by the power of their guide. On the hunt, they would wear the feathers or skin of their guide to empower them.

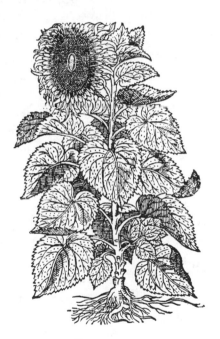

SUNFLOWER

To the North, another animal guide appeared. This one guarded the hunter from evil or self-deception that might bring him harm.

As the fire died and the ritual prayers ended, the hunters gathered objects to make a power shield, or necklace. This represented empowerment and protection offered by animals that appeared in the inner vision. To the Native Americans, hunting was not only a requirement for survival and attunement to nature, it was an art.

◌ *Fresh Game Soup* ◌

The Powahatan tribe of Virginia prepared this stew for Jamestown colonists.

- 1 pound game bird or rabbit
- 2 cups fresh peas
- 2 cups fresh corn
- 3 potatoes, cubed
- 2 onions or garlic cloves
- 2–3 dried bayberry leaves
- 10 dried juniper berries
- 6 tomatoes, chopped
- 1 tablespoon fresh basil or mint
- 4–6 fresh parsley sprigs

Boil the game in a covered pot of water until the meat can be separated from the bone. Return the meat to the pot. Add the remaining ingredients except the tomatoes, basil or mint, and parsley. Cook 30 more minutes. Add the tomatoes and herbs. Cook 10–15 more minutes. Serve with cornmeal mush, made from cornmeal and water, flavored with mint leaves or ashes of coltsfoot. Serves 12.

Mescalero Native Americans of the Southwest

From Central Alaska and Western Canada, a fragment of the Athapascan tribe migrated to the Southwest, arriving in New Mexico and Arizona between A.D. 1000 and A.D. 1200. The Tewa Native Americans named them "Apache," meaning enemy or stranger. The Apache were always warlike and were the last Native Americans to be put on reservations.

During this time, the Apaches divided into at least nine groups. In the eastern southwest area, the Jicarillo, Kiowa, Mescalero, Chiricahua, and Lipan roamed as buffalo hunters and cattlemen. They herded horses, sheep, and cattle from fleeing Spaniards. The most famous Chiricahua Native American is Geronimo. In the west, the Apaches became semi-nomadic, while trading, raiding, and growing the three sisters. Raiding provided clothing, tools, guns, and food. Horses were eaten because they were of no importance in the craggy White Mountains.

The women learned to plant gardens and dig crude irrigation ditches from the neighboring Pima, whom the Apaches raided and victimized.

The earth laughs at him who calls a place his own.

—Hindustani saying

~

Once the gardens were established, the elders tended the crops while the women scouted surrounding areas for wild vegetables and the highly prized agave plant.

Agave, known in Mexico as the century plant, provided the Apache with a nutritious food and many "household" goods. The Mescalero Apaches made a fermented beer-like drink called mescal, from which the name Mescalero was derived.

The Mescaleros tapped sap from the base of the long, flowering stalk. "Pulque" was then fermented and distilled into a beer of low alcoholic content. As they saturated their bodies with beer, they believed the rains would saturate their soil.

At the base of the flowering stalk, a large bud, or heart, was hacked out with wooden spades and roasted in earthen ovens for several days. The baked flower bud was either eaten or dried and pounded into a flour for later use. The yellow agave flower blooms in the Mojave Desert from late May through July. After blooming, the dried plant yields twine, shelter, dye, and soap for nomadic Apaches. To Apaches, the agave gave not only food and shelter, but song for pleasure. The Native Americans used hollow agave stalks as fiddles, called *tsii edo'a'tl*, or "wood that sings." The special power of this instrument was heard at night in love songs.

Native American Teas and Beverages

*W*ild herbal beverages supplied early Americans with much-needed vitamin C to prevent scurvy. Native Americans used tree sap to flavor teas, but preferred bitter tonics to cleanse their system of toxins. Teas were brewed with leaves from the mint family, whose roots were ground and roasted for coffee drinks. When water was unavailable, Native Americans drank the juice from grapevines to quench their thirst. Teas and beverages served an additional benefit as a medicinal tonic.

The Woodland Native Americans made pots from elm bark. They peeled off bark with wedges and chisels, heated sheets of bark over fires, and bent them into shapes. They retained their shape as they cooled and also became watertight, but not fireproof. To avoid burning their pots, the Native Americans filled the pot with water, heated stones in a fire, and dropped them into the water until it boiled.

The garden is the poor man's apothecary.

—Garden proverb

∾ *Bergamot Tea* ∾

Bergamot, or "beebalm" tea, was used by Native Americans to ward off colds and sore throats. *Monarda didyma* is likely to thrive anywhere. It has traveled the Americas with pioneers and Native Americans alike. The large, bright blossoms attract butterflies and pollinators.

Six leaves of this hardy, invasive member of the mint family can be steeped in a cup of boiled water for 15 minutes as an antiseptic tea. The leaves, blossoms, and stem can be brewed to soothe an inflamed throat. American colonists traded their English black tea for Oswego (bergamot) tea during the Boston Tea Party.

∾ *Chicory Tea and Coffee* ∾

The Native Americans brewed chickory root *(Cichorium intybus)* for their morning cup.

Native Americans made a tea from chicory leaves and blossoms to relieve congestion. Two of the large, toothed leaves and striking blue flowers are steeped in 1 cup of boiled water, covered, for 15 minutes. The leaves add a diuretic effect. Large, deep taproots are slowly roasted in a 325 degree oven for 30 minutes to 1 hour and ground for a coffee drink. The bitter root is detoxifying and somewhat laxative. In Louisiana, chicory and coffee are blended equally for a strong cafe au lait.

∾ *Raspberry Leaf Tea* ∾

This raspberry *(Rubus ideaus)* tea prepared pregnant women for delivery and is used today to ease labor.

Several raspberry or blackberry leaves were dried in shade and infused in boiled water. The Native Americans used 2 tablespoons of dried leaves for every 2 cups of boiled water, steeping 20 minutes before serving. This mild tea is beneficial as a sedative and antispasmodic. It was given to pregnant women for an easy delivery and to prevent hemorrhaging. Blackberry leaves were used to alleviate dysentery. The leaves and berries of these plants are also rich in vitamin C and bioflavonoids.

❧ *Dittany Tea* ❧

Dittany *(Cunila origanoides)* tea has a spicy oregano taste.

Many tribes enjoyed a warm infusion of 1 tablespoon of dried dittany leaves steeped in a cup of boiled water for 15 minutes. The Native Americans drank the tea to reduce cold and flu symptoms.

❧ *Elderberry Drink* ❧

Native Americans enjoyed elderberry *(Sambuccus canadensis)* drink to prepare for the cold winter ahead. Elderberry is a native shrub that becomes invasive as an established plant. Native Americans found a use for every part of the bush. Ripe berries were boiled into a syrupy fruit drink sweetened by the sap. It can easily become fermented into a medicinal beverage. The art of fermenting drinks was practiced by most ancient cultures for special elixirs and therapeutic drinks. The dark purple elderberries are available for picking in early autumn.

Twelve of the ripe berries were boiled in one cup of water with a six-inch piece of bark to form a syrupy fruit drink sweetened by the sap.

❧ *Rose Hip Syrup* ❧

Rose hips were eaten raw when food was scarce and made into a delicious tea or syrup when the harvest was bountiful. The dried fruit of several species of old roses, rose hips can be taken during flu and cold season as a preventative. They are high in vitamin C and have diuretic properties. The seeds contain vitamin E. Serve this syrup over ice cream and puddings.

    4 cups crushed, dried rose hips
    4 tablespoons sugar
    1 tablespoon honey

Boil 5 cups of water, add rose hips, and remove from heat. Steep 20 minutes and strain, reserving fluid. Boil the strained pulp again in 2 cups of water. Remove from stove; steep 10 minutes more. Strain and combine with the first liquid. Boil until reduced to half its volume; add sugar and boil 5 more minutes. Remove from stove. Add honey as syrup cools. Store in glass containers and refrigerate. Good for 3 months. Use in moderation: a tablespoon on cold, winter evenings.

Native American Dye Plants

Native Americans were experimenting with dyeing and weaving since A.D. 700. In the early Basketmaker cultures, before cotton and wool were available, yucca and vegetable fibers were used. Wool was introduced to the Native Americans by the Spaniards. The Native Americans immediately went to work weaving and dyeing the wool to make beautiful blankets and shawls. The Navajo Native Americans had perfected the art of dyeing through trial and error. The process was time consuming and labor intensive.

The material was washed with yucca root before dyeing. A handful of fresh or dried pulverized root could clean a pound of material. The dried root was preferred because it would last indefinitely. The Native Americans would rub the roots between their hands under cool water to produce a lather. They would then strain the lather and add heated water to produce a soapy solution. The material would be cleaned and rinsed two or three times before dyeing. Very fine material was spun before cleaning and dyeing and placed on rocks or makeshift screens to dry.

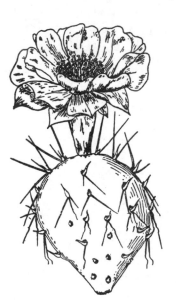

PRICKLY PEAR CACTUS

Color was produced from local plants. A plant's color shade may vary from year to year due to environmental conditions. The same plant grown in another locale may also produce a color variation. Longer boiling times were used to produce deeper colors and shade variations. Material steeped overnight in a dyebath produced deeper colors that remained fast over the years. Berries, blossoms, and cacti that would lose their color if boiled were fermented to produce a natural color. Lighter shades of the same color were produced by dyeing materials in the leftover dyebath.

Most of the materials used were fresh. Fresh plants produce a better color with less material. Any dried plants used were soaked overnight before being made into a dye. The colors remained fast after rinsing several times.

White yarn was produced by dissolving a calcium carbonate white clay into a dye bath. Gypsum was also used to whiten wool and materials. It was toasted in a fire or baked to produce a fine, white powder to be ground and added to a dye bath.

Mordants are agents, usually plants, used to deepen colors. A common mordant is juniper tree needles. The green needles are gathered and burned to produce an ash. These are dissolved in boiled water, strained, and the water used as a mordant. Mordants were not known to be used by the earliest Native American cultures and are unnecessary to hold or produce the color.

Raw alum was also used to fix colors. It can be found in its natural form under rocks where recent water evaporation has occurred in the dry southwest. The alum was either toasted on hot coals first or thrown raw into the dyebath.

The following are some authentic Native American dye recipes created from local herbs.

〜 *Yellow Dye* 〜

Plant: Gaillardia "Indian Blanket" *(Actinea gaillardia)*
Harvest time: June
Material: Fresh flowers, leaves, stems
Vessel: Enamel or granite

Boil 1 pound of fresh material in 5 gallons of water for 2 hours. Strain; add ¼ cup of raw alum to the water. Allow to dissolve by boiling 10 minutes before adding 1 pound of wet yarn. Mix well and boil the yarn for 2 hours. Steep overnight before rinsing several times.

〜 *Light Yellow Dye* 〜

Plant: Wild Celery *(Pseudocymopterus montanus)*
Harvest time: June and July
Material: Fresh flowers, leaves
Vessel: Tin or aluminum

Boil 1 pound of wild celery in 5 gallons of water for 2 hours. Strain; add ¼ cup of raw alum and boil for 10 minutes. Add 1 pound of wet yarn and boil 15 minutes before rinsing.

❧ *Rose Dye* ❧

Plant: Prickly Pear cactus *(Opuntia polycantha)*
Harvest time: September
Material: Fruit, fresh
Vessel: Earthenware or enamel kettle

Note: The Native Americans removed the spines by rubbing the cactus in the sand. Squeeze the juice from 2 pounds of cactus and strain into 3 gallons of water. Add 1 pound of yarn and soak for 1 week in a warm location. Rub the yarn daily. Rinse several times. To deepen the color, repeat the process a second time.

❧ *Purplish Brown Dye* ❧

Plants: Chokecherry *(Prunus malanocarpa)* and
         Wild Plum *(Prunus americana)*
Harvest time: Fall
Material: Fresh bark peeled from roots
Vessel: Earthenware or enamel

Soak 1 pound of each bark in 5 gallons of water overnight. Then boil 2 hours and strain. Add 1 pound of yarn and boil 2 more hours. Steep overnight before rinsing.

❧ *Green Dye* ❧

Plant: Oregon grape *(Berberis aquifolium)*
Harvest time: Fall
Material: Leaves and vines
Vessel: Granite

Boil 4 pounds of vines in 5 gallons of water for 2 hours. Strain; add ¼ cup of raw alum. Boil 10 minutes before adding 1 pound of yarn. Stir and steep overnight before rinsing.

❧ *Tan Dye* ❧

Plant: Indian Paintbrush *(Castilleja integre)*
Harvest time: June, July
Material: Fresh flowers
Vessel: Enamel or granite

Pour cold water to cover 4 pounds of flowers. Soak for 2 days and mash the flowers. Add 1 pound of wet yarn and steep for 1 week, mixing the yarn often. Rinse several times.

❧ *Orange Dye* ❧

Plant: Ground Lichen *(Parmelia molluscula)*
Harvest time: Scraped from underneath sagebrush, especially after a rain
Material: Fresh or dried lichen
Vessel: Earthenware or granite

Boil 1 pound of lichen in 4 gallons of water for 1 hour. Strain; add ¼ of raw alum and boil 15 minutes before adding 1 pound of wet yarn. Boil 30 minutes before rinsing. Boil longer and steep overnight to produce a deeper orange or reddish color.

❧ *Salmon Red Dye* ❧

The Native Americans of New Mexico and Arizona dyed wet yarn in rain water puddles in the red mesas. After a heavy rain, they would collect the reddened water and add ½ pound of wet yarn to 4 gallons of water. They boiled this for 4 hours to produce a salmon red dye.

❧ *Maroon Dye* ❧

The Hopi cooked 2–3 cups of sunflower seeds in 8 cups of boiling water. After about 30 minutes the seeds split open, turning the liquid a bluish maroon color. This would be strained and prepared with wet yarn.

Note: A display of beautiful Navajo blankets is available at the Native American Museum in Santa Fe, New Mexico.

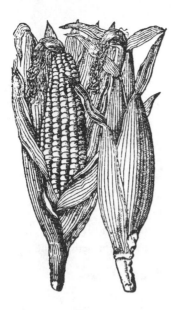

3

Elixirs of the Jaguar People

CORN

All the wonders of Nature, the powers and magical qualities,
are potentials echoing inside of you . . . because you are Nature.

South America, Central America, and Mexico are divided into seven thousand miles of mountains, jungles, and forests that bar civilization and encourage isolation. The cuisine and plant life is as varied as the natural beauty and resources. Here is a unique blend of European, African, and largely Native American heritage. The natives cling tenaciously to indigenous foods and traditions. Traveling and studying in these countries is like hearing a lullaby from the ancient past; even the terrain is a reminder of the transience of time.

Travel has been largely by sea. The terrain is sparsely threaded with torturous roads, often accessible only by ox and cart. These natural boundaries led to isolation among the various countries and inhabitants speaking more than two thousand dialects. The terrain encourages a unique and independent culture and cuisine to develop in each area, called "patrias chicas."

When Spanish and Portuguese adventurers explored the lands, they discovered the homeland of Native American corn. They understood why Native Americans worshiped a corn god who grew maize ten feet tall. Corn flourished in climates and terrain that could not support

The terrain encourages a unique and independent culture and cuisine to develop in each area, called "patrias chicas."

~

To the Mesoamericans, corn represents the seed of eternal life through death.

❧

European wheat. Since corn is the easiest grass to hybridize, Native Americans created hundreds of varieties, some as big as footballs and eaten raw.

Mesoamerican culture revolved around the experience of growing and using corn. Corn was unique to each culture. The Aztecs related to corn as the goddess Xilonen and the god Quetzalcoatl. To the Mayans, corn was one of the twin heroes, Hunahpu, who defeated the Lords of Death. The Incas of Peru embodied corn as Manco-Paca, the son of the Sun, originator of the dynasty of the Royal Lords of Cuzco. The Totonacs of Central America embodied corn as Tzinteotl, the wife of the sun. In North America, the Pawnees called corn the Evening Star, mother of life, who gardened in the sky. To the Mesoamericans, corn represented the seed of eternal life through death.

∽ *Corn Tortillas* ∾

Tortillas are the Mexican "Staff of Life." The production of tortillaria factories is supported by the government.

- 2 cups masa harina corn flour
- 1 teaspoon salt
- 1 cup warm water

Combine flour and salt in a mixing bowl. Add water a little at a time to form a stiff dough (less than 1 cup is acceptable). Divide into 12 pieces. Flatten them into 6-inch circles with a rolling pin or tortilla press. Heat a dry skillet on a medium flame. Fry each tortilla until it bubbles and browns, then turn over and cook 1 more minute. Wrap in a clean cloth and serve warm.

Through innate folk wisdom, Native Americans developed the high-protein bean to supplement their corn diet. Planted in fields next to corn, bacteria on bean roots collected nitrogen to add fertility to the soil, avoiding the soil's depletion by corn as well as completing their dietary requirements.

In Andean valleys of South America, Native Americans developed white potatoes to replace corn and beans, which did not grow well there. For protein, they developed the quinoa, whose seeds provided a rich assortment of nutrients. Squash and pumpkins also thrived in the higher altitudes. Other South American crops are sweet potatoes, manioc, cashew nuts, peanuts, cocoa, chilies, and lima beans that mature into beans as large as pocket watches.

Central and South American countries produce over half the world's coffee. Each person drinks only his or her local coffee several times a day. Coffee is always ground fresh. Peasants often grow and process their own coffee. The first seed was brought to Latin America by a French naval officer in 1720. They soon covered the cool mountain slopes with graceful, dark green glossy leaves.

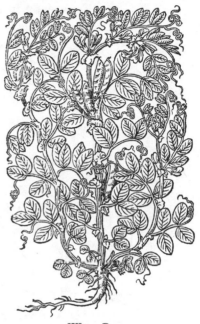

When the trees blossom into fragile, white flowers, a heavy jasmine scent perfumes the air for miles. Beans follow, taking six or seven months to mature. Surrounding the red berries is a tough outer hull and several layers of skin. After a thorough washing, the outer hull is rubbed off and the berries are fermented to loosen inner skins. The beans are dried a little longer than twenty-four hours in machines or up to eight days by sun. Another machine or hand process will remove any inner skin. Only the olive green part is left.

Roasting is done in an iron or clay frying pan over a glowing charcoal pit. They are stirred constantly to brown evenly and release an alluring aroma. Coffee is brewed immediately. Latinos will only roast enough beans for one meal, and they

WILD BEAN

roast them right before brewing their coffee. Demitasse cups of black, sugared, strong coffee are drunk up to twenty times daily. In Mexico and Argentina, green coffee beans are roasted with sugar to provide a caramel coffee flavor. The flavor of coffee will change in different climates and locales. When asked about instant coffee, Latinos reply "no es cafe!" (This is not coffee!)

Chac, The Mayan God of Rain

*H*idden in the jungles of modern Yucatan, Honduras, and Guatemala lie the silent remains of the once-flourishing civilization of the Mayas. The Mayans called themselves "the people of the wood," or Popal Vuh, in memory of their cultural past, having spent several thousand years nomadically wandering through the rain forests.

For centuries after the introduction of agriculture, the Mayan religion and cultural myths slowly evolved. According to the sacred Mayan book, the Popal Vuh, the creator, Hunab Ku ("one god") created the Maya from corn. Throughout their history, every religious and dietary ceremony involved maize. The umbilical cord was cut over a maize cob and maize dough was placed into a deceased Mayan's mouth before burial. Maize was the staple crop of the Maya, like rice in the East and wheat in Europe.

Through the invention of nixtamalization, between 1500 B.C. and 1200 B.C., the Mayans were able to grind their maize easier and raise their protein assimilation. Nixtamalization is a process which begins by soaking ripe maize and then cooking it with lime or wood ashes. The soft grain is then ground and made into a variety of maize dishes, such as tortillas, and

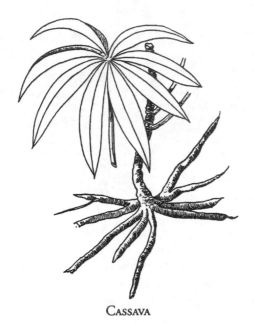

CASSAVA

drinks, such as balché, a fermented maize drink. A standard recipe calls for eight parts water, six parts maize, and up to two parts lime or wood ashes. A larger amount of wood ashes created tortillas with a harder shell to dip into a pot of beans cooked with epazote. Dietary deficiency diseases, such as pellagra, a B_1 thiamine deficiency disease, and kwashiorkor, a protein deficiency disease, did not exist where nixtamalization was used. The civilization expanded as their health improved.

To celebrate the miracle of corn, a ceremonial bread was made for the rain god, Chac. Chac was the most important deity of the Maya, who sent rain to fertilize and bless the crops. Every year the Mayans flocked to the huge ceremonial temples to honor Chac and celebrate the mysteries of Mother Nature: rain, sunlight, planting, and harvesting, which kept their world in balance. For the celebration, they prepared a ceremonial bread made of thirteen layers of maize dough sprinkled with toasted, ground squash seeds and black beans. The thirteen layers of dough represented thirteen levels in the Mayan heavens . . . and the largest tamale on earth! Pieces of dough were dipped into a broth made of water, ground chilies, and epazote, a recipe known to cure a cold and strengthen a weak heart. This recipe is still enjoyed by Mexicans today.

In addition to corn, the Mayans grew sweet manioc or cassava root, jicama, squash, sweet potatoes, and beans. They were boiled and eaten as side dishes with the main dish of maize. The vegetables were seasoned with native onion greens, chayote shoots, native tomatoes, ground squash seeds, and epazote. Honey was gathered to sweeten squash and sweet potatoes. Ground squash seeds and honey were toasted and prepared as a pre-Columbian praline.

Guacamole was prepared from mashed avocados and seasoned with onions, tomatoes, and American coriander leaves *(Eryngium foetidum).* The Mayan tomato is a small, green fruit that grows out of a papery husk. It is a totally different species than the modern genus *Physalis.*

Chocolate, derived from the Mesoamerican *Theobroma* cacao, was the favorite beverage of the Mayans. They learned to process the beans from their ancestors, the Olmecs, the first inhabitants of America. The ripe pods were fermented a few days to allow the seeds to be removed and dried. Next the seeds were toasted, peeled, and ground on a metate (a three-legged stone used to grind seeds with a handstone, or mano) with a small fire under it. The ground seeds were then boiled in water and beaten with a stick to produce a foam on top. The foam was the best part of the drink and a sign of quality to the consumer. Chilies were ground and added to hot, foaming chocolate to season the bitter beverage, which was often cooked with maize to make a spicy gruel. Cacao beans were often stored with *Tagetes lucida,* the Mexican marigold mint that has an anise aroma, to flavor the raw or toasted beans. A relative of black pepper *(Piper nigrum)* is the Mexican species *Piper amalago.* These flowers were stored with the cacao beans to add a spicy flavor and the leaves of this plant are still used in this way by Mexicans today.

Many of these Mayan foods, fertilized and blessed by Chac, the rain god, have spread throughout the world to become part of our culinary heritage. So much of their mythology has been lost or forgotten, but their recipes continue to be cooked in our kitchens.

᧞ *Cassava Cakes* ᧞

Cassava is a tropical root plant that was a staple of the Mayans of Mexico. We enjoy it today as tapioca.

- 2 cups grated, peeled cassava, moistened with water and squeezed dry
- 3 eggs or egg whites
- 2 tablespoons lime zest
- ⅛ teaspoon allspice
- 2 tablespoons cilantro, finely minced
- ½ cup cornmeal
- 3 tablespoons vegetable or sesame oil

Combine cassava, 2 of the eggs or egg whites, lime zest, allspice, and cilantro. Shape into small, flat cakes and dip in remaining egg or egg white, then roll in the cornmeal. Heat the oil in a skillet over medium heat. Fry the cakes until well-browned on both sides. Drain and serve warm. Serves 6.

The Chosen People of Huitzilopochtli

*B*y the year 1168, a new barbarian migration entered the Valley of Mexico from the north. These fearless Nahua-speaking people had been chosen by their god Huitzilopochtli to leave their Aztlan homeland in northwest Mexico to rule the world. They were to settle where they found a cactus growing out from a rock supporting an eagle holding a serpent. This was their promised land of water and abundance, Tenochtitlan, Mexico City.

The Aztec were the first complete urban culture of the New World. When Spanish conquistadors arrived in 1519, they found a culture rich in herbal flora. They were so impressed with the beauty of the gardens, they were spared of destruction. The gardens and flora were still growing in 1570 when the King of Spain, Phillip II, sent his physician to catalog and draw the Aztec flora.

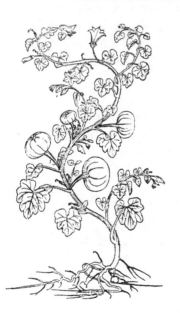

PUMPKIN

Many of the plants used in ancient times continue to grow in Mexico today. Maize, beans, capsicum pepper, cilantro, agave, pineapple, pumpkin, peanuts, avocado, cocoa, sweet potatoes, and vanilla name a few of the rich supplies available to the natives. The Conquistadors enjoyed an Aztec chili sauce made with cocoa beans, called molé. They learned to soak corn kernels and unslaked lime in water and grind it into a paste to cook tortillas over a fire, like the natives of prehistoric times. The Spanish introduced sugar for cocoa, garlic, onions, cinnamon, and rice to Mexico. They taught the Mexicans to fry beans, and introduced the potato and red tomato to Europe from its origin in the New World.

The Aztecs produced the first herbal, with colored pigment drawings of Mexican herbs and a commentary on their medicinal uses. Thirteen chapters outlined the medicinal uses of local plants and gave an herbal remedy for every known ailment. It was preserved and translated at the request of the son of the first Spanish viceroy of the New World, who is also believed to have introduced cloves, ginger, pepper, and other spices to the conquered land.

From the Aztec herbal, known as the *Bandianus Manuscript,* the Native American culture comes to life in a series of simple remedies. Yarrow *(achillea millefolium)* was used as a hemostatic astringent. Mexican marigold mint *(tagetes lucida)* was used in human sacrifices and chocolate drinks. The agave plant, so sacred to all the Latin and Mexican American cultures, was used for treating wounds. The prickly pear cactus *(opuntia* species) was combined with thistle and sedum to treat burns.

These remedies may have been used during the last siege of Tenochtitlan. The Native Americans fought almost to the last man in a battle that lasted eighty-five days. Since the thirteenth of August 1521, only slums remain where the Aztec nation bled to death. Their spirit lives through their own song:

> We only came to sleep
> We only came to dream
> It is not true, no, it is not true
> That we came to live on the earth.
> We are changed into the grass of springtime
> Our hearts will grow green again
> And they will open their petals
> But our body is like a rose tree:
> It puts forth flowers and then withers.

Their herbal remains . . .

Mexican Cuisine

The richness of the Mayan and Aztec cuisine is apparent throughout Mexican cooking today. They eat the same foods, seasoned with the same herbs and spices that flavored their ancestors' foods in centuries past. Their genius lies in time-honored recipes that evolved as slowly as their culture.

How to Handle Chilies

Everything I know about handling chilies, I learned the hard way!

CLEAN FRESH CHILIES in cold water only (hot water produces irritating fumes). While rinsing under cold running water, pull out the stem and break the chili in half. Rinse or brush out the seeds. Soak fresh chilies in cold water 1 hour to remove any intense heat.

DRIED: Tear dried chilies into pieces. Cover them in boiled water and steep for 30 minutes.

CANNED: Rinse in cold water. Stem and seed.

Note: After handling chilies, thoroughly wash your hands with soapy water and rinse with cold water. Be sure to scrub under your nails with a nail scrub brush to remove all volatile oils released from the chilies. The volatile oils will burn skin on contact.

Salsas

Salsas, the ancient flavoring of Mesoamerican cuisine, retain their popularity today.

✑ *Salsa Verde* ✑

Enjoy this green sauce as a side dish with guacamole and tortillas.

- 1 (10-ounce) can Mexican green tomatoes, drained
- 2 serrano chilies (canned green chilies), chopped
- 1 garlic clove
- 1 small onion
  coriander and/or cilantro leaves to taste
  salt and pepper to taste

Blend the above ingredients a few seconds only. This may be lightly seasoned with a no-salt herbal blend (page 287) and freshly ground pepper.

✑ *Salsa de Chili Rojo* ✑

Try this red sauce as a dip with raw vegetables and tortilla chips, and have lots of ice water available to drink.

- 4 ancho chilies
- 1 large onion
- 2 large tomatoes, peeled and seeded
- 1 garlic clove
- 1 tablespoon oil
- 6 parsley sprigs, finely chopped
- ½ teaspoon sugar
  salt and pepper to taste
- 1 tablespoon red wine vinegar
- 3 tablespoons olive oil
- 6 pequin chilies, optional

Combine chilies with onion, tomatoes, and garlic clove, and purée in a blender. Heat oil in a skillet and add purée, stirring constantly for five minutes. Add parsley sprigs, sugar, salt, and pepper to taste. Stir in red wine vinegar and olive oil. Add pequin chilies if you like it HOT.

Sauces

An ancient way to flavor fish, sauces such as the following will enhance any fish or seafood meal.

❧ *Old Sour* ❧

Old Sour is a seasoning for fish and seafood made from fresh limes. This is a favorite seasoning in several Latin and American cuisines.

    2 cups freshly squeezed lime juice
    1 tablespoon salt

Add salt to lime juice and allow to set 1 hour. Strain through double layers of cheesecloth and bottle. Store in a dark, cool place for one month before serving on fish. Do not refrigerate.

❧ *Hot Pepper Lemon Sauce* ❧

This is a baste enjoyed on fish in Mexican, Central American, and South American cuisines along coastal areas. It gives the fish a meaty flavor.

       Juice of 1 lemon (about 2 tablespoons)
    2–4 chilies, seeded and chopped
      6 tablespoons grated onion
      ¼ teaspoon minced garlic
      ¼ fresh lemon or lime, sliced
      5 geranium leaves, minced
      2 pounds fresh fish

Combine all but the fish and let stand, covered, at room temperature for 2 hours before serving. Baste on fish before grilling.

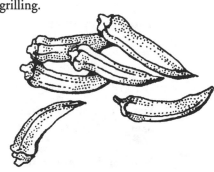

CHILIES

Herbal Teas

Herbal teas are prepared as simple remedies for common complaints. They are rarely served with meals or drunk for pleasure.

❧ *Horchata: Almond and Melon Seed Tea* ☙

A delicious and nutritious milk substitute that can be prepared in minutes.

- ½ cup melon seeds, dried
- ½ cup blanched almonds
- 1 cup sugar
  zest of 1 lime

Pulverize the seeds and almonds in a blender. Combine this mixture with 6 cups of water, sugar, and lime zest in a pitcher and allow to steep 4 hours. Strain through a muslin cloth, squeezing out all the milk. Serves 6.

❧ *Té de Yerba Buena: Yerba Buena Tea* ☙

Yerba buena is a favorite mint of the Mexicans. They drink it to comfort their stomach, reduce fever, and soothe colic.

- 2 tablespoons fresh or 1 tablespoon dried yerba buena leaves
- 4 teaspoons sugar

Boil 4 cups of water in a glass or porcelain pan. Remove from heat. Add yerba buena leaves and steep, covered, for 10 minutes. Strain and serve 4. The Mexicans dissolve 1 teaspoon of sugar in each cup of tea.

❧ *Té de Canela: Cinnamon Tea* ☙

The Mexicans drink cinnamon tea to promote cardiovascular strength.

- 4 cinnamon sticks
  orange zest to taste
- 1 tablespoon sugar, optional

Simmer cinnamon sticks in 5 cups of water for 15 minutes. Add the orange zest or a tablespoon of sugar, if desired. Strain and serve 4.

Herbal Tea Remedies

The Mexicans believe in simple remedies made from local, fresh herbs and spices. Simmer 1 teaspoon of herb in 1 cup of water for 10–15 minutes. Strain and drink, sweeten, if necessary, or follow specific directions.

HERB	PREPARATION
Anise	For stomach cramps and flatulence, crush 1 teaspoon and simmer in 1 cup of water as directed.
Artemisia	For colic, steep 1 teaspoon of leaves in 1 cup of water. Apply locally as a compress. Artemisia, especially the root, is considered toxic by other cultures when taken internally. Dilute the tea in a bathtub of water and enjoy a relaxing soak instead.
Artichoke	For common liver complaints, bilious flatulence and even jaundice, the leaves are cooked in water to cover for 15 minutes and the juice drunk.
Asafoetida	For a digestant to reduce flatulence, simmer ¼ teaspoon in 1 cup of water for 5 minutes and drink. It is also taken as a tea for anger. Not recommended for children, elderly, or those with inflammatory intestinal disease.
Boldo	For diabetes or gallbladder indications of clay-like stool, simmer 1 teaspoon of boldo leaves in 1 cup of water for 15 minutes. Strain and drink
Borage	To reduce fever, steep 1 tablespoon of chopped leaves in 1 cup of boiled water and drink.
Cedar	For colds and flu, steep ½ teaspoon of cedar berries in boiled water for 10 minutes and drink for colds and flu. Consider making this into a topical compress. Apply to the forehead, chest, or throat.
Chamomile	For stomachaches and colds, steep 1 teaspoon of flowers in 1 cup of water for 10 minutes and drink. Inhale the steam from the tea for bronchitis.
Cinnamon	For coughs, simmer ½ cinnamon stick in 1 cup of water for 10 minutes.
Clove	For toothaches, apply a few drops of clove oil to sterile gauze and apply locally. To make clove oil, steep ¼ teaspoon of crushed whole cloves in 3 tablespoons of heated vegetable oil for 5 minutes. Strain and apply locally.
Corn silk	For a diuretic, steep 1 tablespoon of corn silk in 1 cup of boiled water for 10 minutes, before straining. Drink 1 cup.
Jasmine	To reduce stress, steep 1 teaspoon of jasmine flowers in 1 cup of boiled water for 10 minutes and drink. This may be combined with ½ teaspoon of chamomile flowers.

Cocina Costarriqueña: The Costa Rican Kitchen

Costa Rican cuisine is exclusively Spanish and Native American in origin. This small Central American country has 125 miles of coastline along the Caribbean and 600 miles of Pacific coast, giving it the name "rich coast." The land offers dense jungles, active volcanoes, and miles of banana, plantain, coffee, palm, and sugar cane farms. Commercial industry, other than farming, is nonexistent. Tourism and farm export are the mainstay of the economy.

The cocina costarriqueña features an abundance of fresh local seafood. We caught swordfish only a few miles away from the Osa Peninsula rainforest, near the port of Golfito. The taste of pure food is incomparable. The natives fry fish or grill it. There are no markets or stores in the countryside. They walk to the coast and bring home dinner. Chickens are raised by the natives for eggs and meat. There are no refrigerators or freezers in their homes. Everything is prepared fresh daily. The natives I visited had a beautiful turkey, but the women did not want to eat it because it also served as their watch dog. Chicken and eggs are fried in vegetable oil, along with yucca flowers growing nearby.

Beef is raised by farmers in the mountains and along the seacoasts. Many farmers own much of the countryside leading to the virgin western coasts. Europeans are quickly buying these virgin lands to build resorts and cabanas. Farmers there are still using carts drawn by oxen over a land that has never been touched by civilization before.

Although the cattle are skinny, the flavor of the beef is good. The natives fry beef in vegetable oil or lard. Recent data reveals an unusually high incidence of stomach cancer in Costa Rica, due to cattle being grazed on land previously sprayed with DDT. Since the Western world has banned DDT, suppliers have shipped it to third world countries. DDT finds its way back to our tables from food exported from these countries. We buy most of our beef for fast food restaurants from Central America.

Throughout Costa Rica, local black beans and rice are a staple. The Ticos (Costa Ricans) have no original national dishes. Their cuisine has been borrowed from other South American, Central American, and Spanish cuisine. During one of my visits, I met a New York chef brought to San Jose to create a unique national cuisine. Hired by a famous restaurant in San Jose to entice tourists and Ticos alike to enjoy local foods with a new taste, he developed sauces for a variety of fresh fish entrées using local, organically grown herbs such as basil, oregano, rosemary, marjoram, and thyme. He also introduced several pastas with light, aromatic sauces made with lime, mango, and a hint of cayenne. These creations brought clientele back again and again, encouraging other chefs to create new delicacies of their own. What impressed me the most was that the New York chef was also beginning a trend to grow herbs locally, without chemicals, to flavor these new entrées. He believes the flavor of the herbs is enhanced by using only organic amendments and the fresh taste is enhanced by abstaining from pesticides. I hope the Ticos will also be flavoring their beans and rice with organically grown herbs.

The natives with access to land can grow beans and rice. Tortillas are made from locally grown corn, a variety with large, white kernels. The processing is done by hand, for the natives have plenty of time. There are no jobs or industry, so they must catch, grow, and harvest their meals from scratch. In areas like Limón, plantains and local fruit are the mainstay of the diet.

Food is seasoned with chilies, salt, and ginger. They grow lemon grass for tea and a lemonade drink. Onion, garlic, and tomatoes are grown in northern higher altitudes where coffee is grown. The jungle is too hot and humid for herbs and vegetables that thrive in the hottest climates. The high humidity encourages rust and fungal growth on agricultural crops, creating a persistent problem for farmers.

Many tropical fruit trees grow wild in the cloud forests, the mountainous part of a rain forest that has a canopy of cloud cover hovering over the highest elevation. The lush tropical climate is ideal for mango and papaya trees. The mango trees house parrots and tropical birds, who feast off the fruit. Avocados, oranges, limes, and the thorny peach palm, pejibaye, grow almost everywhere. Coconuts offer a refreshing juice and fruit where it is too hot for bananas to thrive.

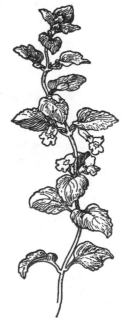

Yerba Buena

Mango Salsa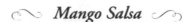

Mango trees are prolific in the western coast of Guanacasta, the Costa Rican jungle. Parrots, howler monkeys, wasps, and Ticos alike are nourished by mangoes.

- 3 large, ripe, peeled and diced mangoes
- 2 tablespoons diced onion or garlic
- 1 chili pepper (poblano or serrano), seeded and diced
- 2 tablespoons fresh lime juice
- 1 cup chopped cilantro or fennel leaves
  salt to taste or 1 teaspoon no-salt herbal blend (page 287)

Combine and serve. Yields 2 cups.

Mango Swordfish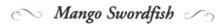

Mango salsa is served in restaurants as a condiment with fresh, succulent, grilled swordfish.

Four 6-ounce steaks serve four. To grill swordfish, brush with olive oil and place on a hot grill. Turn every 2 minutes until done. Steaks will be firm and translucent in the center. Serve with a tablespoon or two of mango salsa on each fish.

Papaya Honey

The Costa Ricans eat this plain or with tortillas and meat. Papaya is an excellent digestive aid for proteins, such as beef, chicken, and fish.

- 2 cups peeled and diced papaya
- ¼ cup honey or sugar (Latinos use sugar because it is more available)
- ¼ cup freshly squeezed lime juice

Rub the papaya through a sieve and blend the lime juice and honey. Yields 2 cups.

Coconut Cream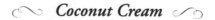

Coconut juice is a favorite roadside beverage in Costa Rica.

- 1 fresh coconut
- 1 tablespoon fresh lemon verbena leaves

Take the juice and meat from a fresh coconut, add lemon verbena leaves, and put it through a juicer. A thick, delicious, fresh cream results. Refrigerate for storage.

The Lords of the Andes

The Inca Empire extended over 2,500 miles, running north and south from northern Ecuador to Central Chile. The Incas ruled over six million subjects in a unique totalitarian government of their own invention. Andean civilizations developed over many thousands of years. These ancient farmers survived the March of Tiahuanacan warriors and the rise and fall of the jaguar feline cults. The basic fundamentals of agriculture, irrigation, terracing, and ceramics developed, never to change.

Every act of daily life began with a religious ceremony. At sunrise priests called out to the Sun to bless his children, the Inca. Their creator was known as Viracocha, who taught them only goodness and then walked away on water across the Pacific Ocean. To the Incans, the only direction was east and west, the direction of the Sun, and their leader was the reincarnation of the Sun.

Plant breeding was culturally advanced. Although maize did not reach Peru until thousands of years after Mexican breeding, Inca cultivation rivaled the genius of the Mexicans. Peru does not have a particular growing season, so corn can be grown and harvested throughout the year. The cultivated corn is soft enough to eat without preparation. Cancha is a toasted corn prepared in a special pottery vessel. It was the ration for Incan soldiers in the 1400s and still carried by journeying Peruvians today for a snack. The Native Americans ground cancha with dried vegetables and ají, a Peruvian chili (page 63) to create an instant soup mix. Corn is ground in a simple and unique stone: one side is cut to be curved so the stone rocks easily on a flat surface.

Many regions of the Andes are too cold to grow corn. In these mountainous regions, the Native American potato is the main crop. Almost every shape and color of potatoes are grown there. They have a distinct flavor and dense matter. After the harvest, the greater part is taken to 13,000-foot altitudes and exposed to extremely cold nights until they are freeze-dried into a material as light as cork. The Native Americans call them chuños in their native Quechua language.

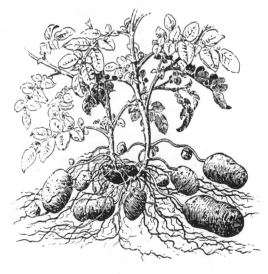

POTATO

⁓ *Papas a la Huancaina* ⁓

Once you taste a Peruvian potato dish, french fries will never be the same.

- ¼ cup fresh lemon or lime juice
- 3 pequin chilies, dried and crumbled
  freshly ground pepper to taste
- 1 large onion, peeled and thinly sliced into rings
- 8 potatoes, boiled and peeled
- ⅓ cup extra virgin olive oil
- 1 cup queso blanco or mozzarella cheese
- ⅔ cup plain yogurt (the Peruvians use heavy cream)
- 1 teaspoon ground turmeric
- 2 teaspoons fresh chilies, chopped and seeded
- ⅓ cup olive oil
  black olives to garnish

Combine lemon juice, dried chilies, and ground pepper in a large bowl. Add onion and marinate at room temperature while the rest of the meal is prepared. Make a sauce by blending (by hand or in a blender) the cheese, yogurt, turmeric, and fresh chilies. Heat olive oil in a heavy 10-inch frying pan. Add the sauce and simmer 5 minutes until the sauce thickens. Pour the sauce over the warm potatoes, sliced or whole. Drain the onions and place over the potatoes with extra strips of fresh chilies. Garnish with black olives. Serves 8.

Pachamanca: Peruvian Earth Oven

A joyous occasion in Andean culture calls for a pachamanca—in the native Inca language of Quechua, an "earth oven." Earth ovens are common in Mesoamerican and South American cuisine. These ancient ovens have existed since people began cooking with fire. It is made by digging a circular three-foot-wide pit in the earth and lining it with stones. After the hole is filled with dry wood and straw, stones are placed on top and a fire is lit. After a few hours, the unburned wood is removed and the pit is lined with aromatic herbs and any available pig, goat, or chicken placed on top. Rice, corn, potatoes, and ají are placed around the meat, and more green leaves are placed on top. Hot stones are placed over everything and the pit is sealed with earth. As the oven cooks, the mound is decorated with flowers as indigenous chants of the ancient Andeans are sung:

> Peacefully, safely sun,
> shine on and illumine the Incas,
> the people, the servants whom you have shepherded
> guard them from sickness and suffering in peace and safety.

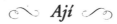

Ají

Ají is an original Incan sauce.

- 1 cup dried chilies, seeded
- 6 tablespoons cold pressed virgin olive oil
- 1 garlic clove
- 1 cup vegetable, beef, or chicken stock

Break dried chilies and remove the seeds. Place in a bowl with 2 cups of boiled water for 2 hours. Drain and discard the water. Combine the chilies with olive oil, garlic, and vegetable, beef, or chicken stock. Purée in a blender for 2 minutes. Yields 2 cups.

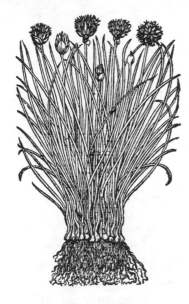

CHIVES

4

Seeds of Freedom

Speak to the earth and it shall teach thee.

—Job 12:8

American colonial cuisine is a blend of Native American foods and traditional English cooking. It quickly became regional and seasonal. Each colony had its specialty, with corn and apple dishes dominating their simple meals. Local Native Americans shared corn seeds and taught the settlers how to grow abundant crops. The gift was returned with apple seeds, which soon grew into orchards dotting the countryside to supplement the lean winter diet of smoked meat and salted fish. Europeans brought seeds of their favorite vegetables and herbs to plant alongside the American corn, beans, and squash.

By 1780, colonists and Native Americans grew every food crop known to the western world. Every settler had a vegetable garden laced with herbs. They cooked with herbs to hide the wild flavor of meat and moldy vegetables and drank beer and wine made from costmary and dandelions. The most popular herbs grown were garlic, onion, sage, rosemary, thyme, and parsley, all of which adapted easily to a variety of colonial soils. Herbs were cooked more often than vegetables and were used along with nutmeg to season meat. Vegetables were grown only as garnishes, the most popular ones being introduced by the local Native

Every settler had a vegetable garden laced with herbs.

⁓

Americans. Many vegetables, like tomatoes, were not cultivated for food until the 1800s because they were believed to be toxic.

Lemon and orange extracts, as well as rose and violet waters, were favorites for flavoring until Thomas Jefferson introduced vanilla in 1789. Since then, only French recipes and flavorings have been acceptable to American cooks.

An American Colonial Kitchen Garden

The kitchen garden was planted outside the back door to produce a variety of seasonal herbs. Plants were selected by usefulness: salad herbs, seasoning herbs, pot herbs for cooking, sweet herbs to be used fresh in seasoning. Tansy was grown close to the door to repel ants and the blooms were hung upside down at the entrance to repel flies. Sweet herbs were dried in the "tin kitchen," a portable oven placed on top of the hearth near the fire. Dried herbs were hung upside down from the kitchen rafters to be saved for winter cooking.

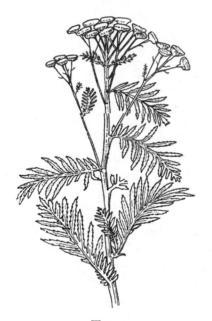

TANSY

The location of the kitchen varied geographically. In the northern colonies, the winter kitchen was built under the house, like a partial basement. During the summer, colonists would construct an outdoor kitchen away from the house. In the south, the kitchen was built as a separate building apart from the house, near the gardens. Since fire was a constant hazard, colonists built separate kitchens whenever land and resources would permit.

Formal gardens were popular with northern colonists. Their straight, linear designs moved the eye quickly, giving a comprehensive effect. Individual plants and colors were not as noticeable as the whole garden. Raised beds were occasionally used for edible beds and dramatic borders. Wood or brick pathways were laid for easy accessibility from the kitchen. Circular gardens with a centerpiece in a square courtyard were popular in southern plantation homes.

Herb gardens were companion planted with vegetables and shaded by nearby cherry or lilac trees. Pink and lavender althea was often grown against the house or fencing for color. Flowers were seeded in any space available to bring pleasure to the eyes and to invite birds and predator insects.

A Colonial Herbal

*H*ere are the favorite herbs and remedies grown and enjoyed by the colonists. Many of the remedies are still useful today.

Angelica archangelica is a hardy biennial native to northern Europe. It was grown against fences or as a background plant, as tall as eight feet. It grew in partial shade and rich soil. Northern colonists used it to flavor jams, rhubarb, cherry, and apple pies. The stalk was used as a straw and the leaves were cooked as greens. A tea was made to alleviate colic and stomachaches. For tea, steep one teaspoon fresh (or one tablespoon dried) angelica leaves in a cup of boiled water for ten minutes, strain, and add honey.

Basil *(Ocimum basilicum)* is an annual that flourishes in full sun and composted soil. It was grown for commercial culinary use in Virginia before the Revolutionary War. It was used in a variety of culinary dishes.

Caraway *(Carum curvi)* is a naturalized biennial in the carrot family, grown by colonists for its seeds. The roots were cooked and eaten like carrots. The seeds were either chewed or added to cheese, fruit, and baked goods as a carminative digestant. Caraway thrives in moist, humus soil and partial sun.

Catnip *(Nepeta cataria)* was brought from England and "escaped handsomely into the wildernesse." It was steeped in wine or mead for contusions, head colds, and stomachaches. Women used catnip in a sitz bath to make them fruitful. Colonists grew catnip along the fences and against the house where it was shaded from the heat.

Chamomile *(Anthemis nobilis)* was brought from Europe for pleasure and medicine. The flowers were cooked in a "posset to provoke sweat and expel colds and aches." A syrup was made with sugar for jaundice and dropsy. The flowers and leaves were made into a decoction for a bath to benefit everyone.

Chives *(Alliums* of garlic and onion) are a hardy perennial grown for culinary and medicinal use, as well as flower arrangements. Garlic and onion were a remedy against every disease and protected children against evil spirits during the night. Chives were gardened in full to partial sun, bordering tomatoes or other vegetables. The flowers were dried for arrangements and the chives garnished vichyssoise.

COSTMARY *(Chrysanthemum balsamita* and *leucanthemum)* was also known to colonists as "Alecost." In the spring, a special ale was brewed with sage. It was blended with sweet herbs to make a "washing water," and the flowers were tied with lavender blooms to bedposts for sweet dreams. Costmary was often mistaken for maudeline, a similar herb. Costmary grows a foot taller and was used as a bookmark in Bibles because of its pleasant aroma.

DILL *(Anethum graveolens)* grows in sunny, well-drained soil as an annual. Dill was enjoyed in stews and pickles, but was especially grown for its tonic purposes. The Norse word *dilla* means "to lull to sleep." It was used as a sleeping tonic and to "stayeth the hiquet" (hiccups). Colonists also believed it would "strengthen" their brain. The Puritans chewed dill seed during long church services to stay awake, reduce hunger, and especially avoid "hiquets." Puritans believed hiccups to be a conflict between spirit and flesh. "Meetin' seeds" kept the secret in the closet!

HYSSOP *(Hyssopus officinalis)* was a popular medicinal herb in new America. It was used as an expectorant in a tea mixed with rue and honey. The leaves were bruised and applied with sugar on "greene wounds," probably staph infections. The leaves were soaked in oil and applied to the head to kill lice. An oil of leaves and flowers was applied to "benumbed joints," probably arthritis. Special application for adders' sting was a compress of bruised hyssop leaves mixed with honey, salt, and cumin seeds.

LAVENDER COTTON *(Santolina chamaecyparissus)* was a favorite border plant in colonial knot gardens. The seeds were eaten to expel worms and the leaves and yellow button blossoms were used in baths and ointments for "cold diseases," such as rheumatic complaints. Lavender cotton is no longer considered safe for internal use.

MARIGOLD *(Calendula officinalis)* was a colonial pot herb added to broths and drinks to "comfort the heart and spirits." A syrup and conserve were made of fresh flowers for the same effect.

MARJORAMS *(Origanum marjorana, vulgare* and *lippia graveolens* as Mexican oregano), sweet or knotted, were grown for culinary and aromatic purposes. Nosegays, sweet powders, sweet bays, and washing water were aromatic uses. It was used to wash sores, heated in wine, and drunk for bites and stings. Sprigs were often seen drying in windows to freshen the air in the house.

Mints (*Mentha* species), especially spearmint, were drunk as a tea to comfort the nerves. Mint boiled in milk was a remedy for lactose intolerance. Leaves were bruised and applied with salt to dog bites. As a culinary herb, it was boiled with fish or dried and added with pennyroyal to puddings and green peas.

Parsley (*Petroselinum hortense*) was grown to cook with meats of every kind. The aromatic flavor removed the wild taste of game meats. The young roots were boiled to remove "obstructions of the liver" and promote urine. The seeds were used with the roots to remove stones, or renal calculi, and possibly gallstones.

Periwinkle (*Vinca minor*) was grown near the garden area as a ground cover. The leaves were bruised and applied locally to stop bleeding. Colonists also believed the wives' tale that eating a few leaves would stop quarreling between a man and his wife. Periwinkle is toxic and is only recommended for topical use.

Purslane (*Portulaca oleracea*) was grown between the herb beds and garden pathways. It was eaten in salads to cool the body during hot weather and increase the appetite during the summer, called a "faint stomacke."

Rose of Sharon (*Althea officinalis* and the marshmallow species) were included in the colonial garden area. It was valued for its "slimy quality" to nullify hard tumors and ease pain as a local compress made from the boiled root.

Rosemary (*Rosmarinus officinalis*) was in every woman's garden, sometimes planted against a brick wall. An oil, "drawn from the heat of the Sunne" of the flowers only, was applied to restore eyesight and remove spots and scars on the skin. First, the flower oil was bottled in glass, "close stopped," and set in hot horse manure for 14 days "to digest." Rosemary compresses and oils were used for the head and heart to relieve painful joints and muscles, or "sinews." Rosemary was often potted and kept inside for the winter.

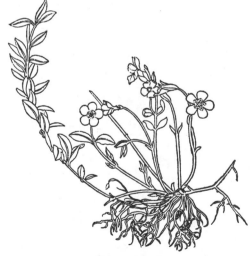

PERIWINKLE

ROSES (*Rosa* species) were grown near the house and gathered for sweet waters, homemade perfumes, and cordials. The hips were gathered in the fall and made into jams and added to meat pies. They were often served at winter meals.

SAGE *(Salvia officinales)* was a favorite culinary and medicinal kitchen herb. For "spring cleaning," colonists fasted on sage with butter and parsley to produce a healthier body. It was brewed into an ale and given to women to facilitate delivery. In the kitchen, it was boiled with a calf's head or minced and cooked with brains to be served in a pepper vinegar sauce. As a tea, sage was used as a gargle and added to baths. Its flowers were also added to salads.

SAVORY (summer and winter, *Satureia hortensis* and *montana*) was used instead of epazote in beans. It was added into meat puddings and sausages or boiled with peas, both being "effectual to expel winde."

THYME *(Thymus vulgaris)* was grown in knot gardens and used for melancholy, splenic diseases, flatulence, and toothaches. The species grown was an upright, wild thyme that survived the cold winters.

Sweet Herbs: "For the Hand or Bosom"

Here is a list of sweet herbs used in early American cuisine. The cook gathered a bouquet from the garden. She made a bouquet for her cooking pot and one to wear in her bosom. Sweet herbs are aromatic, such as rosemary and thyme, and are worn in the bosom of a corset, allowing body heat to release the pleasant scent.

BALM (lemon balm) drunk in wine drives away melancholy.

BASIL'S smell was believed to be good for the heart and head.

BURNET (greater salad burnet) was drunk in claret wine to stop bleeding and added to salads to preserve health.

COAST-MARY (costmary) is a fragrant herb that was used to make ale more nutritious.

CHAMOMILE was a bath herb. The flowers were also boiled to cure colic, colds, and to "bring down stones" in the kidney.

CALAMINT, or "Mountain mint," was eaten with honey to cure shivering and bring out a fever. A decoction was used to bring down a "dead child." Mountain herbs were believed to be much stronger and superior because of where they were grown.

HYSSOP is an expectorant as a tea, often mixed with rue and honey. An oil was made to use for lice.

LAVENDER spikes were made into an oil for cold or numb hands and feet. The flowers were used to perfume linens and clothes.

MARJORAM was used in nosegays, sweet powders, sweet bays, and sweet washing water to comfort the body.

MUSKED CRANESBILL *(Geranium maculatum)* was used to heal open wounds and ulcers as a poultice. Used in baths with balm to strengthen the nerves and as a tea for weak stomach.

MINTS (spearmint, red mint, red apple mint, basil) were used for indigestion as a tea.

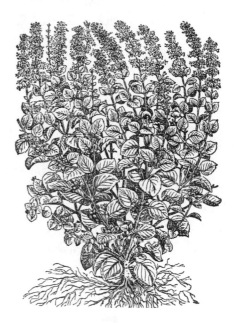

CALAMINT

PENROYAL (pennyroyal), or "Pudding grasse," was added to baths to relieve itching. Only topical use is recommended.

SAGE was served in May with butter and parsley and added to baths and used as a tea for a gargle.

SAVORY (winter and summer) was cooked with meat and added to sausages.

THYME (English hard, French, lemon) was a remedy for whooping cough.

TANSIE (tansy) was made into tansy pancakes. The seed was used to expel worms in children. The flowers were gathered and dried for winter bouquets. Tansy is toxic in large doses. The pancakes were made with only a few fresh leaves for 4–6 servings.

Herbs for Pickled Sallets (Salads)

These herbs were kept in a pickling vinegar of white wine vinegar boiled with sugar and were served in the winter for salads, when settlers were missing the harvest of their vegetable gardens the most.

Burage (Borage) flowers	Onions
Cowslip (Queen Anne's Lace) flowers	Purslaine (Purslane)
Elder buds	Summer Savory
Hartichoaks (Artichokes)	Tarragon
Leekes (Leeks)	

Edible Flowers in a Colonial Kitchen

American colonial housewives used edible flowers of herbs to float in soups, add to salads, and chop into butters. They also decorated their main dishes with a border of herbal flowers. The most popular are listed below.

Anise Hyssop blooms	Fennel and Dill florets
Basil flowers	Mints, Lemon Balm
Bee Balm flowers	Onion and Garlic Chive flowers
Borage	Parsley
Carrot	Sweet Cicily
Dandelion blooms	Thyme
English Lavender blooms	Violets

American Colonial Remedies

Since herbalism was intricately woven into astrology, alchemy, and the Doctrine of Signatures of the Old World, Puritans chose to utilize herbs only through Biblical association. Although diseases afflicting the settlers were the same as the Old Country, the remedies were not. As many Puritans died out, remaining settlers relied on local Native Americans to learn what herbs were edible and which ones were medicinal. Home cures were soon grown in a nearby kitchen garden alongside salad vegetables and apothecary roses. The women were responsible for the health and well-being of the community; as Thomas Tusser writes in *Five Hundred Points of Good Husbandry* (1557):

> Good huswives provide, ere an sickness do come.
> Of sundry good things in her house to have some.
> Good aqua composita and vinegar tart,
> Rose water and treacle to comfort the heart.

> Cold herbs in her garden, for agues that burn,
> That over strong heat, to good temper may turn, . . .
> Conserves of barberry, quinces and such
> With sirops, that easeth the sickly so much.

Diseases affecting settlers included "griping of the belly with fever which turns into a bloody flux" (bloody dysentery, or diarrhea). This, and smallpox, led to high mortality rates in children. Remedies included "sugar and sallet-oyle (salad oil) boiled thick and alltes (aloes) pulverized and taken with the paper (pulp) of an apple." Pleurisies and empyemas (emphysemas) were treated with pulverized coriander seed and drunk in a cup of wine. Onions were roasted, peeled, and boiled with oil and rum to make a compress that sounds good enough to eat.

Colonists were also sufferers of the common cold. They boiled marigolds, sage, and wormwood with "crabsclaws" (a house leek) and drank the resulting concoction. Monkshood was used as a "poison" to relieve pain (in small doses, of course). A water for the eyes (eyewash) was distilled in white wine, steeped with fennel, eyebright, sage, vervain, betony, celandine, cinquefoil, and the "herb of grass," or grace, which is rue. Internally, eyebright was infused with rosemary in white wine to improve vision. Back pain was treated with a syrup of yarrow, borage, or "comphrey," and drunk with brandy and gunpowder. Gunpowder was also applied to the hollow of an aching tooth, while mint leaves were applied to insect stings and chewed for a contraceptive. Sarsaparilla and sassafras were tried for the pox, a venereal disease spread by the Spanish conquistadors, while the Native Americans used *Lobelia syphilitoca,* all to little avail.

Herbs also for man's good: That he may bring out of the earth what may be for their food.

—Puritan psalm

~

A Pioneer's Apothecary

The following authentic remedies were put to the test by American Colonial wives and mothers. They may be reminiscent of remedies your grandmother made.

To RELIEVE BRONCHIAL CONGESTION, make a hot mustard plaster and apply it to the chest or back. First, rub sweet oil (olive oil) on the skin. Then, take a teaspoon of mustard seeds and crush them with a mortar and pestle. Combine with 3 tablespoons of water and 1 egg white, beaten. Apply to a clean cloth, then to the chest or back. Allow to "warm up" and remove after 15 minutes or if the plaster becomes uncomfortable. **Note:** Do not apply to open skin or allow to touch very sensitive skin.

To REMOVE BUNIONS, apply fresh radish juice every day for several days.

To SOFTEN BUNIONS AND CORNS, make a salve from equal amounts of soda ash (baking soda) and render fat (lard). Apply locally at bedtime.

To RELIEVE A COLD, slice open a fresh onion and allow it to sit overnight near the "sick bed."

Boil 1 quart of water, add 1 tablespoon each of sage, thyme, and chamomile flowers, fresh or dried. Allow the steam to rise and inhale the vapors.

Steam 1 tablespoon of freshly grated ginger root in 1 cup of boiled water for 15 minutes. Strain and add 1 tablespoon of filtered honey.

To RELIEVE COLICKY BABIES, make a tea with 1 teaspoon of crushed dill seed and 1 cup of boiled water. Steep 10 minutes; strain. Dip a clean cloth into the tea, and allow the baby to suck on the cloth.

To RELIEVE CONGESTION, steep 1 teaspoon of crushed anise or fennel seed in 1 cup of boiled water for 15 minutes. Strain. Add 1 teaspoon each of honey and cider vinegar.

To REMOVE CORNS, soak ground ivy leaves in cider vinegar overnight. Wrap an ivy leaf around the corn and secure with a clean cloth. Change leaf every day, applying a fresh one.

To RELIEVE A COUGH, squeeze the juice of 1 large onion and add 1 tablespoon of honey. Take 1 teaspoon 3 or 4 times daily. Apply the onion to the chest, "mashing it well."

Mix 2 teaspoons of cider vinegar in water or wine. Sip 1 tablespoon 4 times daily.

Combine 2 tablespoons of honey with 1 tablespoon of grated horseradish root to sooth a cough.

Make a tea of 1 teaspoon grated nutmeg in 1 cup of hot cider. Drink 3 times daily.

To CLEANSE THE DIGESTION SYSTEM, chew on watercress or parsley leaves after a meal.

Drink a cup of chamomile tea.

To RELIEVE DIARRHEA, add 1 drop of cinnamon oil to 1 cup of warm water and sip.

To REDUCE EYESTRAIN, soak a clean cloth (or cotton balls) in a tea made from fresh rosemary leaves. Steep 1 tablespoon in a cup of boiled water for 15 minutes. Strain, apply to a cloth, and lie down, pressing gently while covering the eyes.

To RELIEVE FATIGUE, simmer 1 ginseng root in 2 cups of water for 1 hour, covered. Strain and sip the tea. The root may be boiled again in 1 cup of water and then eaten with honey. (George Washington may have been colonial America's first herbalist. He developed overseas trade with the Chinese for American ginseng, which he learned about from the Native Americans gathering roots in the West Virginia hills.)

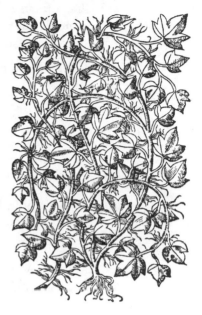

IVY

To RELIEVE A HEADACHE, make a tea from fresh mint, lavender, or rosemary leaves. Steep 2 teaspoons of leaves in 1 cup of boiled water for 15 minutes. Strain and drink or apply as a compress to the forehead and temples.

To RELIEVE HEARTBURN AND INDIGESTION, squeeze the juice from celery and drink it to relieve gas and indigestion.

Make a tea with 1 tablespoon fresh or dried peppermint leaves in 1 cup of boiled water. Strain after 15 minutes and drink 1 cup to relieve gas, indigestion, and nausea.

Make a tea from 1 tablespoon of basil or parsley, steeped in 1 cup of boiled water for 15 minutes. Strain and drink to relieve gas and nausea.

To REDUCE INFLAMED SKIN OR SUNBURNS, apply thin slices of fresh cucumber or potato to affected skin. Bind with a clean cloth.

Cook several lettuce leaves in a few tablespoons of water for 5 minutes. Apply to the skin as it cools.

To ALLEVIATE ITCHING AND INSECT BITES, apply cider vinegar locally. Rinse with salt water.

To RELIEVE RHEUMATISM, simmer ¼ teaspoon of nutmeg in 10 ounces of water for three minutes. Sweeten with honey and drink or apply the tea locally on painful hands.

To RELIEVE A SORE THROAT, combine 1 cup of rose water with 1 tablespoon of mulberry syrup. Drink a swallow 3 times daily.

Simmer 1 tablespoon of chopped licorice root in 1 cup of water for 15 minutes. Strain and drink a swallow three times daily.

Dissolve 1 tablespoon of salt in 1 cup of warm water. Gargle (but do not swallow) the saltwater 3 times daily.

To CLEAN TEETH (REMOVE TARTAR), rub fresh strawberry juice on teeth.

African American Remedies

The African Americans had their own unique remedies. Their circumstances made them very frugal. When illness did occur, they looked for simple solutions to find natural remedies.

COLDS: A plaster of cooked, mashed onions was applied to the chest.

COUGHS: Combine 1 tablespoon honey and 1 tablespoon lemon juice and take it in a shot glass of whiskey.

"BLOOD PRESSURE" HEADACHES (HYPERTENSION): Mash a clove of garlic in a few tablespoons of cider vinegar. Drink a tablespoon for a headache or after eating fatty meats.

INJURY FROM A RUSTY NAIL OR OBJECT: Apply a piece of fatty meat and tie it on with a clean rag. This was used to prevent lockjaw and infection.

Look for simple solutions to find natural remedies.

~

MEASLES: Make a tea from 3 corn shucks boiled in 2 cups of water for 1 hour. Add mint leaves and 2 teaspoons of sugar. Steep 10 more minutes before straining and drinking the tea.

MUMPS: Rub the neck up to the ears in sardine oil. Tie the jaws up with a clean rag to prevent the mumps from traveling down into the testicles of young boys.

SORES AND SCRAPES: Apply cobwebs and cover with tallow or lard. The sores will heal within a few days. Wash thoroughly.

CLEANING TEETH AND GUMS: Use a sassafras twig like a toothbrush. Dip the sassafras twig in baking soda and "brush" to whiten teeth.

TENSION AND MALAISE: Drink a shot glass (1 ounce) of homemade brandy made from the following recipe: Boil 2½ pounds of peach pits in 4 cups of water for 1½ hours, stirring often. Allow to cool and set for 3 days until an alcohol smell develops. Store in clean glass jars.

North American Native Weeds

*H*ere are the herbs that were awaiting American colonists with nourishing and healing roots, berries, and leaves. Like the colonists, they learned to survive in adverse circumstances.

BERRIES *(Rubus* species) grew wild throughout the colonies, foretelling the fertility of the soil. Native Americans and settlers enjoyed them for medicine and pleasure.

BARBERRY *(Berberis vulgaris)* leaves and berries were enjoyed in sauces. As a medicine, the leaves were bruised and applied topically to wounds, and the berries were crushed and cooked with the dried leaves to reduce fever. Native Americans prepared a tea from the dried roots as a tonic for fatigue.

BAYBERRY *(Myrica pensylvania)* was known to colonists as candleberry. Settlers made candles from the wax of the berries. They boiled the berries to allow the wax to float to the top and skimmed it as it hardened.

BEARBERRY *(Arctostaphylos uva ursi)* was also known as whortleberry. A cold water infusion was used to treat kidney and bladder complaints. Native Americans also used the bruised, dampened leaves to keep poison ivy from spreading and to reduce swelling in sprained muscles.

BILBERRY *(Vaccinium)* was a forerunner of the huckleberry and was cooked in meat pies.

BLACKBERRIES *(Rubus* species and dewberries) were known as bramble bushes. The dried leaves were made into a tea for "stomache augue" and dysentery. The berries were eaten in a variety of dishes.

BLOODROOT *(Sanguinaria canadensis)* is a native red dye plant introduced to settlers by Native Americans. It has been used as a powerful emetic and expectorant for pulmonary consumption. The sap was used externally for skin cancers. **Note:** Bloodroot is a very toxic alkaloid herb. Nausea, vomiting, and headaches may occur with ingestion.

BLUEBERRIES *(Vaccinium)* were baked in puddings and eaten to cool the body of fever and searing pain. The leaves were dried and blended with other herbs as a tea.

*A*lready the old things are being lost. . . . It is well that they should be put down, that our children, when they are like white people, can know what were their father's ways.

—Chief Eagle
of the Pawnee

~

BOUNCING BET *(Saponaria officinalis)*, known as soapwort, is a lathering cleanser. The leaves, roots, and stems contain saponins for washing clothes and cleaning wounds and sores. Soapwort is related to the dianthus family of pinks. Their pretty pink flowers are aromatic at night. For a delicate soap, simmer 2 ounces of soapwort in 2 cups of water for 10 minutes. Allow to cool before straining.

BURDOCK *(Artium lappa)* is a naturalized, fast-growing biennial with large, egg-shaped leaves and a long taproot. Burdock roots were boiled in 2 cups of water and used as a compress for skin complaints.

CHERRIES *(Prunus virginiana,* chokecherry, and *Prunus pensylvanica,* pin cherry) are natives to North America. They make a good cough medicine. Cherries grew in thickets and woods. The Native Americans made teas with the stems and pounded, dried, and cooked the cherries in pancakes.

CHICORY *(Cichorium intybus)* is closely related to endive. It grows 3 feet tall with angular dandelion-toothed leaves. The stems blossom into beautiful clusters of sky blue flowers that open and close daily on their own time schedule. The leaves are eaten in salads or cooked with greens for kidney complaints. The roots are laxative, and are cooked like carrots or roasted and served as coffee. Water distilled from the flowers was used to bathe inflamed eyes.

Dogs and cats eat couchgrass as a preventative and cure-all.

CHICKWEED *(Stellaria media)* is an annual with tiny, white, star-shaped flowers that produce an abundance of seeds. It is eaten as a salad herb, cooked as a vegetable, and made into a poultice for abscesses. As the seeds attached to traveler's shoes, chickweed became naturalized all over the world, even at the Arctic circle.

CLOVER *(Trifolium pratense)* was used to reduce acidity and increase the assimilation of iron. The flowers were brewed for tea to relieve whooping cough.

COUCHGRASS *(Agropyron repens)* is a creeping rhizome that has naturalized worldwide. It is an important anti-erosion weed also known as dog grass. Dogs and cats eat it as a preventative and cure-all. Native Americans and colonists made a tea from the root to reduce cystitis, gout, gravel, kidney stones, and rheumatism. It will certainly alleviate prostatitis as well.

CRANBERRIES *(Vaccinium oxycoceus)* were boiled to take away the "heate of burning agues" (fevers). Colonists boiled cranberries with sugar to keep them from spoiling and make their taste palatable.

CURRANTS *(Ribes rubrum)* were used extensively by the colonists for puddings and meat pies.

DANDELION *(Taraxacum officinale)* is a medicinal and culinary weed. The leaves are eaten in salad, brewed for wine and beer, and have a bitter and diuretic effect. The roots are laxative and can be eaten raw, cooked like carrots, or roasted and ground for coffee.

DAYLILIES *(Hemerocallis liliacea)* were enjoyed by the Native Americans in soups and salads. The flowers were steamed or fried and eaten as a vegetable. The tubers were picked in the fall when they were most nutritious and boiled or eaten raw like radishes.

DOCK *(Rumex acetosella,* sorrel and *crispus,* yellowdock) is known as a sour dock. The leaves are long, pointed, or rounded. It can be served in a salad or cooked as a green. Settlers boiled them with meat to produce a better flavor. The roots were boiled in vinegar to relieve itching and "cure freckles."

ELDERBERRIES *(Sambucus canadensis)* were made into jams, wines, and jellies, and used in a darkening hair rinse. The Shakers used elderberries for cold and cough remedies.

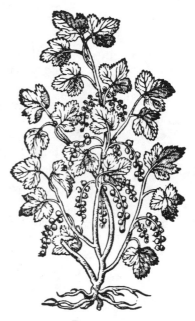

CURRANTS

EPAZOTE *(Chenopodium ambrosioides)* is an annual that reseeds prolifically and grows wild in Mexico and Texas. Migrating birds probably scattered seeds north as far as Albany. Soon colonists found it growing wild in their gardens. Although it was used in bean dishes in the Southwest, it never became popular in the colonies. The Puritans were opposed to the pungent odor, and did not understand that epazote reduced the flatulent properties in beans. It is growing wild in American colonial gardens, parks, and museums in New York. Nicknames for epazote are pigweed, wormseed, or Jerusalem oak.

To make a "safe" pot of beans, cook 1 tablespoon of fresh or reconstituted epazote leaves for each cup of dried beans.

LAMB'S QUARTERS *(Chenopodium album)* is a 3-foot annual with pale green flower clusters. The powdery white undersides of the leaves were dried and ground into flour by the Native Americans and colonists. Also known as goosefoot, it was also eaten as a salad vegetable and is related to spinach and Swiss chard.

LICORICE *(Glycyrrhiza glabra)* is an ancient root grown by colonists. Its wild form, *Galium circaezans,* has been used as a food and medicine for centuries. Colonists combined it with hyssop water for asthma and upper respiratory complaints. Pioneers and travelers used it to reduce thirst on long journeys. As a general tonic, medicinal ales were brewed with anise, sassafras, fennel, and licorice.

MALLOWS *(Althea officinalis)* are in the marshmallow family. Colonists grew hollyhocks and rose of Sharon near their gardens as medicinal herbs. The leaves were bruised and applied to hard tumors. Roots were dug, boiled, and the water drunk for constipation and stomach ailments. French mallow leaves were stewed and eaten as pot herbs.

MULLEIN *(Verbascum thapsus)* is a 5- to 6-foot biennial with clusters of bright yellow flowers. Colonists dipped it to make candles and made a tea of the leaves and flowers for lung complaints and gout. One ounce was steeped in 2 cups of water for 15 minutes and strained through cheesecloth to catch the fine hairs. Its slightly sedative effect is good to reduce coughs.

NETTLE *(Urtica dioica)* is an ancient remedy to counteract poisonous mushrooms and stings. Young nettle shoots were creamed, added to salads, and enjoyed as a wine by settlers. Nettle is not recommended for those with kidney and urinary disorders.

OXEYE DAISY *(Chrysanthemum leucanthemum)* is a common wild plant that flourishes prolifically in pastures. Colonists used the flowers like chamomile for skin problems and as a tea for nervousness.

POTENTILLA *(cinquefoil)* or silverweed was used by the Colonists, who bruised the leaves and applied them to external ulcers. The plant has five finger-like leaves. Its unusual shape made it popular in love potions and charms. Colonists tinctured the leaves in wine to relieve gout and cancerous tumors. An infusion of leaves was added to a bath to relieve "bleeding piles" (hemorrhoids).

PURSLANE *(Portulaca oleracea)* was enjoyed as a salad and pot herb. The bruised leaves were applied to gouty pains and inflamed eyes. A tincture was used to reduce fevers and coughs. A soup was made with peas, edible flowers, and purslane leaves. The hard stems were pickled with ginger root and peppercorns.

TANSY *(Tanacetum vulgare)* was a favorite early American weed. It was used in springtime remedies after a winter diet of salted meat and fish. Colonial women laid the bruised leaves on their abdomen during pregnancy to avoid miscarriage. Women desiring children would drink beer boiled with tansy leaves. Tansy is toxic in large doses. Only small amounts (2 leaves in a 4–6 person serving) should be ingested.

WILD CARROT *(Daucus carota)* is Queen Anne's Lace. It grows wild in meadows, beautifying them with flowering fields of lacy, white umbelliferae flowers. The roots and seeds were boiled by settlers and eaten to "promote urine and expel winde." The leaves were applied with honey to clean runny sores.

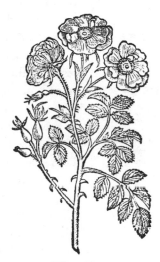

WILD ROSE *(Rosa rugosa)* is a single, magenta-colored rose with dark green leaves that have a hairy underside. It is a very prickly bush that expands by suckering, growing a secondary side or branch root, creating a natural border on fences and near colonial gardens. The hips were brewed into wine and syrup for use during the winter. Dried petals were steeped in teas and fresh roses were made into simple confections.

WILD ROSE

∾ *Rose Confection* ⁀

Colonists added rose confection to puddings or ate it like candy.

- 2 tablespoons fresh rose petals
- 6 tablespoons sugar

Pound the petals of fresh roses with a mortar and pestle until a pulp is formed. For each tablespoon of roses, add 3 tablespoons of sugar. Beat until blended into a smooth paste and seal in sterile glass containers.

Variations: Add any of the following to the rose petals: 1 tablespoon fresh lemon verbena leaves; 1 teaspoon fresh lavender leaves; or ⅔ teaspoon fresh spearmint leaves.

The Cooks of Freedom

The frugal age of colonial cooking led to regional specialties from each of the thirteen colonies. Cooking became a real challenge of the imagination in the chilly isolation of the New England shores. Freedom first brewed on the open hearth over a fire made from a bed of hot coals, where an open fireplace soon became "an altar of patriotism." Food-conscious cooks preparing native foods grown on virgin soil were mistaken by their English countrymen as "cider drinkers" who ate "heathen foods cooked on ashes."

New England cuisine featured the fruits of local natural resources, the results of the length of their growing season as well as the opportunity to trade. Coastal sea trade brought a variety of exotic spices from the East. The most popular was nutmeg, believed to be therapeutic. It was added to meats, pies, and beverages. New Englanders learned to make milk-based chowders when clean water was scarce, and to lighten coarse wheat flour cakes with the invention of pearlash. Since making baker's yeast was an exact and often difficult process, pioneer American women created pearlash, a soda salt obtained from potash leached from the wood ashes in their fireplaces. Pearlash became known as baking powder in the nineteenth century. Any extra wood ash was readily applied to their kitchen garden soil.

Herbs were cultivated to create original American recipes designed to hide the bland and sometimes moldy taste of food. Freedom cooks were too thrifty to trade their tasty cod and giant crabs for herbs they could easily grow outside their kitchen. Due to the high price of paper, recipes were shared by memorizing and repeating them to each new generation. Recipes were simple, like adding fresh mint to cook peas, and rose petals and peach leaves to apple pies. When unexpected company arrived, crushed juniper berries and ground pine needles were added to poultry stuffing, and water to stews.

Good food became the most important contribution of colonial hospitality. Each American colony developed unique cuisine from local produce and catches. From the tidewaters of Chesapeake Bay, Maryland provided Maninose soft-shelled crabs, oysters, fish, and clams. The rocky soil provided blackberries and blueberries for preserves and pies. During the weekly biscuit baking, children were taught to beat dough with a flat stick until it blistered. The "beaten biscuit" was created to keep from molding in the coastal high humidity.

Along the Delaware Bay, Native Americans first navigated boats upriver to Philadelphia to trade with other colonists and foreign lands. The original settlers of Delaware were Swedish, who built the first log

Let your prayers for a good crop be short, and your hoeing be long.

—American Colonial garden proverb

cabins and carefully roasted fish on planks before open fires. They settled in the dense forests on the Naticoke hunting grounds, where high mortality rates quickly reduced their population. What remains of their culture are stories of snowy sleigh rides on Christmas Eve, eggnog served on New Year's Day and Easter, and a local drink of beer and rum called manatham.

In Pennsylvania, English colonists were joined by descendants of the German-Swiss borders. The Pennsylvania Dutchmen cleared land in the black walnut forests and established farms growing wheat, oats, barley, and buckwheat in the limestone soil near the French Huguenots and Quakers. The Pennsylvania Dutch were renowned as gourmet cooks throughout the colonies. They created Pepper Pot Soup to feed the Continental Army and introduced Scrapple, made from fried cornmeal mush and ground pork. They initiated the first American mid-morning coffee break and fried doughnuts, later known as the danish, to accompany it. The Pennsylvania Dutch habit of dunking doughnuts in hot coffee every morning became a popular American tradition after the Boston Tea Party, when the British departed. Benjamin Franklin celebrated both occasions with the invention of the drip coffee pot. Their cuisine soon spread through the colonies, adding dumplings, German-style sausage, and vinegar dressings to the list of national foods.

Fresh fruit and vegetables were provided by New Jersey, soon to be known as the "Garden State." They shipped fresh produce to nearby Pennsylvania and New York, and provided the Continental Army with Fort Morris Turtle Soup, seasoned with fresh onions, parsley, and thyme. Long before the Revolution, New Jersey had become famous for a sauce made with wild cranberries, created for the whalers to prevent scurvy. Today, socials still offer colonial cuisine, such as Native American clam bakes, oyster pies, and soft molasses cookies.

New York's bays and rivers provided a variety of sea life. The fishing season began in March, when the shad appeared in the freshwater rivers. These were soon followed by the sturgeon, oyster, sea bass, salmon, crab, and six-foot lobsters. Oysters were then pickled and exported to Barbados as a delicacy. The shad were carefully dried and preserved for the winter. The "New Netherlands," settled by the great seafaring Dutchmen, enjoyed bountiful crops in the great valleys of the Mohawk, Herkimer, and Hudson. The Native Americans were friendly and

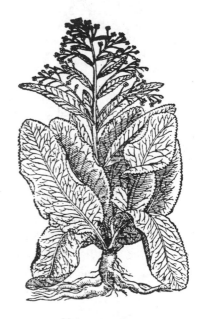

HORSERADISH

taught the colonists to plant in cycles and utilize local herbs and trees for food and medicine. They were amazed to see fruit orchards grow and flourish on the rocky soil now known as Manhattan. The Dykeman cherry originated on the large estate located on what is now 210th Street and Broadway. The original colonial farmhouse and formal gardens have been restored and are administered by the New York Parks and Recreation as a museum called the Dykeman House.

Tea soon became the preferred beverage of the Dutchmen, joined by the Irish, Scottish, and English settlers. It was second only to local brews of rum and beer. Tea and sugar were kept hidden under lock and key, and were served with "split cakes" flavored with cinnamon and spread with butter. Sugar was pressed into cones and cut with special scissors at the table. Fashionable colonists would hold a small piece of sugar in their mouths as they sipped their tea. Cider, squeezed from a horse-drawn press, soon rivaled the popular Albany brewed beer as the national beverage. "Apple holes" (pits dug underground to store apples) appeared as far north as the Catskills and were used to preserve apples for hot milled cider during the winter.

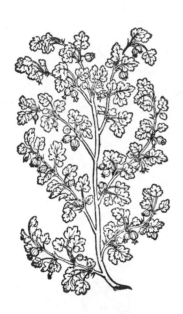

GOOSEBERRIES

In the Tidewaters of Virginia, cooks built their culinary reputation on wild razorback hogs originating from Spain and peanuts introduced to the New World from Africa. The Virginians learned the art of curing and smoking ham from the Native Americans, a process that took eighteen months to complete. A variety of vegetables, herbs, and fruit grew prolifically in the rich, moist soil, where melons and strawberries thrived and wild cuppernong grapes were made into a fine dinner wine. For the aristocracy of Virginia, African-American cooks perfected a deep dish spoon bread, with a lightly browned crust and a rich pudding-like omelette flavored with "yellow buttons" tansy juice. Fresh sturgeon was slowly baked with parsley and sage and served on strawberry leaves. Poultry, mutton, and veal were fried with "all sorts of sweet herbs." Robins were flavored with parsley and thyme, cooked in a pie, and served with corn pudding, fresh black-eyed peas, and pumpkin fritters. In the frontier, opossums were trapped and cooked in pot pies, and bear meat was stewed with wild persimmons. Ash cakes (ashes from an open fire that were mixed with water and pressed into a pancake) were served with a wild blueberry sauce, and wild garlic was cooked in vinegar. Every Virginian had a family recipe for gingerbread. Their recipe made a hard, flat cake that kept well and traveled with the Continental Army until the end of the Revolution.

North Carolinian cuisine was strongly influenced by friendly Native Americans. The land was abundant and fertile. Fresh fish, shellfish, and green turtles were easy to catch. Wild game lived on the largest grapes and wild berries known in the New and Old World. In the fall, Native Americans taught the early settlers how to locate and hunt wild turkey, raccoon, wild boar, opossum, and a variety of local dove and pheasant. In the winter, thousands of ducks and geese found refuge from the Northern climate in the Carolina tidewaters.

The Native Americans smoked thin strips of meat on wood racks over a low fire. They made pemmican to supplement winter supplies by pounding dried meat, adding rendered fat, dried fruit, and oats, wrapping it in a cloth, and dipping it in wax. Surplus peaches were mashed, cooked into a thick paste with sugar, covered and spread into a thin layer and dried in the hot sun for three days to make peach leather. Since the Carolinas were populated with many well-fed grasshoppers, the Native Americans ate them too, fried to produce a nutty flavor.

Because the growing season was twice as long, the Carolinas harvested many times. Succulent green beans and squash grew with corn, Native American-style. Jerusalem artichokes, sweet potatoes, and a variety of greens for pot herbs were grown in kitchen gardens.

A variety of fruits, melons, and wild berries grew in the North Carolina hills. Peaches, plums, figs, cranapples, persimmons, apples, pomegranates, mangoes, and Keiffer pears provided a variety of ciders, pies, preserves, and fresh fruit. Watermelons and banana-cantaloupes were summer favorites, along with currants, dewberries, gooseberries, and cranberries. Hostile Native Americans and pirates hid near the coves where many of the berries grew. These berries were left for the birds, animals, and adventurous travelers.

In all the Southern colonies, drinks were made from local fruit as cordials, wine, and cider. The rule for health was that cider was for drinking and water was only for washing. The Native Americans only drank the water if it was boiled first and steeped with fresh or dried herbs.

In South Carolina, rice was served three times daily or grace was not even spoken. Carolina gold rice seed arrived in 1685 from Madagascar and was cultivated by African slaves. The situation was ripe for an aristocracy of plantation owners to farm hundreds of acres of rice for export.

Cuisine was strongly influenced by friendly Native Americans.

‿

African-American cooks created a large variety of rice dishes over an open hearth fire, complimented by shrimp, Bulls' Bay oysters, pork, hominy, sweet potatoes, and sausages. A traditional plantation breakfast was sautéed shrimp and hominy. French Huguenots introduced their cuisine, adding wine, rues, and French bread to the menu. Fruit, melon ices, and sherbets were served with mint julep on hot summer days. Poke salad, salsify tops, ramp, watercress, and nasturtium flowers were served with salted meats and pickled vegetables for a summer salad. Since olive trees did not grow in South Carolina, an oil was made from pounding "bene," or sesame, seeds that were brought to the colonists by Africans.

The colonists never lost their connection with Mother Nature.

∾

During the American Revolution, the rice crop was exported by the British Army to England, leaving no seeds for future crops. Thomas Jefferson smuggled rice seed from Italy to allow South Carolina to produce the rice they loved so much.

In 1733, Georgia became the last of the original thirteen colonies. Women imported from Europe to be wed to settlers learned to cook from the Native Americans. As eggs and milk became abundantly available, the cooks added them to Native American corn recipes. Large bake ovens were built next to the open fire or near the chimney to bake delicious breads from local rye and oats. Georgians cultivated pimiento peppers for seasoning and developed paper shell pecans to complement a large variety of fruit and vegetable recipes. These colonists ate very well, with eight to fifteen different dishes served in one meal.

The colonists who first settled North America possessed rare qualities of stamina and a great love of the land. Through generations their achievements brought them wealth, fame, and power, yet they never lost their connection with Mother Nature and hospitality for their neighbor.

An American Colonial Cookbook

The first American cookbook, *American Cookery*, was written by "an American orphan," Amelia Simmons. It was published in Connecticut in 1796 and became an instant success. The work is unique in utilizing Native American foods, such as "Indian meal" (cornmeal), pumpkin, Jerusalem artichokes, and maple syrup. The author recommended the use of pearlash from wood ashes to leaven cakes and cookies, the forerunner of baking powder. American words such as molasses replaced the traditional British treacle, and native traditions replaced the formal British way of eating. Corn was eaten off the cob, "like playing a harmonica," and sweet dough was fried in hog fat and called a doughnut.

Recipes were given for pickling watermelon rind and for a sauce of cranberries made to serve with roasted turkey. Nutmeg was used to flavor meats and game, as well as desserts. Instructions were given on how to grow and use kitchen herbs: parsley, sage, thyme, garlic, rosemary, savory, sweet marjoram, and onion. Food was prepared in a very large open fireplace or brick oven, until Dr. Benjamin Franklin invented the Dutch oven. These black kettles with fitted lids stood on four short legs in the fireplace's hot coals and enabled cooks to bake "johnny cakes," bread, and beans. The first American iron box stoves were cast in 1765 at the Mary Ann Furnace in Pennsylvania, but were not readily available in American kitchens until after 1820.

Original American Colonial Recipes

Reading these recipes reminds me of learning to cook with my mom . . . take a little of this and add it to a little of that!

❧ *American Citron* ❧

Pickled watermelon rind was served during the winter months when fresh food was scarce. This recipe is from *American Cookery* by Amelia Simmons.

"Take the rine of a large watermelon . . . cut it into small pieces, take two pounds of loaf sugar, one pint of water, put it all into a kettle, let it boil gently for four hours, then put it in pots for use."

❧ *American Colonial Gingerbread* ❧

During the Revolution, gingerbread was hard and would keep for years. It was a staple for British and American soldiers alike. Original recipes call for grated nutmeg, ginger, and fresh cream, and were served to Lafayette by General Washington. This recipe is from *The Art of Cookery Made Plain and Easy by a Lady* (London, 1760) by Hannah Glasse.

"Take three pounds of flour, one pound of sugar, one pound of butter rubbed in very fine, two ounces of ginger beat fine, a large nutmeg grated, then take a pound of molasses, a quarter pint of cream, make them warm together, and make up the bread stiff; roll it out, and make it up into thin cakes; cut them out with a teacup, or small glass, or roll them round like nuts, and bake them on tin plates in a slack oven."

∾ *A Colonial Thanksgiving Turkey* ∽

This eighteenth-century southern recipe is still enjoyed in Virginia on Thanksgiving Day.

"Stuffing: Soak 1 large loaf of stale bread in milk to moisten. Add salt, pepper, ½ teaspoon each of thyme and marjoram, three sprigs of chopped parsley, 1 onion finely chopped, 2 stalks of celery, 12 olives stoned and cut and 1 pound of sausage cooked in a skillet. Knead and add 1 pound of roast chestnuts cut in two. Stuff your turkey, sew it, truss it well. This will fill a ten- or twelve-pound turkey.

"Put it up to the fire and allow 25 minutes per pound. Roast slowly at first and be often basted with butter on a fork. Dredge it with flour just before taking it up, and let it brown."

∾ *Colonial Herb Stuffing* ∽

Colonists enjoyed this stuffing in hens, turkeys, and game birds.

- 1 teaspoon sage
- 1 tablespoon each sweet herbs: sweet marjoram, mint, basil, thyme
- 1 lemon rind
- ½ teaspoon fresh grated nutmeg
- ½ teaspoon each salt and pepper
- 4 cups stale bread cubes, optional*

Combine and mix well. *No bread was mentioned in the original recipe.

∾ *And the Gravy . . .* ∽

From Marion Cabell Tyree, *Housekeeping in Old Virginia*, 1879.

"The giblets ought to be boyled tender. Use the water for gravy, adding a little of the turkey trimmings, seasoning with pepper, salt and sweet herbs, and thickening with a little flour and water, mixed smoothly. Place it where it will boyl."

∾ *Homemade Bitters to Improve Digestion* ∽

From the cookbook of Miss Margaret Prentis, 1832.

"Set into 1 gallon of brandy, 4 ounces of dried cut orange peel, 4 ounces of dried gentian finely cut, 2 ounces of whole cardamom seed. After 3 weeks, take 1 jiggerful with the evening meal."

❧ *Dandelion Wine* ❧

In colonial times, dandelion wine was brewed every summer. It was made by the barrel in a community project. The children were sent out in groups to scour the countryside for every yellow bloom. Here is an eighteenth-century recipe found in Salem, Massachusetts.

"Boil 4 quarts of water. Add 2 quarts of dandelion flowers and allow to steep 3 days. Stir daily. Then strain, add 5 pounds of sugar, 3 oranges and thinly sliced lemons and 1 yeast cake dissolved in warm water. Steep 3 more days and strain. Leave for 4 weeks, strain and add ½ pint of good whiskey. Bottle and add 3 raisins to each bottle."

❧ *Homemade Soup Powder* ❧

Shakers were the first to advertise using herbs in homemade recipes such as this soup powder. From Miss Beecher, 1859, the Colonial Williamsburg foundation library.

"Dry and pound 1 ounce of lemon peel, basil, thyme, sweet marjoram, summer savory, a few celery seeds and 2 ounces of parsley. Bottle tight to season soup or sauces."

❧ *Homemade Stock for Herb Soup* ❧

From *The Lady's Companion*, 1753.

"Get chervil, beets, chard, spinach, "sellery" leeks, a bunch of sweet herbs, two large crusts of bread, butter, a little salt in a moderate quantity of water. Boil them an hour and a half, strain out the liquor through a sieve and it will be good stock for soup."

❧ *Syrup of Roses* ❧

Rose syrup flavored sweet breads and cakes served at mid-afternoon teas. From Elizabeth Monroe, 1800 (from *Historic Food Programs*, Colonial Williamsburg foundation).

"Steep 3 pounds of fresh damask roses in a gallon of warm water 8 hours. Use an earthen glazed pot with a narrow mouth and secure a lid very tightly. After 8 hours, squeeze out the roses, reheat the water and steep 3 more pounds of fresh roses for 8 hours. Press the roses very hard and remove. To one quart of liquid, boil 4 pounds of sugar to make a syrup."

❧ *Syrup of Violets* ❧

Martha Washington served violet syrup to delegates from many governments who dined with the Washingtons at their ten-course meals. From *Martha Washington's Booke of Cookery*, 1770.

"Boil 3 pounds of sugar in 2 cups of water for 10 minutes. Remove any scum. Crush 1 pound of violets in a mortar, add to syrup and cook until it loses color. Strain and bottle in glass when cool."

The Marriage of French and Virginian Cuisine

He that plants trees loves others besides himself.

—Old English garden proverb

Thomas Jefferson introduced French cuisine to America. He brought his servant, James Hemings, with him in 1784 when he set sail to become the American ambassador to France. While Jefferson negotiated treaties, Hemings quickly learned French cuisine as well as mastering the language. Jefferson smuggled seeds and knowledge about herb gardening to enhance his chef's table. He brought back a waffle iron from Holland and a "cream machine for ice," introducing ice cream to America. His successful experimentation with animal and plant husbandry and culinary hospitality gave him the name "father of his country's cuisine."

The advent of the French Revolution and soon-to-be famous Delmonico restaurants soon flooded the new country with French "specialities." French chefs immigrated first to the Gulf of Mexico ports and then to New Orleans to blend with the French Canadian Cajuns, creating authentic Creole cuisine.

Jefferson continued to enjoy southern cooking, as well as French cuisine. During his 1800 campaign for the Presidency, Jefferson's rival claimed Thomas was unqualified for the White House because he was "raised wholly on hoe cake made of coarse ground Southern corn, bacon and hominy."

❧ *Rice "Woffles"* ❧

This is a waffle recipe enjoyed by Thomas Jefferson. From Mary Randolph, *The Virginia Housewife*, 1831.

"Boil two gills (1 cup) of rice quite soft, mix it with three gills (1½ cups) of flour, a little salt, 2 ounces of melted butter, 2 eggs beaten well, and milk to make a thick batter—beat it till very light, and bake it in woffle irons."

❧ *Tansy Pudding* ❧

Tansy pudding was a favorite southern recipe. When you try it, you will have a new appreciation of your tansy. From *MacKenzie's 5,000 Receipts*,* 1829. **Receipts* is a colonial name for recipes.

"Blanch and pound ¼ pound of almonds. Put them in a stew pan with a gill (½ cup) of syrup of roses (page 89), the crumbs of a French roll, some grated nutmeg, half a glass of brandy, 2 tablespoons of tansy juice (pressed from fresh leaves), 3 ounces of fresh butter and some slices of citron. Pour over it a pint and a half of boiling cream or milk, sweeten and when cold, mix it; add the juice of a lemon and 8 beaten eggs. It may either be boiled or baked."

❧ *Redeye Gravy* ❧

Virginia Ham is not complete without a serving of redeye gravy. From Patricia B. Mitchell, *Cooking in the Young Republic,* 1992; also in *American Food: The Gastronomic Story* by Evan Jones, 1975.

"Fry slices of country ham, draining off the excess grease. Add a little water to the drippings. Scrape the water and drippings together with a spatula and add a tablespoon of strong coffee. Boil and serve with sliced ham."

❧ *Cherry Delmonico* ❧

This recipe was served to Thomas Jefferson in 1784. From Delmonico's restaurant, *Thomas Jefferson American Heritage Cookbook* by Marshall Fishwick, 1964.

"Drain thoroughly a can of large, red, sweet pitted cherries. Put a blanched almond in place of the pit. Arrange nests of crisp, fresh watercress on chilled plates. Line each nest with mayonnaise and fill each with 3 stuffed cherries, rolled in softened cream cheese. Dust with a pinch of paprika blended with cinnamon."

∿ *American Ice Cream* ∿

Ice cream was introduced to the colonists by the French in the mid-eighteenth century. Here is an original recipe from the *Journal of William Black,* Pennsylvania Magazine of History and Biography, 1744.

"Mash (or purée) 12 stoned apricots and combine 6 ounces of sugar and 1 pint of scalding cream. Place in a tin or pewter container and pack in a tub of ice and salt."

Modern adaptation: This would taste great with a tablespoon of finely minced fresh lemon verbena.

∿ *Martha Washington's Fricassee* ∿

Martha Washington stayed at her husband's side through the entire Revolutionary War. Here is a recipe from her kitchen that she likely served the General and his guests, from Rosemary Brandau, *Historic Food Programs,* Colonial Williamsburg Foundation.

"After the chickens are cut in small pieces (bone and chop 1 chicken), season them with clove, mace, nutmeg, and pepper beat small together and some salt (½ teaspoon each mace, nutmeg, ground cloves, salt and pepper). Then fry them a little in sweet butter (combine spices, season and fry chicken in ¼ pound of butter). Then beat 3 or 4 egge youlks with a little white wine and sweet herbs minced small put into eggs and wine and give them another fry together. (Beat egg yolks, ¼ cup white wine and 1 teaspoon parsley, marjoram, and thyme combined. Stir into frying pan over low heat). And put into them a little strong broth, some gravie, a little vinegar, a slice of lemon minced. Give all a fry together, then dish it up. Garnish with grapes or barberries." (Add ½ cup of chicken broth and ½ cup chicken gravy. Stir until thickened. Add chicken, 1 tablespoon of vinegar and 1 lemon slice, minced. Cook a few minutes longer and dish it up.) Serves 4.

Of Piñons and Peppers

When the Spanish arrived in America over three hundred years go, they brought with them figs and unforgettable barbecue sauces. Their most famous contribution was the chili pepper, or *capsicum.* Combined and cooked with tomatoes, Creole cuisine was born. Although chili peppers are prevalent in East Indian and Chinese Szechwan food, they were only accepted in the Southwest and California during Spanish rule. American

Colonial Puritans forbade their use because they were believed to excite passion. In actuality, chilies could have enlivened the northern boiled dinners and created internal warmth during cold winter months.

The Spanish found another herb to balance the heat of chilies: Yerba buena. Also known as the good herb, it is a native mint that balances and accents hot Creole cooking. Other herbs were used to accent meats and stews. Juniper berries were cooked with lamb to enhance flavor. Dried safflower blooms were substituted for Old World saffron, and garlic and olives were grown to enhance fish and poultry dishes. Tomatoes were introduced as a safe vegetable to stew with onions in beef dishes.

The Pueblo Native Americans introduced native piñon nuts to the Spaniards. A staple for the Native Americans, piñons soon became a connoisseur's delight. Spanish cooks made a light chicken broth and blended cream and piñons with coriander, mint, and scallions in a unique Spanish version of a vichyssoise.

The rivers of our soul spring from the same well.

—Pochii (Chinese poet), 772-846

～

Soul Food

Many African Americans were poor and free after the Civil War. Sharecropping provided only necessities for African-American families. These farmers lived in the south and paid half of their crop to the landowner. Even though life was hard, African-American cooks served delicious meals from their home garden. The women would can their surplus vegetables and sell them to the townsfolk for extra money.

Many African Americans in the north and south turned to cooking as a livelihood. Their recipes were handed down to each new generation, but the source stayed the same: the land.

African Americans always provided their own fresh, organic food. They had fruit and nut trees, vegetable gardens, and their own chickens and hogs for slaughter. They also enjoyed fresh catches from local streams, rivers, and the ocean. The children were given a bucket at a young age and taught to find crawfish. Dinner was as close as their backyard or a nearby waterway. They would gather wild greens, onions, berries, and grapes. Melons grew in sandy soil in the south, providing Mother Nature's relief from the sweltering summer heat.

Greens were believed to be the most healing food. They were served liberally throughout the year as they became available. Sour milk, greens, and cornmeal were the basics for many dinner meals. Collards, mustard, and turnip greens were eaten as "muscle food," while poke weed, wild onion, and garlic chives were made into a salad.

Fresh "Choke" Pie

Jerusalem artichokes are a Native American food low in carbohydrates and a good substitute for potatoes.

- 4 medium "chokes" (Jerusalem artichokes)
- 2 fresh eggs
- ½ cup evaporated milk
- 1 tablespoon cinnamon or nutmeg
- 1 tablespoon baking powder
- 1 cup raw sugar
- 1 9-inch pie crust (graham cracker is ⅓ lower in fat than regular pie crust made with butter)

Boil chokes in water to cover until tender. Drain and mash. Add eggs, milk, spice, and baking powder and mix. Stir in the sugar. Pour into a pie crust. Bake at 350 degrees for 45 minutes. Serves 6.

Berry Cobbler

This dessert is worth the effort for a berry hunt.

- 4 cups fresh dewberries or blackberries
- 1 cup raw sugar
- 2 teaspoons vanilla extract
- 1 tablespoon lemon balm or lemon verbena
- ½ stick unsalted butter (4 tablespoons)
- 1 (8-inch) pie crust

Combine the berries, sugar, vanilla, and lemon. Add the butter in small pieces. Pour the mixture into a greased 8-inch baking dish. Put the crust on top and bake at 375 degrees for 30–45 minutes until the crust browns.

Homemade Pork and Sage Sausage

Sage enhances the flavor and helps to digest pork.

- 5 pounds lean ground pork or ground venison
- 4 teaspoons no-salt herbal blend (page 287)
- ½ cup ground, dried sage
- ¼–½ cup crushed hot pepper, more if desired

Combine and mix thoroughly. Divide into patties and cook in a frying pan until done or freeze the patties for later use.

❧ *Homemade Cooked Greens* ❧

You'll look forward to eating greens when you cook them like the African Americans do.

    2 quarts mustard, collards, dandelion, turnip,
        lamb's quarters, and sorrel greens (any edible greens will work)
    1 teaspoon salt (or vegetable no-salt herbal blend, page 287)
    8 slices salt pork or 2 ham hocks, already cooked
    2 teaspoons sugar
    2 tablespoons butter or ghee (page 183)

Wash greens by soaking them in cool water sprinkled with salt for 10 minutes. The salt will make any soil sink to the bottom of the container. Rinse the greens at least twice. Remove any stems. Add the greens to the cooked salt pork or ham hocks. Add sugar and butter and simmer in a covered pot 15–20 minutes, allowing its own gravy to form. Serves 4.

❧ *Red Beans with Rice* ❧

The homemade sausage and chili is a staple of Cajun cooking.

      1 pound dried red kidney beans
        Several pieces salt pork
      4 tablespoons butter or ghee (page 183)
      1 teaspoon salt, optional
      1 teaspoon sugar
      4 whole bay leaves
      2 pounds homemade sausage
      2 small onions, chopped
      2 bell peppers, chopped
      1 chili, chopped or ½ teaspoon chili powder
      3 teaspoons cumin
      2 garlic cloves
      1 teaspoon peppercorns
      1 teaspoon dried sage
    2–3 tablespoons oil

Soak beans in water to cover for 30 minutes and drain. In another pot, simmer salt pork in 3 quarts of water for 30 minutes. Add beans, butter, salt, sugar, and bay leaves. Cover and simmer 1½ hours. Cook sausage in a separate pot. Strain and chop into several pieces. Sauté onion, peppers, chili, cumin, garlic, peppercorns, and sage in oil. Add the sausage and cook 10 minutes to blend flavors. Add the cooked beans and cook another 20 minutes, stirring several times. Serve over rice. Serves 6–8.

∾ *Steamed Rice* ∾

African Americans use vinegar to whiten rice.

2 cups rice
2 tablespoons vinegar

Cook rice and vinegar in 3½ cups of water. When most of the water cooks out, about 25 minutes, uncover and lower the heat until the rice is dry and fluffy. Serves 6–8.

∾ *Boiled Crayfish (Crawfish)* ∾

Get a bucket to gather crawfish in a bayou.

2 dozen crawfish
1 red chili pepper, seeded and chopped
2 whole bay leaves
1 teaspoon whole allspice
2 tablespoons butter
1 tablespoon salt

Boil crawfish in water to cover containing chili pepper, bay leaves, allspice, butter, and salt. Crawfish will cook in 15–20 minutes. Strain and serve with crackers, cornbread, and fried green tomatoes.

∾ *Fried Green Tomatoes* ∾

An original recipe. African Americans picked the green tomatoes off their vines as winter approached, almost like a celebration for winter to come. They knew winter eating could be lean so they made use of every available food.

4 green tomatoes, sliced ½-inch thick
2 cups white cornmeal
    salt and pepper to taste

Dredge each tomato slice in white cornmeal and fry them in hot oil until golden brown. Salt and pepper before serving. Serves 4.

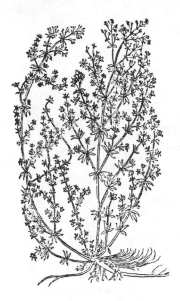

5

Medieval Knowledge of Simples

SWEET WOODRUFF

Beauty hath pierced me with her golden shaft.

—Ms. of Benedictbeuren

During the Dark Ages and medieval times, the cultivation of herb gardens was perpetuated by monks and crones, female herbalists living outside of the villages. Herbs were initially forbidden by the church, as illness was believed to be the punishment for sins. Herbs were considered evil because of their association with pagan Nature rites. However, the Benedictine monks made a vow to take care of the common people and continued to grow herbs under the protection of the monastery walls and orchards. Large gardens were nurtured to produce medicinal herbal apothecaries for the surrounding community.

The Benedictine monks at Monte Cassino, Italy, owned the only library of herbal manuscripts. The Benedictine library accumulated the ancient knowledge of Persian, Roman, and Greek herbalists, as well as their experiential knowledge from cultivation and experimentation. The knowledge eventually became available to the public through the invention of the printing press in the fifteenth century. It was always common knowledge to the crones and peasants.

By the 1600s, commoners began growing their own herb gardens. The gardens were designed to be near the house and open to the north and east for the winds. Soon a traditional knot pattern became the layout of

Herbs were considered evil because of their association with pagan Nature rites.

~

choice. The knot garden was a large rectangle divided into four quarters. The paths led to a central theme at the midpoint, usually a fountain, sundial, or well for watering, "for its purity gives much pleasure."

After the War of the Roses (1455–1485), peace blanketed England. Nobleman and commoner alike began to grow herbs and roses that transmitted fragrance and beauty. Each quarter of the knot garden contained a collection of plants: medicinal, culinary, fragrant, religious, or magical. As the garden design evolved, intertwined rows of herbs were laid out in a symmetrical design. The ribbons of herbs would form knots, or interconnected wheels. The patterns were kept visible by pruning low-growing herbs. Borders were of one hedge plant, often boxwood, later becoming a commonality in knot gardens. Patterns were dramatized by filling the spaces between plants with gravel or bouquets of low-growing, bright flowers. In this symmetrical enclosure of beautiful, aromatic herbs lay the peace of tranquility.

Every morning and evening, a visit was made to the garden; the poet Ausonius reflects here on newly blown roses:

> And I was walking in my formal garden,
> To freshen me, before the day grew old. . . .
> O Earth, to give a flower so brief a grace!
> As long as a day is long, so long the life of a rose.
> The golden sun at morning sees her born,
> And late at eve returning finds her old.
> Wise is she, that hath so soon to die,
> And lives her life in some succeeding rose.
> O maid, while youth is with the rose and thee,
> Pluck thou the rose: life is as swift for thee.

A Time to Gather Herbs

During medieval times, plants were gathered at the "moment of their full maturity and their greatest vigour." Observance and attunement to nature set the time of harvest. The gatherer was expected to harvest only in a proper state of mind, with malice toward none, to save the purity of the herb. Herbs could only be gathered on sunny days when the dew did not appear on the leaves and flowers, for dampness would almost assuredly lose the virtues of their pleasure.

Medieval Medicine

Medieval Europe accepted a theory of health developed from the ancient Greeks and refined by Persians and Arabic Muslim traditions. Their original theory can be traced to the Indian Upanashad of the first millennium. Here, it was stated that the constitution, health, personality, and morals of a child were determined by the mother's diet and milk during pregnancy and infancy. After infancy, health could be moderated only through nutrition and balance of the four bodily "humors" (bodily fluids). The four humor theory was extracted from the Indo-Chinese five element theory of wood, fire, earth, metal, and water. It was first recorded by the Grecian Empedocles during the fifth century B.C. and perfected by the famous Greek physician and teacher, Galen. The four humors classified temperament as blood, bile, phlegm, and black bile. Subsequent diseases occurred from eating foods that aggravated these humors. Foods were classified by energy patterns: hot, hot and moist, cold and dry, and cold and moist. From this, it is easy to recognize how herbs and spices could be used to modify the temperance of the food or person. In fact, for a few thousand years, Ayurvedic Indian physicians had been successfully treating patients by utilizing their "tridosha," or three humor system, bringing the body, mind, and spirit into balance.

Experts in the use of medicine are inferior to those who recommend proper diet.

—Culpepper, *The English Physitian*, 1652

The four humor theory of medieval Europe was never successfully developed. The foods were not fully classified and the scarcity and lack of variety offered few substitutions. Salted and dried foods, cabbage, beans, and onion were all the main Medieval diet and were all hot foods. Fresh fruits were cold because of their juices and mistakenly considered unhealthy for the ill, elderly, and children. The difference between the Eastern and Western systems is that Western perception is objective and relies on reason. Eastern perception relies on fate and a subjective intuitive feeling developing into wisdom and understanding. The West questions and leads; the East knows and follows the path of least resistance.

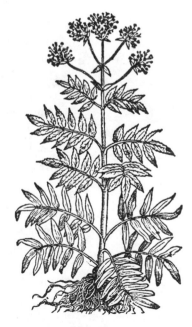

VALERIAN

A Medieval Herbal

In the knowledge of simples, wherein the manifold wisdom of God is wonderfully to be seen, one thing would carefully be observed; which is to know what herbs may be used instead of drugs of the same nature and to make the garden the shop. For home-bred medicines are both more easy for the Parson's purse and more familiar for all men's bodies. So where the apothecary useth for loosing, rhubarb, or for binding, bolearmena, the Parson useth damask or white roses for the one and plantain, shepherd's purse, knotgrass, for the other, and that with better success. . . The Parson's wife prefers not the city, but her gardens and fields [of] hyssop, valerian, yarrow and St. John's wort made into a salve; and elder, camomile, mallows and comphrey made into a poultice have done great and rare cures.

—George Herbert (seventeenth-century English poet),
Country Parson

ANISE *(Pimpinella anisum)* was a favorite medieval herb for curing a variety of ailments. Its properties were digestant, diuretic, carminative (or "good against belching"), corrected bad breath, "ingendreth milke," and "stirreth up bodily lust." The seeds were chewed for a sweeter breath, to quench thirst, and to aid those who were short-winded. Roasted seeds, dried by the fire and taken with honey, cleared the lungs. For a cough, the roasted seeds were eaten with bitter almonds. A tea made with anise and hyssop was gargled with honey and vinegar for Quincy sore throat, or tonsillitis (*Quincy sore throat* is an old-fashioned term for tonsillitis with pus pockets on the tonsils. This is before the germ theory, so we don't know if it was strep).

APPLE *(Malus* species) was baked for pies, cooked with sugar, cinnamon, or ginger, and roasted in the winter to be dropped in a cup of warm ale or wine. Traditionally, Pippin apple juice (from the Pippin variety of apples) was given to melancholy people. The pulp was made into a compress for hot swellings or used in an ointment to "smooth the skin." Raw apples were combined with camphor and buttermilk and applied to smallpox scars. Then the individual was given saffron milk to drink. The roasted pulp was made into a frothy water to be drunk by the quart for gonorrhea. Undesirable apples were made into cider.

BALM, or LEMON BALM *(Melissa officinales)*, was rubbed on green (infectious) wounds and steeped in ale to sedate the sudden passions of the heart. The leaves were also rubbed on bee hives to keep the bees together and to attract more bees.

BETONY *(Stachys officinalis)* flowers were made into a headache remedy. A conserve type of jam was made with flowering stalks. The leaves prevented "sower belchings," and often were dried and powdered to be taken with meat.

CHAMOMILE *(Anthemis noblis)* was drunk for colic, headaches, stones, and "coldness in the stomach." A bath in chamomile water was used to "produce a sweat." For a "megram," or migraine, a handful each of chamomile flowers, sage, mugwort, and gentian cooked in honey was applied to the head as a compress.

CLARY *(Salvia sclarea)* seed was taken powdered and mixed with honey "to clear the sight." The seed was pounded and steeped into a "slimy substance" to dissolve swelling in the joints and draw out splinters. Clary leaves were fried in a cream egg batter and eaten with sweetened lemon juice.

CLOTBUR *(Articum lappa and minus)*, or burdock, roots were pounded with salt to draw out venomous wounds, and the juice of the leaves were cooked with honey for cystitis. Compresses of burdock were applied to the navel to prevent a miscarriage.

CLOVE GILLYFLOWERS *(Dianthus caryophyllus)* were as popular as roses. They were grown en masse for pleasure to attract the "colibuy," or hummingbird, and made into a syrup to "expel fever and furie." As a nosegay, they were recommended to guard against the plague. Red was considered the most medicinal.

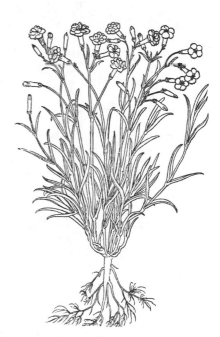

CLOVE GILLYFLOWERS

COLUMBINE *(Aquilegia* species) was grown for pleasure and for "women in travail" (women having labor pains). There was some experimentation for a jaundice and kidney stone remedy with a syrup made from the blooms.

COWSLIP *(Primula* species) is the common primrose. It was used for facials and eaten in salads, being hardy only in more temperate climates.

CRESS: gardencress, watercress, and wintercress *(Lepidium sativum, Nasturtium officinale, Barbarea vulgaris)* were eaten with bread and butter, tarragon, and rocket and salad herbs to prevent scurvy. The seeds were used for sciatica, pounded and applied with malt and vinegar as a compress. As a blood coagulant, the seeds were given to those who suffered from accidents to reduce bruising and hemorrhaging. The boiled leaves were made into a compress for inflamed breasts and testicles.

EYEBRIGHT *(Euphrasia officinalis)* was used to preserve eyesight and clear cataracts. The leaves were pounded, then either pressed onto the eyelids, distilled and dropped into the eyes, or steeped in white wine or strong beer and drunk.

Clove

Gillyflowers

were made

into a syrup

to "expel fever

and furie."

~

FEATHERFEW or FEVERFEW *(Chrysanthemum parthenium)* was powdered and drunk in wine for vertigo, melancholy, and as "the housewife's aspirin." Both leaves and flowers were used. For toothaches, it was bagged, soaked in hot rum, and applied to the tooth.

FLAX *(Linum usitatissimum)* was believed to have the same properties as fenugreek seeds, an analgesic (painkiller) during medieval times. The seeds were powdered and cooked with violet leaves, mallows, and chickweed, held in hog fat, and applied warm to swellings.

GENTIAN *(Gentiana crinata;* in North America, *Gentian officinalis)* was taken as a purge with anise seeds and rhubarb. It is mentioned as one of the herbs for migraines (see *chamomile).* As a bitter, it was prescribed for many stomach and liver complaints, but not recommended during pregnancy.

HEMP *(Cannabis sativa)* was given to hens to lay more eggs. Only the seeds were added as a food.

HOPS *(Humulus lupulus)* strobiles were harvested in late summer and brewed in a beer "to keep the bodie in health." Bread was made by boiling hops in potato water and letting it ferment, then a little yeast and flowers were added. As a medicine, hops were decocted to cleanse the blood and "loosen the belly" (reduce spasms and alleviate cramps).

HORSETAIL *(Equisetum hyemale),* known as "pewterwoort," was used as a scouring agent for pewter in the kitchen. It was also used for kidney and lung ailments when boiled in wine.

HYSSOP *(Hyssopus officinales)* was medicine for a cut or green wound, being "bruised with sugar and applyed." It was decocted in oil and applied locally to kill lice and abate "benumbed joints" with rheumatic pain. A cough remedy was made with hyssop, rue, and honey. A steam from hyssop boiled in water was funneled into the ears to reduce inflammation and "singing noises," or tinnitis.

LAVENDER *(Lavendula spica)* was distilled and applied to the temples for "light" migraines. The flowers, "the blewe part," were powdered and drunk in distilled water to quiet the "panting and passion of the heart." The oil, called oil of spike, was applied locally for palsy, trembling and shaking of the limbs. The dried blooms were sniffed to "comfort and dry up [decongest] the moisture of a cold braine" (believing a cold brain was waterlogged). A gargle, made from a tea, was used for laryngitis.

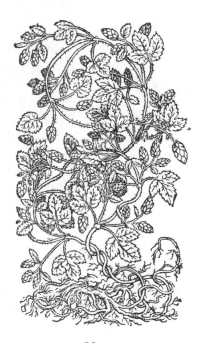

HOPS

LAVENDER COTTON *(Santolina chamaecyparissus)* was a favorite border plant in knot gardens. The seeds were decocted and drunk to drive out intestinal parasites as well as to cure scabs and itches. **Note:** Only local application is advised today.

LETTUCE *(Lactuca sativa)* was boiled and the juice applied to the forehead with rose oil to induce sleep and relieve headaches. Applied to the heart, it would cure lust . . . sometimes it was also applied to other body parts!

LILY OF THE VALLEY *(Convallaria majalis)* flowers were steeped in wine and a spoonful was taken for gout. It was also used to restore speech by comforting the heart. Today it is considered toxic and is not recommended for ingestion.

LOVAGE *(Ligusticum officinale)* was also known as ligusticum. The seeds were used like pepper to season meats. A distillation was used to clear the eyes and reduce fevers. Locally, lovage was used to remove freckles and boils.

LUNGWORT *(Pulmonaria officinalis)* was called autumn gentian. The leaves and flowers were applied to the chest for those "who spit blood" (tuberculosis or other lung disease sufferers). It was also enjoyed as a pot herb (an herb eaten as a vegetable).

MARIGOLD *(Calendula officinalis)* was made into a conserve with sugar or pounded and steeped in vinegar or ale. It was taken to break the fast in the morning as a preventative for the plague. Only true calendula was used, never African marigolds. They were named *merrigoulds,* because their golden color shone in the garden. The flowers were often cooked in broths to "comfort the hearte and spirit."

MUGWORT *(Artemisia vulgaris)* was a remedy for migraines, hysteria, and used as a blood cleanser. Boiled in honey with gentian, chamomile, and sage, it was applied locally for headaches. For hysteria, mugwort was boiled in old ale with fennel and red stem applemint and drunk warm. It was tied to the waist of travelers to protect them from wild beasts and weariness and applied to the female body to cure many feminine disorders, such as sterility and miscarriage. **Note:** Artemisias are recommended for external use only today.

PENNYROYAL (PENNIE ROYALL) *(Mentha pulegium)* was also known as "Pudding grasse" and "pepper worte." It was used to bring down a stillborn child and relieve cramping. It was taken with honey to clear the chest of congestion, and with honey and aloe to clear the colon. For gout and rheumatic pain, "pepper worte" leaves were bruised and added to "old hog's lard" and applied locally for four hours on men and two hours on women. Then the area was bathed in wine and oil, and wrapped in woolens to "sweat a little." The herb is considered too hot and bitter to use internally for those with "weak and tender stomaches." **Note:** Pennyroyal is not recommended for internal use.

RUE *(Ruta graveolens)* was used as a remedy boiled in oil, juice, wine, or honey. The seeds were drunk in wine to antidote poisons; the leaves to counteract the plague and clear dimness of vision. Rue was used to "provoke urine and expel afterbirth." As a poultice, it was used for nosebleeds, warts, gout, colic, and earaches. Only domestic rue was used as a remedy, "but beware of the too frequent or overmuch use thereof." **Note:** Rue should be avoided during pregnancy and lactation.

SHEPHERD'S PURSE *(Capsella bursa pastoris)* "stayeth bleeding in any part of the body . . . drunke . . . pultesse [poultice] or in bath" (Gerard). An ointment was especially used for head wounds and the juice was used for toothaches and dropped into the ears for inflammation.

SOUTHERNWOOD *(Artemisia abrotanum)* was pounded and steeped in wine to cure talking in one's sleep. Tops boiled and added to wine cured shortness of breath, abated sciatica pain, stopped baldness, and killed intestinal worms. Lavender cotton was considered the female species and often grown nearby. Both species were used in ointments to prevent "the French disease" (syphyllis). Only topical use is recommended.

SPEEDWELL *(Veronica officinalis)* was decocted and drunk in wine to stop the spreading of sores, pox, and measles. Rubbed on, it could heal wounds that would otherwise be amputated.

VERVAIN *(Verbena officinalis)* was used to strengthen the womb. It was hung around the neck or extracted as a juice to prevent dreams. Since vervain grew all over the garden, it was believed to cure everything.

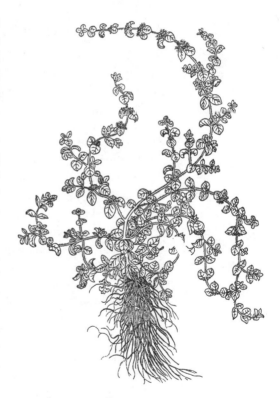

PENNYROYAL

VIOLET *(Viola odorata)* was taken with sugar for all inflammations, especially affecting the lungs and chest. Dry violets were combined with medicines to strengthen the heart. A decoction was made by boiling sugar to a "meane thicknesse" and adding violets "upon a gentle fire to simmer." Violets were added three or four more times until the purple syrup became infused with the aroma of fresh violets. It was used as a children's cough syrup and to ease Quincy sore throats. Also, a nosegay of violets, because of their fragrance and fragility, was considered a very special gift.

WORMWOOD *(Artemisia absinthum)* was taken for internal bleeding, worms, "stinking breath," and all putrifications of the body. Steeped in vinegar, wormwood was an antidote for mushroom poisoning. It is toxic and no longer used internally.

YARROW *(Achillea millefolium)* was a popular hemostatic. Women who suffered from profuse menses bathed in it. The dried, ground leaves were powdered and snorted to relieve migraines, and a rinse was used to "stayeth the shedding of hair." For a backache, yarrow was steeped in brandy with comfrey or borage and drunk with gunpowder. Hardening of the veins or varicosities was treated with wine, honey, and yarrow leaf juice taken warm.

A Medieval Garden at The Cloisters

In the northwest corner of Manhattan Island, a branch of the New York Metropolitan Museum of Art has reconstructed a medieval monastery and herb garden overlooking the Hudson River in Fort Tyron Park. The building is designed from twelfth-century European architecture, and is best known for its unicorn tapestries woven in 1500, stained glass windows, and panel paintings.

A cloister is a covered walkway with access to an open courtyard leading to another building. In the museum, each cloister leads to another gallery of art. The medieval herb garden is tucked in the back part of the cloisters overlooking the Hudson River.

The garden is a collection of herbs grown in medieval monasteries. Its gardeners are researchers who reference each herb. Many of the plants come alive in the individual tapestries and paintings displayed in each cloister. The raised beds are designed for culinary, dye, medicinal, and aromatic herbs. There are topiary container plants and wattle fences woven from branches and twigs. Quince trees are used to center small theme gardens, where a large variety of herbs are grown. The herbs were chosen from old herbals and Charlemagne's imperial gardens. More research on medieval herbs and their uses are available through the New York Botanical Garden research library.

ℋere are a few of the plants tucked away in the beds at the Cloister herb garden. Over 250 varieties of herbs and flowers are blooming there through the work of a dedicated team of gracious gardeners.

ANGELICA *(archangelica)* was grown in monasteries to ward off evil spirits and was believed to be the great protector from the plague. Monks grew it for carmelite water and liquors as an after-dinner digestant. A decoction of the root was made in wine to reduce fevers with chills, or "cold shivering agues," while the green root, still full of juice, helped asthmatics. The green, young stalks were candied and eaten to aid digestion. Angelica is a biennial umbelliferae propagated from seed and grown in light shade. It prefers moist, rich soil. **Note:** Angelica is toxic raw and must be cooked or tinctured before ingesting.

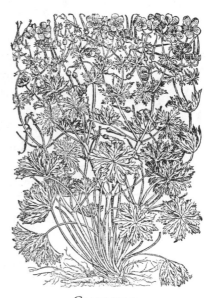

CRANESBILL

BLACK MUSTARD *(Brassica nigra)* was grown for a salad green, and its seeds were pounded into a condiment. External applications were used to reduce pain and increase circulation. Monks preferred the black variety because it was valued during biblical times. Mustard is a cruciferae, grown from seed as an annual in composted soil where it can self-sow.

COSTMARY *(Chrysanthemum balsamita)* was introduced to Europe in the sixteenth century from the Orient. Monks used it to mark their Bibles and brew their beer. As an external compress, it was applied as a salve to ulcers and boils. Costmary is a compositae from the daisy family. It is a hardy perennial propagated by division in the early spring. Costmary spreads easily in a sunny location and self-mulches.

CRANESBILL *(Geranium pratense* and *robertianum)* was named after Robert, Abbot of Molesme, an eleventh-century saint. Monks grew this hardy perennial as a topical astringent. Cranesbill grows well from seed in light shade. Harvest the leaves and use fresh as an astringent hemostatic.

Quince trees were grown as topiaries and center trees in medieval gardens.

~

LENTEN ROSE *(Helleborus officinalis)* was grown as a cardiotonic and narcotic drug. Although the rhizome is very toxic, the plant is enjoyed for its beauty. It blooms throughout the Lenten season; monks grew it to remind them of Christ's purity and trials. The Lenten Rose is a ranunculae native to the Caucasus, Greece, and Turkey. It prefers shade in the mountainous woods of Europe. The large, bell-shaped white flowers have no scent, but are irresistible to touch. It is a hardy perennial propagated by division and grown in moist, rich soil.

OUR LADY'S BEDSTRAW *(Galium verum)* is a biblical herb said to be used by Mary to freshen the Christ child's bed. It is a soporific that releases a light aroma to encourage sleep. Monks stuffed their pillows and beds with the honey scented, yellow flowers. Also referred to as "cheese rennet," monks also used the green part of the plant to curdle milk for cheese from the enzyme parachymozine. As a dye plant, it was used to color cheese and fabric red. The roots were made into a red dye, while the leaves and stems produced a yellow dye. Externally, the leaves were used as a compress to treat skin problems. The flowering stems were infused as a tea for kidney disorders. Lady's bedstraw is a rubiaceae with creeping rhizomes, and propagates by division. Grow this perennial in light shade and loamy soil.

QUINCE *(Cydonia oblonga),* the "apple of Cydonia," originated in the Near East and Central Asia. Monks grew this deciduous rose tree for its nutritious fruit. The fruit was dried to treat digestive complaints and sore throats. The uncrushed seeds were infused for coughs, gastritis, and enteritis. The crushed seeds are toxic. Quince trees were grown as topiaries and center trees in medieval gardens. The fruit is tastiest when grown in warm regions.

RAMPION *(Campanula)* is best known as a salad green in the fairy tale of Rapunzel (the man would gather rampion for his pregnant wife by night. The couple kept Rapunzel locked in a tower). The medieval monks grew rampion for salad greens. Rampion enjoys humid, cool climates and composted, well-mulched soil. Propagate from seed.

SWEET CICILY *(Myrrhis odorata)* was grown as a preventative for the plague and as a digestant. The roots were boiled for antiseptic liquor and cough medicine. Sweet Cicily enjoys cold weather and requires freeze and thaw periods to propagate from seed. Monks grew this umbelliferae in shade and sowed seeds in the fall.

VALERIAN *(Valeriana officinalis)* was also known as "garden heliotrope" and "all heal." The wild species is indigenous to Europe. The root was distilled by monks to provoke urine, counteract jaundice and poison, and alleviate "pain in the sides." It was also used as a medicine for epilepsy and tuberculosis. The leaves were bruised and used to heal ulcers and mouth ulcers. Monks dedicated this great herb to the Virgin Mary, otherwise called Setewall, during medieval times. It is worth mentioning that wild valerian did not smell like old dirty socks like the dried root used today. Wild valerian may be the Biblical plant called spikenard, another reason monks would prefer it in their gardens. Valerian is best propagated in the spring or fall by division and replaced every three years. It enjoys sun or part shade and rich soil. **Note:** Please contact your health care practitioner before using this internally. Valerian is not recommended for those using antidepressants.

WOAD *(Isatis tinctoria)* produced a blue dye. The leaves could be used externally to stop bleeding. Woad is a biennial cruciferae of the mustard family. It is grown from seed and the leaves harvested for dye the second year before blossoming in June. Woad was combined with Dyer's greenwood *(Genista tinctoria)* to produce a beautiful green dye.

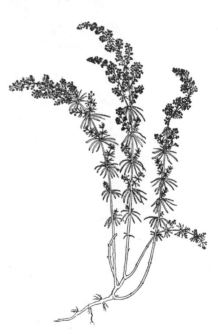

OUR LADY'S BEDSTRAW

Medieval Cuisine

Medieval cuisine was rather bland, with very few choices for the menus. Meats and fish were often preserved by salting, especially during the winter and early spring. Food was too scarce to keep animals alive during the winter. The diet consisted mainly of dried beans, onions, and cabbage, three good reasons digestant herbs and spices were so popular. Bread was offered at every meal with pudding and gruel made from whole grains, or almond milk and egg yolks when hens were laying. Starchy and salty dishes were well seasoned with every available herb and spice.

> Take and boil a good piece of pork. . . then take it up and chop it as small as you may; then take cloves and mace, and chop forth withall, and also chop forth with raisins of Corinth; then take it and roll it as round as you may, . . . then lay them in a dish by themselves; then make a good almond milk, and blend it with flour and rice, and let it boil well, but look that it be quite runny; . . . lay five pumpes (meatballs) in a dish and pour the pottage thereon. And if you will, set on every pumpe a flower, and over them strew on sugar enough and mace: and serve them forth.
>
> —Thomas Austin, *Two Fifteenth Century Cookery Books,*
> London, 1888

Dried fish was served regularly in medieval homes. Country folk seasoned fish with mustard or vinegar, while the wealthy seasoned with a variety of spices and dried fruit. By the fourteenth century, professional "saucemakers" were in vogue. There were several sauces available:

> Green sauce of ginger, cloves, cardamom and green herbs . . . yellow sauce of ginger and saffron . . . [but the favorite was] carmeline sauce with cinnamon and varying spices . . . pound ginger, plenty of cinnamon, cloves, mace, long pepper, cardamom . . . then squeeze out bread soaked in vinegar and strain it all together and salt it just right.
>
> —Taillevent, *Le Viandier,* Paris, 1892

Several dishes were served at the same time. Diners dug in with their fingers where a "first come, first serve" rule prevailed (forks were not in fashion until well into the eighteenth century). Napkins were another oddity. Diners were requested not to scratch for lice or fleas nor to blow their noses with their fingers during the meal. Putting meat back into the main dish after eating of it was also frowned upon. Discards were supposed to be thrown on the floor for the dogs, who were waiting on a carpet of southernwood to abate the odor and the fleas. Bon appetit!

Finger Bowls

Toward the end of a formal dinner, a finger bowl was scented with a bouquet of sweet-smelling herbs and flowers floating in the water. To prepare your own finger bowls, make a bouquet from any of the following: lemon verbena, rose petals, violets, scented geranium leaves, sweet marjoram, lavender, honeysuckles, basils, rosemary, mints, lemon balm.

Herbal Wine Flavorings

Water was not safe for drinking purposes in medieval times. Wines, ales, and liqueurs were brewed with herbs for flavoring and to "maketh the hearte merry." Here are a few examples of herbal additions to wines and other brews. To enjoy these flavors today, steep a few fresh leaves in a 4-ounce glass of wine or ale.

ANGELICA leaves imparted a muscatel flavor.

BERGAMOT leaves and flowers enhanced a sharp, clear taste.

BORAGE flowers were steeped in wine for courage.

CLARY SAGE leaves are so large only a few small pieces could be steeped to promote a relaxing, euphoric feeling. Steeping a few flowers is easier.

LEMON BALM drunk in wine deterred the bites of venomous beasts and drove away melancholy by comforting the heart.

MINT leaves were steeped to enhance digestion.

SALAD BURNET leaves were steeped in wine to lift flagging spirits.

SWEET WOODRUFF leaves were steeped to enhance relaxation.

Flowers were also steeped in brandy and liqueurs for one month to impart flavor for a romantic evening. To 4 cups of brandy or liqueur, steep I cup of fresh rose petals, dianthus flowers, or violets. A combination of all three is delightful.

⟡ *Latti di Mandorla: Almond Milk* ⟡

In medieval times, chefs needed to substitute cow's milk during the Lenten fasting season. They used a Middle Eastern almond milk recipe from ancient times, from which this recipe is adapted. *Latte di Mandorla* is an Italian translation of "milk of almonds."

1½ cups ground almonds
3¾ cups water
4 cups sugar
2 tablespoons rose or orange blossom water

Place ground almonds in a bag of layered cheesecloth. Tie the top, leaving room for the almonds to move. Soak the almonds in water 1 hour, squeezing the bag every 15 minutes to collect the milk. As the water is squeezed out, a milky, fragrant substance will come out from the almonds. Repeat the process as long as the milk can be produced. Then pour the milk into a saucepan, add the sugar and boil gently only to dissolve the sugar. Allow the syrup to thicken and coat the back of a spoon. Remove from heat and add flower water. Bottle when cool. Use as a milk substitute in cooking or serve as a cold drink.

Favorite Medieval Strewing Herbs

And let the ground whereas her foot shall tread, be strewed with fragrant flowers all along . . .

—Edmund Spenser

In medieval Europe, herbal paths were not only sown near the gardens, but also brought inside to cover floors with a sweet, refreshing blanket of strewing herbs. This custom was introduced to Europe by the conquering Romans and the Persians before them. Banquets and processions were occasions for scattering herbs and flowers for officials to walk on. The aroma was so pleasing that chamber rooms and parlors were soon covered with fresh herbs when visitors arrived. The coronation of Tudor kings and queens began with the strewing of sweet flag and meadowsweet. Church floors and pews were laced with local flowering herbs for fragrance and to reduce disease. Herbs were also burned to repel insects and reduce the stench from the lack of sanitation. In contrast, rushes (fibrous herbs) and straw were used to cover walkways and entrances during rainy and adverse weather as a nonfragrant floormat.

Today, herbs can be simmered in an open pot to freshen a room or strewn on the carpet before vacuuming. A few drops of essential oil can be dropped on a moist sponge or cotton ball and laid on a table to quickly freshen a room. Cooking angelica, anise, or fennel seeds in an ungreased frying pan will also quickly release a purifying scent. Bowls of fresh herbs can be placed in spring water near entrances and in the kitchen and bathrooms for a refreshing finger bath during hot summer days.

FAVORITE MEDIEVAL STREWING HERBS

Basil leaves and flowers*	Mints
Bay leaves, fresh	Myrtle
Chamomile leaves	Roses
Fennel	Sage
Fleabane*	Sweet Flag
Germander	Sweet Woodruff
Hops	Tansy*
Hyssop	Thyme
Juniper and pine needles	Winter Savory
Lavender leaves and flowers	Wormwood*
Lemon Balm	Violets
Marjoram	Vervain**
Meadowsweet	

* used as an insecticide
** steeped in water and sprinkled in the dining areas to make the guests merry

The tradition of burning aromatic herbs was once the most popular way to cleanse a room of odors and guard against plagues. Herbs were burned in an open hearth fireplace or made into incense.

∾ *Soul-Soothing Incense* ∾

Relax with this potpourri after a stressful day and sleep well!

   12 dried lavender stems, flowers removed*
    1 tablespoon saltpeter (potassium nitrate, available from a pharmacy)

Soak the lavender stems in a solution of saltpeter and 1 cup of warm water for 30 minutes. Remove stems and dry completely. Place the stems in a glass jar of sand. When lit, they will burn like incense.

*Use the lavender flowers in potpourri or simmer them in water to release their aroma.

Herbs to Lay Among Linens

COSTMARY: Lay fresh leaves between layers of linen and bed sheets for a sweet balsam scent.

FEVERFEW: Place flowers and leaves in cabinets and drawers to repel insects.

HYSSOP: Lay fresh sprigs between sheets and clothes for a very fresh scent and antiseptic effect.

LAVENDER: Hang flowering sprigs upside down in closets and lay sprigs in drawers to deter moths.

LAVENDER COTTON: Combine flowering sprigs with rosemary, thyme, or lavender to deter moths. Place in drawers or hang in closets.

MUGWORT: Tie sprigs and hang in closets to deter moths. Place among woolens for storage.

ROSEMARY: Place flowering stalks among clothes and between pages of books to deter moths and silverfish.

SOUTHERNWOOD: Hang sprays in closets to deter moths.

SWEET WOODRUFF: Lay fresh leaves in drawers and between clothes to impart a fresh hay-like scent.

TANSY: Hang flowering sprigs in doorways to deter flies.

THYME: Place sprigs among winter clothes to freshen and in drawers to overcome musty odors.

∾ *Scented Washing Water* ∾

Sweet waters were used to give clothes an aromatic fragrance. This recipe uses soapwort and sweet herbs to wash your linens in place of a detergent. Use it to handwash an undergarment.

- 2 ounces soapwort roots and stems
- 2 cups distilled water
- 4 ounces sweet herbs (any of the following): rosemary, lavender, rose petals, Sweet Annie, lemon thyme, scented geraniums, chamomile, lemon grass, mints

Simmer soapwort in distilled water for 5 minutes. Add sweet herbs. Cover and allow to cool. Strain, squeezing out any liquid from the stems and roots.

⮜ *Homemade Rosewater* ⮞

Rosewater was worn by men and women during Medieval times as a sign of wealth and a romantic heart. As a variation, rosewater may be held in the same amount of denatured alcohol instead of glycerin to make a refreshing cologne.

      2 cups fresh, fragrant rose petals
    3–4 cups distilled water
    ½–1 cup vegetable glycerine, from a health food store or a pharmacy

Simmer rose petals in distilled water, covered, for 30 minutes. Allow to steep, covered, until cool. Strain and squeeze the petals tightly. Add vegetable glycerin and bottle in a clean, airtight container. Shake before splashing on after a bath or shower.

Variation: Add 3 tablespoons of fresh lemon grass to the roses and simmer according to above directions.

⮜ *Elizabethan Talc* ⮞

Talc became popular during the reign of Queen Elizabeth I. People were very conscious of body odor, but rarely bathed. Instead, they would rub their bodies with a powder made of sweet-smelling herbs. The talc was also dusted on their clothes and gloves. Here is a recipe that was fashionable in Elizabethan times, taken from Phillipe Guibert, Physician Regent, Paris.

     2 pounds orris root
     2 ounces dried sweet marjoram
     ½ pound dried rose petals
     2 ounces calamus root
     4 cloves
    $\frac{1}{16}$ ounce musk

Grind orris root into a powder; then finely grind dried sweet marjoram and dried rose petals. With a mortar and pestle, grind calamus root with cloves and musk. Combine and store airtight for up to 1 year.

Symbolism of the Rosary

The rosary represents the circle of wholeness and time in the endless cycle of asceticism. In the Hindu religion, the rosary is an attribute of their gods Shiva, Brahma, and Ganesh. The rosaries have 108 beads made from Tulasi wood. For the Buddhists, the 108 beads represent the 108 Brahmins present at the birth of Buddha.

Christianity envisions the rosary as the mystic rose garden of the Virgin Mary. The rosary has sixty beads, divided into five decants, each with its own mystery of the joys, sorrows, or glories of the Virgin goddess. On large beads, a Pater Noster is recited with a Gloria to the Trinity of the Father, Holy Spirit, and Son. On the smaller beads, Ave Marias are said.

For the Islamic, who recognize Mohammed as the last prophet, ninety-nine beads are numbered on the rosary, each corresponding to a Divine Name or attribute of Allah. The hundredth bead represents the Essence of God, only to be discovered in Paradise. (Taken from *An Illustrated Encyclopedia of Traditional Symbols*, pp. 140–141.)

~ *Medieval Rosary Beads* ~

4 cups rose petals
4 cups distilled water
1 teaspoon sandalwood oil
1 teaspoon rose oil

Finely chop rose petals into an iron pot, adding enough distilled water to cover the petals. Heat, uncovered, for 1 hour without boiling the petals. Cover and leave overnight to set. Repeat the process for 4 more days. Then begin to roll the petals into beads, rubbing your hands with 1 drop each of sandalwood and rose oil first, repeating every 5 beads. Press out any liquid as you roll the beads. Thread with a large needle and thick (or plastic) thread. Allow to dry. Makes 60 beads. Separate every 10 beads with a space and 1 isolated bead.

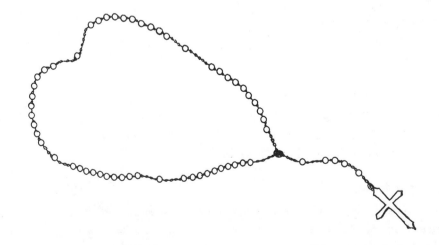

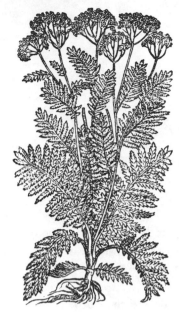

Yarrow

6

Western Folk Wisdom

Whatsoever herb thy power dost produce, give, I pray, with goodwill

to all nations to save them and grant me this my medicine.

—Pagan prayer to the Earth Goddess

Throughout history, every plant known to humanity has been sampled for food or medicine. Ancient cures have evolved and passed on to the next generation for over twenty-five thousand years.

Hippocrates was the first western man to treat medicinal herbs as a science. He is credited with writing the *Materia Medica,* describing over four hundred herbal remedies for common illnesses. He researched herbal cures while traveling to foreign countries, practicing medicine as a Greek physician four hundred years before the birth of Christ. Before Hippocrates established herbal medicine as a legitimate service, medicine and the knowledge of herbs were considered unworthy of a Western scholar. Herbalism was a blend of fantasy, fact, and superstition. People created their own remedies, invoking the gods for a blessing. If the remedy did not work, the ill person would invoke a different god and try another remedy. The panacea for the time was cabbage steeped in wine, either eaten or applied locally as a compress.

Four hundred years later, Dioscorides, another Greek physician, wrote the famous *De Materia Medica,* chronicling over six hundred medicinal

Herbalism

used to be

considered a

blend of

fantasy, fact,

and

superstition.

~

herbs. His work became the foundation for Western herbalists throughout medieval Europe. The Roman army introduced herbs and their medicinal knowledge with each conquest. As the Romans arrived to govern each new country, they brought herbs and built formal gardens for culinary and medicinal pleasure.

As the Dark Ages spread through Europe, the knowledge of how to grow and use herbs was lost. Through neglect, many varieties of herbs died out. Only the escaped and naturalized varieties of herbs survived.

The Roman army introduced herbs and medicinal knowledge with each conquest.

∾

In contrast, Arabic and Eastern countries developed the art of perfumery through the distillation of essential oils and left the West in the dark over the use of medicinal herbs and spices. Their knowledge would return to enlighten the West once more in the Middle Ages through the translations of Constantine the African.

During the Dark Ages, the knowledge of herbs and their beneficial qualities was kept alive by the peasants and traveling monks by word of mouth. These monks later transcribed their knowledge and became the only physicians caring for their monasterial inhabitants. They refined their medical skills through the Dark Ages as they combed the countryside for naturalized herbs to grow in their physic gardens. Herbs were grown for dyes, clothing, antiseptics, digestive and culinary purposes, insect repellents, strewing, medicine, and, of course, for brewing ale and liqueurs.

Flowers were grown in a sacristan garden, used for holy days and church services. Different colors were grown for different occasions. White flowers represented the resurrection of Christ and were cut for all of the sacraments: baptism, confirmation, communion, marriage, church vows, and death. They decorated the altars at Christmas, Easter, Epiphany, and Ascension. Yellow or golden flowers symbolized revealed truth and were used during the feasts of the confessors. Violet was the color for fasting and penitence, adorning the altars during Lent and Advent. Red, the color of Christ's passion, symbolized the bloodshed at Calvary and the Crown of Thorns, as well as zealous faith represented by the fire of Pentecost. Herbal green was the color of immortality, the triumph of spring over winter; during medieval times, green represented the Holy Trinity. Blue symbolized faith and heaven. It became the color of Mary as she represented the queen of Heaven.

Herbs and flowers could only be gathered according to a very strict set of rules. Particular prayers were said as each crop was harvested. Only certain garden tools could be used and each plant was gathered on the saint's day it represented (the saint's day pertained to the time of year the herb or flower was ripe for harvesting). These gardens were the forerunners of medieval pleasure gardens, dotted with a variety of brightly colored flowers and surrounded by kitchen herbs and a vineyard.

Before the Dark Ages descended, the writings of the first century Greek physician, Galen, become popular. He learned herbal remedies during extensive travels and practiced his knowledge when he became the surgeon at the school of gladiators in Pergamos. Those who read and followed his practices became known as Eclectics during the Middle Ages, utilizing herbal and mineral compounds for remedies. Western medical allopathic and holistic homeopathic systems are based on Galen's writings.

After the fall of the Roman Empire, herbal remedies fell out of favor and into the use of pagans. The Christian Church promoted only spiritual cures and penance, for all disease was thought to have been caused by sin. Guilt was deeply ingrained in European culture. Although the cure for sins was prayer, money was accepted for more alms for the poor. The only treatment condoned by the Church was bloodletting, as it symbolized a form of penance similar to the Passion of Christ. Saints were assigned to various parts of the body to be accredited in case one did recuperate.

Herbalism spread to other countries through traveling monks' lore, whereby local myths were blended with the herbal information. In Scotland, the *Leech Book of Bald* described disease to be caused by mischievous elves, who polluted the air with elf shot (created by elves from a bolt of lightening so filled with mischief that none who have survived it dare tell). If prayer did not produce the desired results, the monks charged for their herbal remedies and even performed surgery (for another fee).

As medicine and herbalism went their separate ways, the Doctrine of Signatures became popular. Paracelsus, a Swiss physician and alchemist, theorized that an herb's shape was God's way of guiding believers to gain their healing quality. Thus, the kidney bean dissolved stones and abated urinary complaints, and liverwort healed biliary complaints; in other words, herbs were shaped like the organ they were meant to heal. Herbs were angels in another form, calling forth God's goodness through Mother Nature's bounty. The Doctrine of Signatures became ingrained in Puritan belief and was later brought to America by them to unite with Native American herbalism.

The Doctrine of Signatures stated that herbs were shaped like the organ they were meant to heal.

In the New World, colonists were on their own. The Puritans brought only a few of their favorite herbs. Although Puritans believed in the Doctrine of Signatures, they also believed the "unseen" world was ruled by the devil. Like the early Christians, they believed in prayer for healing and accepted illness as a part of a sinful world. The colonists inhabiting America were determined to leave superstition and all "nonsense" about herbs and medicine behind. They desired a clean slate to start anew.

Many of the less religious settlers followed Culpepper's herbal, originally published in 1652 as *The English Physitian*. Colonists used Culpepper's cures as well as his astrological botany to sow and harvest their crops. The demand for English seeds, roots, and cures continued until many of the European herbs naturalized in America. Settlers continued to learn about Native American herbs and their uses from local tribes. This information was handed down verbally to later generations. Americans shared their knowledge of Native American cures with the Europeans and sent new plants across the ocean to be naturalized in Europe.

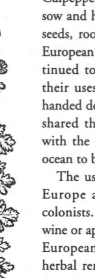

FEVERFEW

The use of gunpowder in remedies originated in Europe and was continued by many American colonists. Sometimes only gunpowder was taken in wine or applied to a tooth to abate pain. Colonists and Europeans alike believed gunpowder activated an herbal remedy. It never caught on with the Native Americans because they did not trust white man's remedies, especially when they did not come from Mother Nature. Since the white man had to write remedies and later read them in books, they must not be of any value.

A popular book of the time was *The Queen's Closet Opened* (1732). It included "incomparable secrets" for medicine, candying, preserving, and cookery. Western herbalists especially liked herbs that were valuable in culinary and medicinal practices, such as "Dr. Aitkinson's Excellent Perfume against the Plague," which states:

> Take angelica roots and dry them a very little in an oven, or by
> the fire; and then bruise them very softly, and lay them in wine
> vinegar to keep, being close covered three or four days, and then
> heat a brick hot, and lay the flame thereon every morning; this
> is excellent to air the house or any clothes, or to breath over in
> the morning . . .

Besides simpling, herbs were employed to balance the four humors, a very acceptable theory passed on through Western medicine since the time of Aristotle. The four elements—earth, fire, air, and water—were affected by hot, cold, dry, and moist conditions. These formed the four humors, or temperaments, of the personality: sanguine, melancholy, choleric, and phlegmatic. Herbs could restore health by having qualities that would restore balance.

With knowledge and faith that everything growing was provided by God for health, Western herbalism flourished into a thriving home industry. Western herbalism is rooted in a self-care system, where necessary items could be grown locally. The most enthusiastic herbalists were women, who used herbs and home remedies to heal their loved ones. They grew them and they brewed them, just like the Native American women. Their tradition lives on . . . .

The Many Faces of Medical Herbalism

A good cook is half a physitian.

—Culpepper,
The English Physitian, 1652

～

All life evolves by adapting to an ever-changing environment. Health is a reflection of homeostasis. The body seeks balance like the thinker seeks peace of mind, affirming the universal, healing principle inherent throughout creation.

Herbal tradition continued as folk remedies, and by the middle of the eighteenth century, European herbal medicine was at its peak. The printing press allowed herbals to be published for all who could read; not only were the monasterial herbals published, but also the works of ancient Greek scholars and modern herbalists. The first edition of the *London Pharmacopoeia* became available by 1618, with many new herbals following.

Herbs were also popular with physicians and available through apothecaries and grocers. Apothecaries imported herbs and spices from all over the world as well as growing local herbs in physic gardens. As the demand for herbs increased, the available information and identity of many herbs became uncertain, confusing even knowledgeable herbalists. The market became clogged with cure-all tonics that combined various chemical compounds and mixtures, some toxic. Red lead, mercury, and arsenic were frequently recommended for internal use in herbal mixtures, often with fatal results.

At the same time, scientific technology and medical therapeutics advanced rapidly with the advent of organic chemistry and anatomy. Research moved toward locating and isolating chemicals to produce an appropriate effect. Morphine, quinine, and strychnine became the miracle drugs of the age (morphine and strychnine are highly toxic). Subsequently, herbal medicine declined as pharmaceuticals increased, although herbs remained the medicine of choice for the country folk.

By 1886, medical licensing was required to practice surgery, pharmacy, and medicine. The apothecaries were not allowed to prescribe herbal or pharmaceutical medicine anymore, and the practice of medicine was solely in the hands of licensed physicians. These physicians were taught only pharmaceutical drugs.

An offshoot of medical herbalism grew into the practice of homeopathy.

∼

An offshoot of medical herbalism grew into the practice of homeopathy. *Organon of Medicine* was published by Samuel Hahnemann in Germany. Hahnemann was known as "the experimenter." He used infinitesimally small dilutions of a substance or herb to cure a "like" condition. Through the law of similars, Hahnemann catalyzed the body's innate healing ability to correct itself. He irritated the immune system just enough to force it into action. For example, he might use a greatly diluted poison to counteract a similar poison overwhelming the immune system. Lead would treat lead poisoning in such a great dilution that no toxic effect was made; as Hahnemann states,

> Homeopathy sheds not a drop of blood, administers no emetics, purgatives, laxatives or diaphoretics, drives off no external affection by external means, prescribes no hot or unknown mineral baths or medicated clysters, applies no Spanish flies or mustard plasters . . . burns not with moxa or red hot iron to the very bone . . . but gives with its own hand its own preparations of simple uncompounded medicines [and] is capable of removing the natural disease in question by similarity . . . in rare and minute form.

In homeopathy, correct treatment enhances the immune system and treats the whole patient. The constitution, state of mind, and emotional well-being are all taken into account in every treatment.

Homeopathy was well accepted by American physicians in the 1800s. They had learned to be open to alternative treatments from living among the Native Americans. However, Hahnemann's dietary suggestions were not popular with Americans. Hahnemann counseled against the use of coffee, tobacco, tea, and alcohol because they negated the subtle healing effects of homeopathic medicines. Americans were too fond of their cordials to change their lifestyles. Doctor Samuel Thompson believed if a small dose of a plant was healing, a lot might be better. This led him and a group of his fellow physicians to dose with tinctures made from the whole herb to catalyze healing and regeneration on a tissue level.

The Thompsonian school of thought is still popular today in Western herbalism. It led us from simpling to combinations of several synergistic herbs that can counteract many negative side effects. Combinations can also work systemically as well as organically to correct imbalances in homeostasis. Herbs heal through the action of volatile oils, chemical compounds, and nutritional ingredients. They offer many of the minerals deficient in Western soil, such as chromium, zinc, and manganese, which catalyze hundreds of enzyme systems in the body. Thompsonian herbalism uses simples and combinations to not only catalyze immunity but also build immunity by chemically acting on a cell, as well as building it through nutrition.

Pioneer Home Remedies of the 1800s

These remedies were published by the friends of the Inglenook Magazine from the farms, homes, and kitchens of the nineteenth-century American in *The Inglenook Doctor Book* (Elgin, IL: Brethren Publishing House, 1903).

Children's Diseases

COLDS. Give onion juice.

COLIC. Steep 1 teacupful of catnip leaves in enough boiling water to cover them completely. Sweeten with a little sugar and give to the child, making sure the temperature is not too hot. Place bottles of warm water around the child and let in plenty of pure air.

COUGH SYRUP. Take one handful of hops, one handful of horehound, and one handful of elecampane root, put in two quarts of water, and boil down to one quart. Strain, add one pound of rock candy, one large piece of grated licorice root, and one-half pound of brown sugar. Heat until dissolved.

CROUP. Take ¼ teaspoon of salt, fill the teaspoon with the juice squeezed from a lemon. It will cut the phlegm and give immediate relief.

For a two- to three-year-old child, give a teaspoonful of elderberry jelly every half hour, more often in severe cases; or stew dried elderberries and sweeten to taste. Give the juice to drink. We have never known this to fail.

Rub rattlesnake oil on the outside of the throat and drop 4 or 5 drops slowly in the mouth.

DIARRHEA. Boil purslane in milk and give to drink. Make a tea from calamus (sweet flag) root. The dose for a one-year-old child is one teaspoonful.

FEBRILE CONVULSIONS AND EPILEPSY. Black cohosh root can be set in a good whiskey for 14 days. Pound 2 ounces of root for every pint of whiskey. Three or four times daily, give 1 teaspoon in sweetened water for adults and 5 drops for children. Too much will produce vomiting.

FEVERS. Give a strong tea of catnip blossoms.

INFANTILE SICKNESS. Take the black soot out of a wood stove, tie in a thin cloth, and put boiling water over it. Given in small doses, this will quiet a small child and cure flesh decay.

NERVOUS STOMACH. Give a mint tea from dried or green leaves, crushed, with a little sugar.

SUMMER CHOLERA. Steep green peach leaves in a little water and drink the tea. Cleanse the bowels after each purging with enemas of sweet milk and warm water. Feed only warm boiled milk and toast, and avoid all greens. For fever, bathe the body, especially the spinal cord, with tepid water. Bathe the spine often, every 15 to 20 minutes, until the fever is reduced. Keep the head cool and the feet and limbs warm.

WORMS. Make a strong sage tea very sweet and give one-half teacupful before breakfast. Add senna leaves to move the bowels freely.

WHOOPING COUGH. Take 1 ounce of boneset, 1 ounce of slippery elm, and 1 ounce of flaxseed, and simmer in 2 cups of water for 1 hour. The dose is 1 teaspoonful three times daily.

Immune and Upper Respiratory Complaints

ASTHMA. Put 4 ounces of pulverized lobelia in a quart of good rum, let it stand nine days, then strain it off. Begin with 2 drops three times a day. **Note:** Lobelia is toxic in large doses. Pioneers only used a few drops when necessary.

A muskrat skin worn over the lungs with the fur side next to the body is certain relief for asthma.

BRONCHITIS. Take 2 ounces each of the following dried herbs: elecampane, comfrey, horehound leaves, and ginger. Add a pleurisy root, dried, and grind in coffee mill. Mix well and use one spoonful to make a pint of tea. Drink often.

DIPHTHERIA. Take sumac berries, boil them in vinegar, sweeten with honey, and gargle and wash the throat every half hour.

Take one ounce of black cohosh, ¼ ounce of blue cohosh and teaspoonful of goldenseal. Put in a quart of water, boil down to one pint, strain, dissolve 1 heaping teaspoon of alum and enough honey to form a syrup. Dose 1 teaspoonful every 5 minutes for 2 hours, then less frequently.

HEAD CONGESTION. Smoke cubeb berries in a clay pipe and swallow the smoke. Dried mullein leaves may be used instead.

PNEUMONIA. Make a tea of pleurisy roots, a handful of sunflower seeds, and a tablespoon of flaxseed. Drink of this very freely. Apply over the lungs a poultice made of equal parts of flaxseed and ground mustard and keep the person warm in bed.

Make a bag of flannel sufficiently large to cover the chest well, fill with hops, dip in hot apple vinegar and apply.

Muskrat skin worn over the lungs is certain relief for asthma.

Eruptive diseases

BOILS. Get flaxseed meal, moisten it, and apply it to the boil, wrapping a bandage around it to keep it in place. Apply moistened flaxseed meal to the boil. Renew it 3 times a day until the boil comes to a head.

HIVES. Take a teaspoonful of flour in a glass of water. Repeat several times a day. Hives are caused by too much acid in the blood and the flour counteracts this.

Take fresh burdock roots, slice in ¼-inch thick pieces. Pour twice as much boiling water over it and let it cool. Drink ½ cupful 3 times a day.

INFLAMMATION OF THE SKIN. Apply the white of fresh egg with the fingers. Allow to dry to let itching subside and inflammation heal.

MEASLES. To bring out measles, give hot tea made of the bark of the blackhaw root *(Viburnum)*.

Give all the cold lemonade the patient can drink to drive away the measles, to check the fever, and to loosen the cough.

SMALLPOX. Dissolve an ounce of cream of tartar in a pint of water and drink at intervals. This will cure smallpox in 3 days and never leave a mark.

SORES. Boil the bulbs of the white lily *(Lilium candidum)* in sweet cream and use as an ointment.

SWELLING OR MUMPS. Stewed pumpkin made into a poultice and renewed every 15 minutes will reduce the worse case of swelling.

Women's Complaints

The following female complaint recipes are from *Dr. Chase's Recipe Book and Household Physician* by A. W. Chase, M.D., Detroit: F. B. Dickerson Co., 1899.

CAKED BREASTS. Take feverfew blossoms or leaves and fry them in fresh lard until crisp. Strain and let cool. Bathe the breast with the lard often and cover with a woolen cloth to keep warm.

HEAVY MENSES WITH CLOTTING. Drink freely of a tea of either pennyroyal, catmint, sage, or the leaves of spruce pine until the discharge is fully established. Strictly avoid the use of all spirituous liquors and keep the bowels well open. **Note:** Pennyroyal tea may be toxic to some individuals when taken "freely." The other herbs mentioned in this remedy are safe.

PAINFUL MENSTRUATION. Apply a hot poultice of hops, tansy, or boneset.

SORE NIPPLES. Use soda and borax, wet, and make a poultice with grated raw carrots.

NIGHT SWEATS. Make sage tea, let it cool, and drink it during the day instead of water.

Stomach and Bowel Complaints

BILIOUS COLIC (GALLSTONES). Take young black walnuts tender enough to slice easily into ¼-inch slices, put in a bottle or jar, and cover with alcohol and let stand for several days. Take a teaspoonful or tablespoonful 3 or 4 times a day when symptoms appear. Continue its use for some time after the attack and it will effect a permanent cure.

CONSTIPATION. Finely chop a half pound of the best prunes and a half pound of the best figs. Add a half ounce of pure senna and enough molasses to make a thick paste. Simmer on the stove about 20 minutes. Eat a half cup daily. **Note:** *Cascara sagrada* is much gentler than senna and a safe substitute.

CRAMPS. Dissolve a half teaspoonful of soda in 2 tablespoons of hot ginger tea.

DIARRHEA. Make a tea of white oak bark, but use it carefully. A tablespoon may be enough, given only when needed.

Take the leaves and roots of berry plants and steep them to make a tea.

EMETIC. Take 1 teaspoon of salt and the same quantity of dry or prepared mustard in a tumbler of warm water till vomiting is produced.

INDIGESTION. Scald mint, put between two cloths, and lay on the stomach.

INFLAMMATORY BOWEL (COLITIS, ILEITIS). Make a strong tea of catnip leaves and add to it the inside bark of the slippery elm tree, cut in very small pieces. **Note:** Marshmallow root can be substituted for slippery elm bark and is not presently an endangered species. A poultice of finely cut tobacco placed on the abdomen will give relief in 30 minutes if the person does not use tobacco otherwise.

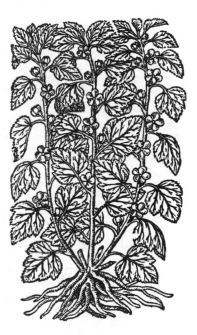

MARSHMALLOW

OVEREATING. Give a tincture of rhubarb. 1 teaspoon for adults, ½ teaspoon for children. **Note:** Rhubarb is best avoided by those with kidney disease.

PILES (HEMORRHOIDS). Drink a tea made from sumac tops. For piles or loss of power in the rectum, fry any quantity of green catnip in unsalted butter or lard (do not scorch it). Strain and cool. Use as an ointment, applying inwardly to the rectum.

STOMACHACHE. Drink a tea made of slippery elm bark.

VOMITING, NAUSEA, SEASICKNESS. Use lemon juice in water freely and plenty of pure air.

Headaches and Nervous Complaints

HEADACHES. Bruise the leaves of horseradish, wet in cold water, and bind on forehead. Wet again when it becomes dry. Keep it on an hour or more.

NERVOUS HEADACHE, INSOMNIA. Drink hops tea, warm.

NEURALGIC HEADACHE. Squeeze the juice of one lemon into a cup of strong coffee and drink.

Aches and Pains

FACIAL NEURALGIA. Make a plaster of ginger and whiskey and apply.

RHEUMATISM. Mix 2 ounces each of black cohosh, burdock seed, juniper berries, sassafras bark, and sulphur in 2 cups of Jamaican rum. Take 1 tablespoon 3 times a day for 10 days, then miss 10 days and take as before. Renew several times by adding more rum.

SPRAINS. Take equal parts of oregano and spirits of camphor, put in a bottle, and shake well. Bathe the affected part well.

STIFF JOINTS. Bathe joint with witch hazel.

Infectious Fevers

CHILLS AND FEVERS. Tea made of mountain sage or salvia used freely.

FEVER. To break up a fever, begin in time and drink very freely of boneset tea.

Neither mosquitoes nor fleas will touch the blood of persons who take sulphur. By putting a little sulphur into the shoes, enough will be absorbed into the system to keep the pests off.

MALARIA. Make a strong tea of mullein root. Drink ⅓ glass every 2 hours until fever breaks. Continue for twenty-eight days to prevent the return of the malady. For obstinate cases, make a tea of peach leaves and lemons.

Urinary Troubles

DROPSY. Take of goldenseal, boneset, and parsley each one ounce, steep and drink between meals.

Get ten cents' worth of juniper berries (probably about 2 ounces) at the drugstore and put them in a pint of liquor. Take 1 tablespoon 3 times daily.

KIDNEY TROUBLE. If the kidneys won't work, use purslane. This can be eaten as greens, salads, or pickles. Where there is inflammation, drink hops tea, warm.

Hearing Troubles

DEAFNESS. Drop rattlesnake oil in the ear once or twice a week.

EARACHES. Dip cotton in molasses, put in the ear and the pain will cease.

Fry sweet clover in unsalted butter. Drop into the ear while melted but not hot.

Dissolve asafoetida in warm water, drop a few drops in the ear and close the ear with cotton.

Skin Afflictions

To make a mustard poultice that does not burn, use the white of an egg instead of vinegar.

BRUISES. Take equal quantities of butter and bread crumbs, mix thoroughly, add a little water, apply as a poultice. This reduces pain and swelling and prevents discoloration.

BURNS, SCALDS, CHAPS. Put the inner bark of elder and a teacupful of fresh unsalted butter in a frying pan and stew slowly for half an hour. Strain and spread on a soft cloth. Apply to affected area.

CALLOUSES. Apply oil of peppermint freely.

CARBUNCLES, BOILS. Prepare oatmeal without salt, add fresh milk until a very soft mass. Bind on the sore. Change often and clean daily with glycerin soap.

CORNS. Keep soft corns sprinkled with dry sulphur and they will disappear.

RINGWORM. Bruise the green leaves or hulls of black walnuts and apply as a poultice.

Bites and Stings

MOSQUITO BITES. Bathe bites with witch hazel.

SNAKEBITE OR ANY POISONOUS BITE. Pound a lot of onions until soft, salt liberally, and bind on as a poultice. Renew often.

Make a strong tea from a large handful of plantain, sweeten to taste, and give freely.

Hygiene

HAIR GROWTH. Use a strong tea of sage for a wash. To prevent hair from falling out, wash the hair in weak salt water.

NETTLE RASH. For nettle rash, bathe with water as hot as can be borne.

PRICKLY HEAT. Rub the eruption with the inside of a watermelon rind.

TOOTHPOWDER. Mix equal parts of powdered orris root and chalk.

Mother Nature's Golden Rule

Health is a product of internal harmony and the expression of vitality.

~

Health is a product of internal harmony and the expression of vitality. Our well-being should be pursued with cautious patience. Tonics are gentle and have been proven effective for thousands of years. They are highly nutritious foods requiring special preparation and application. We should approach these tonics with respect, never abusing their benefits carelessly. Too much of a good thing is still too much! Give your body time to appreciate these new foods, just as you would nurture a child.

Tonic herbs have several properties and may also be indicated when disease is not present. They are excellent choices for preventative measures. Be sure to use them in moderation and observe how your body reacts to the energy. Allow tonic herbs to keep you young and beautiful like Mother Nature herself.

Western Tonics

The closer we live in harmony with Nature, we become available to fulfill our purpose in life. We are a product of heaven and earth and someday will return in kind.

Just as our cells select the nutrients that fulfill their requirements, herbs grow in climate and soil conditions that cause them to thrive. This is Mother Nature's process of natural selection. Herbs grown in an ideal habitat will produce the best medicinal properties. As we become in tune to our needs, we will select the best herbs for our condition. Once we know what our bodies require for greater health, we will likely find an herb growing nearby to fulfill our needs. Like wild creatures, our needs have already been provided for through Mother Nature.

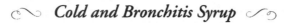

⟨⟩ *Cold and Bronchitis Syrup* ⟨⟩

A Belgian recipe from Simone De Maere.

  1 lemon
  ¼ teaspoon saffron
  1 cup honey

Wash the lemon to remove the wax layer. Then cut it into halves, and cut twice the middle of both halves. Fill those cuts carefully with saffron and tie with a cotton string. Bring its halves securely together. Place both honey and lemon into a pan. Bring to a soft boil at a medium heat. Simmer for 15 minutes. When lemon is tender, place the lemon on a plate and press out all juices. Add this to the honey syrup. Mix well and let cook. Take 1 tablespoon every 4 hours as needed.

⟨⟩ *Cold and Cough Syrup* ⟨⟩

An Belgian elderberry syrup from Simone De Maere.

  1 cup dried elderberries
  1 pound raw sugar

Soak dried berries in 4 cups of water overnight. Drain berries, saving the juice. Discard berries. Heat reserved juice plus sugar to 200 degrees. Boil at medium heat for 10 minutes. Cook in a Crock-Pot for 5–6 hours. Pour into glass bottles. Keep in refrigerator for storing.

Three Principles of Western Herbalism

*W*estern herbalists seek homeostasis in three stages of health. The first is to eliminate any excesses of heat toxins, over-acidity, mucus or fluid through the lungs, colon, kidneys and skin.

Signs of excess conditions include the following:

- Thick discharges that are yellow or green
- Redness of skin or bloody discharges
- High temperature, rapid pulse or breathing
- Acute or sudden onset of illness
- Cloudy or bloody urine
- Heavily coated tongue
- Irritability
- Desire for cold or cold drinks
- Constipation
- Desire not to be touched or to be heavily clothed

Herbs to eliminate excesses are often bitter and detoxifying, laxative, diuretic, or diaphoretic for sweating. Some examples include goldenseal root, aloe vera, white willow bark *(Salix alba)*, gentian *(Gentian officinalis)*, barberry *(Berberis vulgaris)*, dandelion root and leaves, chicory root, uva ursi *(Arctostaphylos uva ursi)*, and burdock seed *(Arctium cappa)*. Many of the herbs that reduce excess move energy down and out. For example, gentian is a bitter digestant, stimulating peristalsis. Goldenseal clears heat from the liver and is anti-inflammatory to the mucosa. Both are slightly laxative. Uva ursi is used for cystitis as a cold infusion. The leaves are soaked in enough water to cover them for several hours, strained and made into a tea, which is diuretic. Burdock seed removes heat and itching from the skin, driving toxins out through the pores. It combines well with dandelion leaves to promote diuresis. Barberry root aids in the treatment of inflammatory arthritis, removing toxins through the colon and skin. Bitters are used for short durations.

Once the excess condition is removed, a Western herbalist tonifies by building a healthier organ, stronger immunity, and balancing the mental/emotional outlook. It may be necessary to stimulate or sedate the system. Stimulation will increase circulation, metabolism, and assimilation of nutrients. This is not recommended after a prolonged illness, inflammatory disease, or skin eruption. Metabolism requires stimulation when the individual complains of the following symptoms:

- Coldness with a slow pulse and shallow breathing
- Chronic illness with low-grade fever, aches, cramps, and spasms of the muscles
- Anemia or a very pale, drawn complexion
- Poor digestion and assimilation with watery stools or undigested food
- Frequent urination with low volume
- Watery discharges
- Emotionally oversensitive and "burned out"
- Responds well to touch and deep massage

Herbs that will build and tonify may include warming, nutritive berries, roots, and herbs like the following.

AMARANTH GRAIN *(Amaranthaceae)*, known as pigweed to Western herbalists, is a staple building food, considered a god by the ancient Aztecs. The leaves are high in vitamins A and C. Leaves and grain are building for convalescents, the elderly, and growing children.

ANGELICA ARCHANGELICA is similar to the Chinese tang kuei *(Angelica sinensis)*. The roots of these herbs are cooked and eaten, or made into a tea to alleviate menstrual and menopausal symptoms. The Chinese also use tang kuei to alleviate constipation and "build the blood" to reduce chronic fatigue. **Note:** Angelica is toxic in its raw state.

ASTRAGALUS YELLOW VETCH *(Astragalus membranicus)* is a fibrous herb without taste. As a tea or in combination with other herbs, it increases vitality as it strengthens immunity. Over a period of time, astragalus improves the tone of prolapsed organs.

CHINESE FOXGLOVE *(Rehmannia glutinosa)* is a famous Chinese herb used for diabetes, anemia, premenstrual and menopausal complaints. It is a relative of the foxglove grown in Western gardens. The root is prepared by steaming and sun drying. The herb looks black and tarry. When cooked, the taste is very sweet and warming. **Note:** The raw, unprepared root is used as an alterative, a blood purifier clearing excess heat.

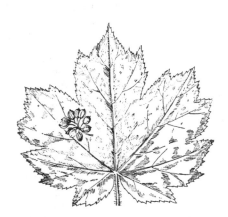

DEVIL'S CLUB

DEVIL'S CLUB *(Oplopanax horridus)* was used by the northwestern Native Americans to regulate blood sugar.

FENNEL *(Foeniculum vulgar)* is sweet and warming. Both seeds and bulb are nutritious. The anise flavor is a stimulating digestant, relieving colic and indigestion. Greeks and Romans made a tea from the seeds to restore clear vision and increase milk for nursing mothers.

GINGER ROOT is a very warming herb used in small amounts to alleviate nausea and cramps and to produce warmth. It can be applied as a warm compress to alleviate pain or taken in combination with other herbs. It is not recommended in large doses for those with low platelet counts or for those who suffer from gastrointestinal disorders.

HAWTHORN BERRIES *(Crataegus oxycantha)* are a sweet, warming cardiac tonic and mild digestant.

LICORICE ROOT is a very nutritive, soothing tonic, beneficial for convalescing and elderly people. The sweet taste comes from fifty molecules of natural sugar abating low blood sugar and low blood pressure. It is helpful for overcoming alcoholic and addictive behavior and builds muscle in children. Licorice root is an intestinal tonic that combines well with marshmallow root. It is not recommended for hypertension.

Tonic herbs
promote
self-healing.

∾

LOVAGE *(Ligusticum officinalis)* promotes digestion, regulates menses, and enhances immunity to viral invasion. The Chinese taught Western herbalists to add it to female tonics to promote vitality and a smooth flow of energy.

MARSHMALLOW ROOT *(Althea officinalis)* is a demulcent nutritive tonic that soothes the intestines and urinary tract.

PAPAYA *(Caricaeae)* is a fruit that contains papain, an enzyme used to digest protein.

SIBERIAN GINSENG *(Eleutherococcus senticosus)* is a close relative of Chinese and American ginsengs. The energy is warm but not as heating as other ginsengs. It is beneficial in balancing blood sugar, improving stamina and immunity, and reducing rheumatic tendencies. It is taken by many travelers to reduce jet lag. Chinese herbalists call it "wu cha seng" and tincture it with honey. Siberian ginseng is an excellent tonic for convalescing and fatigued individuals alone or in combination with other building herbs. According to herbalist Michael Tierra, there are two western herbs similar to Siberian ginseng: spikenard root and devil's club.

SPIKENARD ROOT *(Aralia racemosa)* can be roasted with honey and eaten to reduce rheumatic pain and alleviate female hormonal imbalances. It is a warming herb also used in combination for chronic lung complaints.

SUMA, OR BRAZILIAN GINSENG *(Pfaffia paniculata)*, is a nutritive tonic that enhances immunity and regulates blood sugar. It can be used to increase energy.

Sedation may also aid in tonification. Hyper and environmentally oversensitive individuals may benefit from tonification of the central nervous system. Sedation will reduce environmental sensitivity, spasticity, emotional conflict, pain, and a nervous stomach. Both nervines and demulcents may be used or added to a building tonic. Demulcents, like slippery elm bark, marshmallow root, and flaxseed teas or compresses, may be used to lubricate and sedate the intestines, bronchials, and joints, as well as to fortify the bones and muscles. Mild nervines, such as hops, red raspberry leaves, gotu kola, skullcap, and black cohosh root, reduce spasticity, nervous and emotional reactions.

As an individual becomes stronger, maintenance can be achieved with tonic herbs to promote self-healing. Our bodies know how to heal better than we do. A positive attitude is essential to believe the body can regenerate. It can take one to three years for the body to heal chronic problems. Once the immune system is altered, it is always wise to use small maintenance doses of tonics to balance the endocrine, immune, and neurological centers.

Attunement

*B*efore choosing a tonic for yourself or a loved one, allow yourself to attune to the needs of the recipient. First, choose a tonic that most suits the symptom.

Is the symptom acute or chronic and recurring? Acute symptoms need quick-acting, bitter, sedating, or cooling tonics. Chronic, recurring symptoms require warming and nurturing herbs. Roots and barks often have nurturing qualities. Leaves and flowers are cooling and can reduce the vitality of one with chronic symptoms if used without building roots and soothing barks. Plan a tonic with long-term results for long-term or recurring problems. Stimulating herbs and spices may be used sparingly to allow the system to accept their warmth. Long-term and heavy detoxification is not recommended for chronic disease.

Choose herbs that support the personality and awareness of the recipient. It is normal to have emotional manifestations when the body's chemistry is not in balance. If the individual is displaying anger, choose herbs that will not overstimulate or heat up their system, such as spearmint or chamomile. Do not choose a heating root like ginseng in the combination. If the individual is weepy, choose herbs that promote diuresis. When the kidneys flush, they will move out excess fluids and metabolic wastes. Use the tonic long enough to achieve the desired effect. Longer duration is only acceptable for longevity tonics recommended by an experienced practitioner. If someone tells you "it's natural, it can't hurt you," run home and make a tension-reliever tea. You probably know more about herbs and have been blessed with greater common sense.

Become acquainted with as many herbs as you can grow organically or obtain locally. It is better to be well-acquainted with a few herbs than to know little about many. When in doubt, use local compresses, external applications, and aromasignatures before ingesting a questionable tonic.

Choose herbs that support the personality and awareness of the recipient.

~

Hearsay and what works for your neighbor is not the safest way to choose a tonic. We wouldn't think of sharing a prescription drug. Make sure you use tonics as a food and not a drug. Each individual has a body that knows how to heal itself. Give yourself that chance as you enjoy the rapport you will experience from growing organic herbs and cooking a tonic as an elixir for radiant health.

Preparing Western Tonics

*E*ach

*individual has
a body that
knows how to
heal itself.*

∼

Tonics can safely be used once a day, several times a week. As your body regenerates, once or twice a week will be sufficient. Tonics are foods and should be rotated and used in moderation.

Use glassware or porcelain to cook herbal tonics and bottled water. As you learn the energy and property of individual herbs, you can combine them into tonics to renew the dynamic life force within you. Combining herbs is like making a casserole. Look for the synergistic qualities of herbs and you will become a powerful mediator of Mother Nature's secrets. Here are some examples of tonics for health and pleasure. Make half-doses to begin with to ensure you can handle the energy. **Note:** Please check with your physician before starting a tonic.

๑๑ *Pain, Spasm, and Cramp Tonic* ๑๑

Drink this tonic to abate headaches, tension, muscle spasms, and intestinal cramps. Ginger and cinnamon should be omitted if any inflammatory bowel or gastritis is involved. This tonic may also be used as a compress.

- 4 tablespoons cramp bark *(Viburnum opulis)* or blackhaw *(Viburnum prunifolium)*
- 1 (¼-inch) slice fresh ginger root or ½ cinnamon stick
- 1 ounce chamomile flowers

Simmer cramp bark or blackhaw and ginger or cinnamon in 2 cups of water for 20 minutes, covered. Turn off the heat and add chamomile flowers. Cover. Allow to cool 15 minutes. Strain and sip a half cup every half hour as needed to abate symptoms.

๑๑ *PMS Tonic* ๑๑

This tonic will quickly reduce painful menstruation.

Add 2 tablespoons wild yam root *(Dioscorea villosa)* to the above pain, spasm, and cramp tonic and simmer for 20 minutes.

❧ *Headache Tonic* ❧

Make this tonic before a headache starts. Freeze it in ice trays and heat one or two cubes when a headache occurs. Chamomile flowers can be substituted for any of the following herbs.

    1 tablespoon skullcap *(Scutellaria laterifolia)*
    1 tablespoon passionflower *(Passiflora incarnata)*
    1 tablespoon wood betony leaves *(Betonica officinalis)*
    1 tablespoon hops *(Humulus lupulus)*

Boil 2 cups of water, turn off heat, and add the above herbs. Cover and steep 10 minutes before straining and drinking a half cup at a time.

❧ *Energy Tonic* ❧

Drink this in the midafternoon when your energy levels begin to slide.

    1 American ginseng root *(Panax quinquefolium)*
    1 teaspoon fenugreek seeds *(Trigonella foenumgraecum)*
    1 (¼-inch) slice ginger root or 1 piece licorice root

Simmer in 2 cups of water for 1 hour, covered. Strain and drink a half cup for a morning or a mid-afternoon boost. **Note:** Ginseng and ginger are not recommended for inflammatory disease or for women on estrogen blockers. Licorice root is not recommended for hypertensives.

❧ *Mild Energy Tonic for Fatigue* ❧

This is an excellent tonic for travelers or those recuperating from chronic illness or surgery.

    1 tablespoon Siberian ginseng root *(Eleutherococcus senticosus)*
    1 tablespoon ho shou wu (foti) *(Polygonum multiflorum)*
    1 codonopsis dang shen root *(Codonopsis pilosula)*
    2 slices (or 2 tablespoons ground root) astragalus yellow vetch
        (Astragalus mongolicus or *membranicus)*
    1 tablespoon suma root (optional)

Simmer all in 2 cups of water, covered, for 1½ hours, or tincture in brandy to cover for 1 month. Drink ½ cup of tea daily or dilute 1 teaspoon of tincture in boiled water. It is safe for elderly folks and children in half-doses. For elderly folks, drink ¼ cup of tea twice daily. Children over 10 years old may drink 1 teaspoon to 1 tablespoon of diluted tea daily for 1 to 2 weeks of the month. If suma and Siberian ginseng are not available as roots, use a tablespoon of dried herbs or buy a tincture (an alcoholic tincture of these roots is often available in health food stores) and add a few drops to your tea.

❧ *Tonic for the Elderly* ❧

Drink this tonic daily and feel young again.

- 1 tablespoon hawthorn berries *(Crataegus* species) to enhance the cardiovascular system and regulate blood pressure
- 1 2½- to 3-year-old echinacea root to enhance immunity
- 1 teaspoon parsley root to support kidney function
- 1 teaspoon licorice root, optional (not recommended for hypertension), ginger root may be substituted
- 1 dandelion root to enhance bowel function
- 1 tablespoon gotu kola leaves (fresh is best) or 1 tablespoon basil leaves or flowers

Simmer hawthorn, echinacea, parsley, licorice, and dandelion in 2 cups of water for 30 minutes, covered. Remove from heat and add gotu kola or basil. Steep, covered, for 10 more minutes. Strain and sip one cup daily.

❧ *Rheumatism Tonic* ❧

Enjoy this tonic and feel the bounce return to your step.

- 1 tablespoon devil's claw *(Harpagophytum procumbens)*; this anti-inflammatory root can be fresh or powdered
- 1 teaspoon yucca root *(Yucca* species), dried and split; yucca root is a safe steroid of vegetable origin (powdered is acceptable)
- 1 teaspoon black cohosh root *(Cimicifuga racemosa)* to reduce pain and sedate the central nervous system
- ⅛ teaspoon ginger may be added to disperse heat, optional
- 1 tablespoon wild yam root *(Dioscorea villosa),* optional

Simmer in 2 cups of water for 30 minutes. Strain and sip up to half a cup daily. You may also drink half a cup of a pain tonic as necessary. Reduce or delete ginger if the tonic is too hot and stimulating. For rheumatoid arthritis, add wild yam root.

❧ *Flu Tonic* ❧

Drink this tonic at the onset of chills or flu symptoms every thirty to sixty minutes.

- 1 teaspoon dried citrus peel

Simmer citrus peel in 1 cup of water for 5 minutes. Allow to cool before straining and drinking. Drink 2–3 times during onset of symptoms, then change to the cold and fever tonic (page 139).

⌒ *Cold and Fever Tonic* ⌒

Tonics are generally not recommended in acute disease. This tonic is meant to be taken at the onset of symptoms and repeated every few hours until symptoms abate. It is very safe for children and adults.

- 4 tablespoons spearmint leaves
- 1 tablespoon yarrow flowers
- 1 tablespoon basil or elder flowers
- 1 tablespoon lemon balm leaves

In 2 cups of boiled water, steep the above herbs for 15 minutes, covered. Strain and serve warm or cool. Drink half a cup at a time.

⌒ *Sinus and Allergy Tonic* ⌒

This tea may also be used as a gargle for sore and tickling throats or as a compress on the forehead to relieve a stuffy head.

- 1 teaspoon thyme leaves
- 1 teaspoon sage leaves
- 1 teaspoon lavender leaves

Steep the above herbs in 2 cups of boiled water for 10–15 minutes. Strain and drink 1 cup to relieve sinus congestion.

⌒ *Lung Tonic* ⌒

Native Americans of the Midwest used this tonic to alleviate bronchial coughs and congestion.

- 2 tablespoons pleurisy root *(Asclepias tuberosa)*
- 1 tablespoon mullein root *(Verbascum thaspus)*
- 2 tablespoons elecampane root *(Inula helinium)*
- 1 tablespoon cramp bark *(Viburnum opulis)* or
  blackhaw *(Viburnum prunifolium)*
- 1 teaspoon licorice root or ginger
- 2 tablespoons osha root *(Ligusticum porteri),* optional;
  take only if there is congestion or a productive cough
- 2 tablespoons yucca, dried and split, optional;
  take only if there is wheezing

Simmer in 2 cups of water, covered, for 15 minutes. Strain when cool and drink half a cup daily to facilitate the lungs or drink half a cup three times daily to alleviate congestion. For wheezing, add dried and split yucca, and add half a cup to coffee or drink alone up to 3 times daily.

Relaxation Tonic

This is a soothing tea to enjoy when the mind can't slow down.

- 2 tablespoons hops *(Humulus lupulus)*
- 2 tablespoons chamomile flowers
- 2 tablespoons lemon balm or spearmint leaves
  (peppermint is too stimulating)
- 1 teaspoon chopped lavender leaves

Steep in 2 cups of boiled water, covered. Strain after 10–15 minutes and drink half a cup to 1 cup to relax.

Nobody Loves Me Tonic

When life has let you down and no one seems to care, have a cup of tea and wait for things to come your way.

- 1 tablespoon skullcap leaves and flowers *(Scutellaria laterifolia)*
- 1 tablespoon passionflower *(Passiflora incarnata)*
- 1 teaspoon lavender flowers and leaves
- 1 teaspoon chamomile flowers
- 1 tablespoon lemon grass

Combine all and steep in 2 cups of boiled water, covered, 15 minutes. Strain and surrender.

Stabilizing Tonic

This tonic helps you to get centered and focused.

- 1 tablespoon lemon grass
- 1 teaspoon chamomile flowers

Steep in 1 cup of boiled water for 10 to 15 minutes. Strain and sip ½–1 cup and feel the power of a balanced mind.

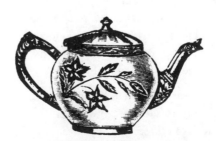

❧ *Colitis and Irritable Bowel Tonic* ❧

Drink this tonic to relax the bowel and reduce inflammation.

    1 tablespoon black cohosh root
    1 tablespoon marshmallow root *(Althea officinalis)*
    1 tablespoon cramp bark or blackhaw bark
    1 tablespoon chamomile flowers
    1 tablespoon shepherd's purse *(Capsella bursa pastoris)*, optional
    1 tablespoon sliced licorice root, optional

Simmer roots and bark in 2 cups of water for 20 minutes, covered. Remove from heat, add chamomile flowers, and steep 10 more minutes before straining. Drink half a cup as needed. Add shepherd's purse if bleeding occurs and see your doctor immediately. Add licorice root only when hypertension or edema is not a problem.

❧ *Cystitis and Soothing Bladder Tonic* ❧

The flaxseed will make this tonic congeal into a gelatin you can eat with a spoon.

    1 tablespoon flaxseed, whole
    1 tablespoon marshmallow root
    1 tablespoon parsley root
    1 tablespoon cramp bark
    ½ cup fresh parsley leaves

Simmer flaxseed, marshmallow, parsley root and cramp bark in 2 cups of water for 20 minutes. Remove from heat and steep fresh parsley leaves for 10 minutes before straining. Sip half a cup every thirty minutes to abate symptoms. Apply the discarded herbs as a compress to the lower abdomen in a clean cloth while they are warm.

❧ *Non-Irritating Laxative and Liver Tonic* ❧

This tonic works on the most stubborn cases of constipation.

    1 tablespoon dandelion roots

Simmer dandelion roots pulled from your yard for 10 minutes. Strain and eat the roots like carrots. The juice may also be ingested for chronic constipation. Work with digestants and blood builder tonics. Cook with the dandelion roots to avoid future problems (powdered roots can be purchased at health food stores as a substitute).

⤳ *Male Prostate and Bladder Tonic* ⤲

Saw palmetto berries were used by Western herbalists for building and toning muscles, reducing male pattern baldness and impotence due to chronic prostatitis. Fenugreek seeds were used by Western herbalists to reduce impotence, balance blood sugar, and abate male pattern baldness. Fenugreek was introduced to the West by the Arabic traders in the Mediterranean. This tonic is very successful at lowering PSA blood levels, which are markers of prostatic tumor growth.

> 1 tablespoon saw palmetto berries *(Serrenoa serrulata)*
> 1 tablespoon fenugreek seeds
> 1 tablespoon parsley root
> 1 tablespoon echinacea root
> 1 tablespoon marshmallow root
> 1 tablespoon goldenseal root, optional; use to reduce inflammation
> 4 tablespoons fresh dandelion leaves

Simmer in 2 cups of water for 30 minutes, covered. Remove from heat and steep dandelion leaves for 15 minutes before straining. Drink ½–1 cup daily. When inflammation has gone down, discontinue goldenseal. Consider a building tonic, such as the energy tonic for fatigue, at breakfast or lunch.

⤳ *Kidney Cleansing Tonic* ⤲

This tonic is both stimulating and soothing to enhance function and drainage.

> 2 tablespoons dandelion root
> 2 tablespoons parsley root
> 2 tablespoons marshmallow root
> 4 tablespoons fresh dandelion leaves
> 4 tablespoons fresh parsley or cilantro leaves
> 2 tablespoons goldenseal root, optional, for inflammation

Simmer roots in 2 cups of water for 20 minutes. Remove from heat and steep dandelion and parsley or cilantro leaves for 15 minutes before straining. When inflammation has gone down, discontinue goldenseal. Drink ½–1 cup daily and stay close to home. A kidney tonic is best taken once a week and then once a month after the first week of usage.

⮌ *Stimulating Digestant Tonic* ⮎

Drink this tonic when your food sits on your stomach or you have overeaten.

½ teaspoon freshly ground ginger
½ teaspoon freshly ground cardamom
½ teaspoon freshly ground cinnamon
½ teaspoon freshly ground cloves
½ teaspoon freshly grated citrus peel

Simmer in 2 cups of water for 10 minutes. Strain and drink half a cup with a meal. This tonic is not recommended for tender tummies and intestinal inflammatory disease.

⮌ *Mild Digestant Tonic* ⮎

This tonic is refreshing and mildly stimulating for circulation and digestion—your tummy will thank you.

½ teaspoon hawthorn berries
½ teaspoon anise or fennel seeds
1 ounce fresh mint leaves
1 ounce fresh gotu kola leaves
1 ounce fresh rose petals
1 teaspoon lemon balm, lemon grass, or lemon thyme

Simmer berries and seeds in 2 cups of water for 10 minutes. Remove from heat and steep mint, gotu kola, rose petals, and lemon balm, lemon grass, or lemon thyme. Strain after 10 minutes and sip with a meal or as an after-dinner tonic. Dilute by half for children and elderly.

⮌ *Soothing Intestinal Tonic* ⮎

This tonic is helpful for rumbling tummies and diarrhea. For chronic conditions, consult a physician.

2 tablespoons wild yam root *(Dioscorea villosa)*
2 tablespoons marshmallow root
2 tablespoons kudzu root *(Puerariae lobata)*
2 tablespoons dried lotus root, available at Oriental markets
2 tablespoons powdered carob, available at health markets

Simmer in 2 cups of water for 15 minutes. Strain and sip half a cup.

❧ *Blood Tonic* ❧

This tonic is excellent for women of all ages, elderly people, those with chronic debilitated conditions, and for those who are recuperating from a long-term illness. Those who use energy tonics often should balance it with a nurturing blood tonic.

- 2 tablespoons lotus seed *(Nelumbiun nuciferae)*
- 2 tablespoons hawthorn berries *(Crataegus* species)
- 1 tablespoon yellowdock root *(Rumex* species)
- 6 jujube red dates *(Zizyphus sativa)*
- 1 tang kuei root *(Angelica sinensis)*
- 1 tablespoon Chinese foxglove *(Rehmannia glutinosa)*, prepared
- 2 tablespoons dark grapes or raisins
- 1 tablespoon lycee berries *(Lycium chinensis)*, or matrimony vine berries
- 1 tablespoon blackstrap molasses

Choose 3–4 herbs from the above list and simmer in 2 cups of water for 30 minutes, covered. Strain and add 1 tablespoon or less of blackstrap molasses and drink 1 cup daily. Reduce or delete the molasses if hypoglycemia is a concern.

❧ *Tonic for Coldness* ❧

This tonic is helpful for those who suffer during cold weather conditions or cold hands and feet. It is not recommended during pregnancy.

- 2 tablespoons celery seed
- 2 tablespoons ginger root

Simmer in 2 cups of water for 10 minutes. Strain and sip half a cup to enhance peripheral circulation. For those with gastrointestinal inflammation, use this tonic as a foot bath.

❧ *Tonic to Enhance Collagen Synthesis* ❧

Collagen is the interconnecting skin that holds our organs in place and keeps our external skin from sagging.

- 2 tablespoons rose hips
- 2 tablespoons black currant berries *(Ribes rubrum)*
- 2 tablespoons raisins
- 2 tablespoons gelatin or donkey hides glue, from Oriental pharmacy

Simmer rose hips, berries, and raisins in 2 cups of water for 20 minutes. Strain and dissolve gelatin or donkey hides glue into it. Drink half a cup daily and eat the raisins.

❧ *Blood Sugar Stabilizing Tonic* ❧

Drink this tonic to avoid sinking spells of low energy and the urge to raid the candy machine.

- 2 tablespoons suma root *(Pfaffia paniculata)*. This is known as "Brazilian ginseng," and increases energy as well as regulates blood sugar
- 2 tablespoons fenugreek seeds
- ½ teaspoon or 2 slices of licorice or ginger root (licorice root is not recommended for hypertension and edema)
- 2 tablespoons ho shou wu (foti) *(Polygonum multiflorum)*
- 2 tablespoons Chinese foxglove *(Rehmannia glutinosa)*, prepared

Simmer in 2 cups of water for 30 minutes. Strain and drink half a cup twice daily or as desired.

❧ *Clear Vision Tonic* ❧

This is a valuable tonic for tired eyes and blurry vision.

- 2 tablespoons fennel seeds
- 2 tablespoons eyebright *(Euphrasia officinalis)*
- 2 tablespoons bilberry powder *(Vaccinium myrtellus)*
- 2 tablespoons gotu kola leaves, optional

Simmer in 2 cups of water for 15 minutes. Strain and drink half a cup daily. Two tablespoons of gotu kola leaves may be steeped for 10 minutes after the tonic has been simmered to increase circulation from the carotids.

❧ *Liver Tonic* ❧

Western herbalists recommended a liver cleanser as a spring tonic.

- 2 tablespoons wild yam root
- 2 tablespoons milk thistle globes *(Silybum marianum)*
- 2 tablespoons Oregon graperoot *(Mahonia repens)*
- 2 tablespoons dandelion root
- 2 tablespoons chicory root
- 2 tablespoons goldenseal root, optional

Simmer in 2 cups of water for 20 minutes. Strain and alternate with the kidney tonic (page 142) ½–1 cup daily. Goldenseal root may lower blood sugar and may be deleted from this remedy.

❧ *Tonic for Sleepless Nights* ❧

This tonic may also help alleviate migraine headaches, anxiety, insomnia, and tension.

- 2 tablespoons valerian root *(Valeriana officinalis)*
- 2 tablespoons peony root *(Paeonia alba)*
- 5 jujube red dates *(Zizyphus)*, available at Oriental markets
- ¼ teaspoon (1 slice) licorice root *(Glycyrrhiza glabra* species), optional

Simmer in 2 cups of water for 20 minutes. Remove from heat and steep for 10 minutes with:

- 2 tablespoons skullcap *(Scutellaria)* or passionflower
- 2 tablespoons chamomile flowers
- 2 tablespoons lemon grass

Strain, drink ½–1 cup, and get ready for a good night's sleep. Delete licorice root if hypertension or edema are present.

❧ *Safe Delivery Tonic* ❧

This tonic may arrest heavy bleeding and "secure the fetus" for a safe delivery. Also, it may be used during menopause when those cranky days occur.

- 2 tablespoons lotus seeds *(Nelumbium nuciferae)*
- 2 tablespoons skullcap leaves and flowers
- 1 tablespoon rose petals
- 1 tablespoon lemon grass

Simmer lotus seeds in 2 cups of water for 20 minutes (also known as lotus nodes, they are available from Oriental markets and are edible when cooked). Remove from heat and add skullcap leaves and flowers, rose petals, and lemon grass. Steep for 10 minutes, covered. Strain and drink half a cup daily or as needed. Consult with your midwife or physician before using herbal tonics.

❧ *Nursing Tonic* ❧

Here is a simple tea to enhance the flow of mother's milk.

- 1 tablespoon crushed fennel seeds
- 1 tablespoon red raspberry leaves
- 2 tablespoons chopped borage leaves

In 2 cups of boiled water, steep the above herbs for 15 minutes. Strain and drink half a cup daily.

Longevity Tonic

This tonic is good for women of any age. It will increase energy and strengthen immunity. The combination may also regulate blood sugar and female hormones from menses through menopause. The herbs may be tinctured in brandy for three weeks instead of cooking.

- 1 small tang kuei root
- 2 tablespoons suma
- 2 tablespoons Siberian ginseng or ho shou wu (foti)
- 5 jujube red dates
- 2 tablespoons Bupleurum falcatum, available at a Chinese market
- ¼ teaspoon (1 slice) ginger root or licorice root

Simmer in 2 cups of water for 30 minutes, covered or in a ginseng cooker. Strain when cold and drink half a cup daily or as needed for energy. Delete tang kuei if estrogen blockers are being prescribed by your physician.

Rejuvenating Menopause Tonic

This combination is beneficial for those who suffer from heat flashes. It is slightly estrogenic, but it is not estrogen replacement therapy. Be sure to check with your physician as an estrogen deficiency may lead to osteoporosis or heart disease. These herbs can be tinctured in 2–3 cups of brandy for 1 month.

- 2 tablespoons black cohosh root
- 2 small tang kuei roots
- 1 tablespoon wild yam root
- 1 tablespoon chasteberries
- ¼ teaspoon (¼ slice) ginger root or licorice root

Dilute a teaspoon of the tincture daily or simmer in 2 cups of water, covered, for 30 minutes. Strain when cool and sip ½ cup daily or as needed to reduce feelings of heat, heaviness, and emotional instability. This combination will also work to alleviate many symptoms of PMS and may help restore prolapsed organs. Delete tang kuei if estrogen blockers are being prescribed by your physician.

∾ *Energizing Tonic* ∾

This tonic will increase energy and enhance digestion.

- 1 tablespoon fresh peppermint leaves
- 1 tablespoon lemon grass leaves
- 1 teaspoon suma, optional

Steep peppermint and lemon grass leaves in 2 cups of boiled water for 15 minutes, covered. Strain and drink warm or cold. **Optional:** Suma may be steeped in the combination for an extra boost.

∾ *Delayed Menses Tonic* ∾

Here's an excellent tonic to bring on the inevitable, alleviating that heavy, bloated feeling of "dense clouds, no rain."

- 2 tablespoons black cohosh root
- 2 tablespoons wild yam root
- 2 tablespoons parsley root
- 2 tablespoons chamomile flowers
- 2 tablespoons lemon balm leaves

Simmer cohosh, yam, and parsley roots in 2 cups of water, covered, for 20 minutes. Remove from heat and steep chamomile flowers and lemon balm leaves for 10 minutes before straining. Drink 1–3 cups daily until menses begin.

∾ *Water Tonic* ∾

This tonic can be made from herbs growing in your backyard. It will reduce bloating through diuresis.

- 2 tablespoons fresh parsley leaves
- 2 tablespoons dandelion leaves
- 2 tablespoons chicory leaves
- 2 tablespoons corn silk from fresh corn

Steep a combination of available herbs in 2 cups of boiled water for 15 minutes, covered. Strain and drink 1 cup daily. **Note:** Corn silk is the fibrous, hairy material next to the fresh corn on the cob that we usually discard. Next time you shuck fresh corn, dry this material, store it in a closed container, and use it for a gentle diuretic tea. Any of these herbs may produce a diuretic tea.

❧ *Nausea and Morning Sickness Tonic* ❧

Have a pitcher of this tea placed next to a plate of crackers to sedate the stomach.

- 1 tablespoon lemon grass
- ¼ inch fresh or ⅛ teaspoon powdered ginger root
- 1 teaspoon chamomile flowers

Steep the above herbs for 15 minutes in 2 cups of boiled water. Strain and sip half a cup daily.

❧ *Hormonal Headache Tonic* ❧

This tonic will calm the storm you feel brewing in your head.

- 2 tablespoons cramp bark
- 2 tablespoons chasteberries *(Vitex)*
- 2 tablespoons wild yam
- 2 tablespoons black cohosh root, optional

Simmer in 2 cups of water for 30 minutes, covered. Remove from heat and steep the following herbs for 15 minutes before straining:

- 1 tablespoon chamomile flowers
- 1 tablespoon passionflower
- 1 tablespoon lavender leaves and flowers

Drink half a cup every hour until headache abates.

❧ *Tension Reliever Tonic* ❧

For headaches, tense shoulders, and symptoms of stress.

- 1 tablespoon passionflower leaves and flowers
- 1 teaspoon black cohosh root, optional

Steep passion flower leaves and flowers in 1 cup of boiled water for 15 minutes, covered. Strain and drink warm. Depending on how stressful the day has been, you may want to try something a little stronger: simmer black cohosh root in 1 cup of water for 15 minutes, covered. Strain, add to passionflower tea, and get ready for bed.

Compresses to Complement Tonics

Compresses may be used to complement tonics, nurturing the immune system through the skin.

❧ *Rosemary Compress for Headaches* ❧

Enjoy this compress to reduce stressful headaches or to relax after an afternoon of gardening.

4 ounces rosemary, fresh or dried

Steep rosemary in 2 cups of boiled water for 20 minutes, covered. Strain and apply on a clean cloth to the forehead or back of the neck.

❧ *Compress for Varicosities* ❧

This external compress will increase circulation to the affected veins as well as astringe and decompress them.

- 2 tablespoons witch hazel bark *(Haemelis virginiana)*
- 2 tablespoons marigold flowers *(Tagetes* species)
- 2 tablespoons yarrow leaves *(Achilles millifollium)*
- 2 tablespoons comfrey leaves or root *(Symphytum officinale)*
- 2 tablespoons burnet root *(Arcticum lappa)*
- 2 tablespoons horse chestnut *(Aesculus hippocastanum),* optional

Steep in 2 cups of boiled water for 20 minutes. Cool, strain and refrigerate to apply cold. To improve the integrity of the veins, drink 1 cup of hawthornberry tea several times weekly and eat buckwheat often. Consider using the tonic for the elderly (page 138) in addition to the blood tonic (page 144).

❧ *Ginger Compress* ❧

An external application can be safe and effective for cramps, nausea, and pain. This compress is not recommended during heavy bleeding.

2 tablespoons ginger root or powder

Steep ginger root or powder in 2 cups of boiled water for 15-20 minutes. Keep the decoction covered until ready to use. Dip a clean cloth or washcloth into the tonic, squeeze out any excess liquid and apply warm to the abdomen. Reapply every 15 minutes as necessary. This tonic will bring on menses as a topical emmenagogue.

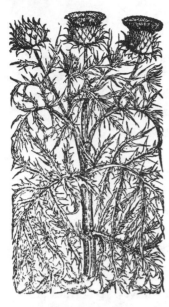

CARDOON

7

The Land of 1,000 Flavors

Someday after we have mastered the winds, the waves, the tides and gravity,
we shall harness for God the energies of love. Then, for the second time in
the history of the world, we will have discovered fire.

—Teilhard de Chardin

The Mediterranean people are seafaring adventurers who have utilized the medicinal properties of an abundant source of herbs since antiquity. The following are some of the herbs native to their lands.

A Mediterranean Herbal

Mediterraneans have utilized medicinal herbs since antiquity.

ARTICHOKES *(Cynara scolymus)*. A thistle that was eaten as a natural deodorant, "against the rank smell of armholes." The root was "boyled and drunke" as a diuretic that cleaned out the kidneys and "sendeth forth plenty of stinking urine." The buds were steeped in wine and eaten to "stir up the lust of the body," possibly after the deodorant took effect.

BASIL *(Ocimum basilicum)*. Originated in India, where it is considered a sacred herb. It is made into a tea to reduce fever, and cuttings are kept in water to reduce viral disease and malefic odors. In Mediterranean countries, it is used as a digestive aid and carminative, either in cuisine or steeped in a good red wine. Basil leaves are eaten alone to counteract poisons and scorpion stings. "They of Africke affirm that those who have been stung by a scorpion eat basil, they feel no pain." Since rue will not grow near basil, other Europeans were hesitant to use it internally.

BAY *(Laurus nobilis)*. Sacred to Apollo, the Sun God of the ancient Greeks. In Europe, bay leaves were burned to kill plague germs and protect against evils: "neither witch nor devil, thunder nor lightning will hurt a man where a bay tree is." The leaves are steeped in oil to use as an antiseptic, analgesic poultice for sprains.

BORAGE *(Borago officinalis)*. Referred to by ancient Greeks as "lingua bubula," an herb with "rough and hairie" leaves. Its virtues are many: courage, joy, merriment, exhilaration, and "making the mind glad." The ancients grew at least three varieties of borage, one with "blew floures," one with white flowers, and one that lived through the winter. As a medicinal herb, the leaves are eaten raw after an illness to clean the blood, or washed and applied to bruises and abrasions as a poultice. The leaves and flowers are steeped in wine to drive away melancholy. Flowers are made into conserves to alleviate hoarseness. Roots are dug and cleaned, steeped in a little oil, and applied to green wounds (staph or gangrenous infections).

CARDOON *(Cynara cardunculus)*. Like artichokes, cardoons are related to the thistle family. They grow freely throughout the Mediterranean. The Roman soldiers learned about their culinary value from the Jewish people.

CILANTRO *(Coriandrum sativum)*. A "very stinking herbe" that the Portuguese eat in abundance. They love the bitter taste and use it as a blood purifier, blood thinner, and natural detoxifier. It is usually ingested as a food, but a tea of fresh leaves can be taken as a diuretic.

CUCUMBER *(Cucumis sativus)*. "Good for the other parts troubled with heat." "Cowcumbers" would be eaten and applied externally for "red and shining fierie noses, as red as red roses," "pumples," and "ulcers of the bladder," or cystitis. Externally, the skin was first bathed in a decoction of white vinegar, apple cores, iris roots, camphor, almonds, and lemons, and "set in the sun for ten days." As a food, these Mediterranean melons would "unstop the liver," which indicates they were eaten for a gallstone cleanse.

Cucumbers can be applied externally for "red and shining fierie noses, as red as red roses."

DILL *(Anethum graveolens)*. Believed to strengthen the brain. The seeds are decocted to increase milk in women and "seed" in men. An oil made of seeds boiled or "sunned" increases digestion, eases pain, provokes lust, and induces sleep, preferably in that order. A vapor is made for aromatherapy by boiling dill seed in wine with wormwood branches and roses for those who found internal use of the decocted seed too stimulating, to calm colicky babies, and to stay hiccups.

DITTANY *(Origanum dictamnus)*. Known as Dittany of Crete and Dittany of Candie. Shepherds learned that goats could heal wounds by eating the leaves and tiny flowers of this wild herb. Herders would ingest and later make compresses of the leaves to heal open wounds. The strong flavor is very sharp and biting.

FENNEL *(Foeniculum dulce)*. Eaten and decocted to "fill women's breasts with milk," as well as clear the liver, kidneys, and lungs of obstructions and stones. Fish was considered safe to eat when cooked with fennel leaves. Fennel seeds were chewed to sweeten the breath and improve digestion. Seeds were used in desserts and baked goods for the dual pleasure of digestant and a delicious finale for a meal. Eating fennel was believed to strengthen the eyes.

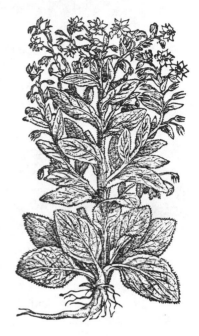

BORAGE

GARLIC *(Allium sativum)*. A remedy for all diseases and eaten often by those with strong stomachs. Cumin or fennel seeds were chewed after meals to "remove the disagreeable smell from the breath." A tea was made to break up kidney stones and to alleviate prostatitis and difficult urination. Garlic was made into an ear oil or applied, mashed, to an aching ear. Similar practices healed bronchitis by applying garlic compresses to the chest. The mashed clove was bound to the feet of those suffering from smallpox, or dipped in honey and put into the ear to relieve headaches and "comfort the brain." Garlic was not given to those suffering from depression or melancholy unless it was worn as a charm against infection, stagnant water, or "poyson," because it was considered a very hot, strong herb.

HYSSOP *(Hyssopus officinalis).* A holy herb of the Israelites that has antiseptic qualities. Mediterraneans combined it with garlic to alleviate
the croup, and mixed it with figs to expel worms and "loosen the
belly." Hyssop was used as a cleaning agent in sick rooms and hung
at entrances to prevent plague and illness.

LAVENDER *(Lavendula officinalis).* Worn under hats or entwined in the
hair to prevent headaches and tension from the intensity of the sun.
The floral water and oil was used to prevent fainting and alleviate
nervous ticks.

LEMON BALM *(Melissa officinales).* A favorite of the ancient Greeks, it was
used externally to alleviate toothaches and dress "green wounds."
Steeped in wine, it was believed to be healthy for the heart and an
antidote for melancholy. Lemon balm grew wild on the mountain-
sides, a free spirit in the first democracy.

*Rosemary
quickens the
senses and
increases
memory.*

❧

MARJORAM *(Origanum vulgare).* Grows wild on Grecian hillsides and has
a sharp, biting taste. A decoction was used to promote menses and
increase urination. The juice was combined in milk and put into the
ears to reduce pain. Combined with vinegar, marjoram helped the
spleen and diseases of the blood, and with wine, marjoram allayed
nausea, restored a normal appetite, and encouraged speech for those
who stuttered. It was strewn in houses to drive away snakes and used
as a remedy for venomous bites and stings as a local compress. In the
Mediterranean, marjoram includes the species of oregano and what
was later cultivated as sweet, knotted marjoram.

MINTS *(Mentha* species). Believed to exhilarate the mind and alleviate
nervous disorders. Compresses were applied to the forehead to alleviate headaches. It was laid upon insect stings and put into inflamed
ears mixed with honey and water. As a digestive aid, mints were
taken with milk to keep it from curdling in the stomach.

PARSLEY *(Petroselinum hortense).* Used as a diuretic. The seeds were used
to dissolve stones, bring on menses, deliver an afterbirth, and alleviate dropsy. As a poultice, the seeds were pounded and applied to old
sores and to the stomach for colic. A good amount of leaves were
stewed with mutton to make it more digestible.

POPPY *(Papaver somniferum).* Used as an analgesic for pain, gout, and as
a sleeping aid. The heads and leaves were boiled in water with a little
sugar or sweetening agent to make a syrup. An oil was made and put
into the hollow of a tooth for pain. A floral water was drunk for
pleurisy or a compress made to apply to the chest to aid breathing.

ROSEMARY *(Rosmarinus officinalis)*. The remedy for quickening the senses and increasing memory. The leaves and branches were burned in houses to clean the air. Rosemary tea was a remedy for gallstones and jaundice and was often cooked with meats to make them more digestible. Rosemary leaves were used in preserving meats as an antioxidant preservative. The flower water was sprinkled on the head "to cool the brain" and relieve headaches.

ROSES *(Rosa* species). A symbol of heavenly perfection and earthly passion. The flower represented time and eternity, life, death and the afterlife, fertility and virginity. The rose garden is a symbol of Paradise, the place of the mystic marriage and the union of opposites. The essential oil was first distilled by the Arabs. Mediterraneans use roses as a food, an essence for aromatherapy, and a medicine for building the blood. The buds were applied locally or cooked with honey to arrest bleeding. The ends of the petals were made into a water for weak eyes. A conserve of roses was eaten to strengthen the heart. Red roses were generally used for medicinal purposes.

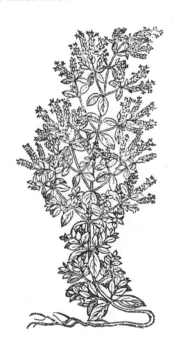

SAGE *(Salvia officinalis)*. Growing in the garden was a sign of prosperity. The leaves were made into a tea to stop premature labor and used later to stop the flow of milk when it was time to wean the baby. Added to wine, sage was a blood tonic that also stopped the spitting of blood and stitching pains in the side. Mediterraneans cooked their beans with sage as a digestant. A decoction made of sage leaves steeped in red wine or dark ale was applied to the hair as a darkening agent. The Mediterraneans were more interested in looking good during social festivities than in long-term cures or preventative remedies. Most of their tonics were about clearing heat from the blood. If that did not work, they were likely to lose interest and just drink some good wine.

MARJORAM

SORREL *(Rumex acetosa)*. One of the five bitter herbs of Passover. It is still eaten by the world's Jews in remembrance of the bitter cup Life sometimes serves us. Sorrel is incorporated into a wonderful soup, Shav, made with the Jewish contribution to health, chicken broth. Bitter herbs, especially greens, are tonic and detoxifying to the liver, clearing heat from the blood and promoting proper digestion.

THYME *(Thymus serpyllus* and *Thymus vulgaris)*. An antiseptic herb used by Mediterraneans to bring out a sweat, reducing fevers, flu, and viral invasion. It was especially useful in melancholic, splenic diseases recognized today as chronic fatigue syndrome. Thyme was used as a remedy for whooping cough and generally applied as a poultice for any lung complaint. Mediterraneans were unlikely to run out of garlic and thyme for health and cooking. A combination of the two herbs was thought to be strong and odorous enough to combat any disease.

VIOLETS *(Viola odorata)*. Birthed from the blood of the god Attis, violets became a symbol of modesty and virtue in Christianity. Violets best describe the Mediterranean people's hidden virtues. Although their hospitality and love of festivity is what is displayed to the public, they remain humble to their values and Creator.

Mediterranean Flavors

*M*editerranean people love to eat. A sunny climate encourages many social outings where food is served. The Greeks invented the sack lunch to share during the open air amphitheater. Olive oil predominates the taste of vegetable, grain, and fish entrées. Fresh herbs and spices flavor every meal, combined to promote digestion and robust health.

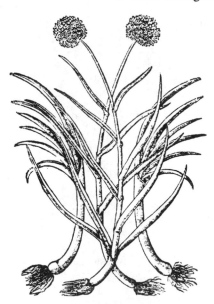

LEEKS

The Mediterraneans and their food have been influenced by every culture through trade or conquest. The area includes geographical, climatic, social, and national contrasts. It includes both the birthplace of civilization and the battleground of the philosophies and religions dominant in modern thinking.

Many of the peoples inhabiting the Mediterranean coast are a mix of races, nationalities, and religions. Yet they are linked by culinary preferences. The Oriental area and Arab natives inhabit Syria, Lebanon, Egypt, Iran, Turkey, Iraq, Saudi Arabia, Yemen, and Sudan. Greece is related through the Ottoman rule. The North African countries of Tunisia, Algeria, and Morocco are related through

Phoenician and Arab traders, who also inhabited Sicily. The Muslim Moors of North Africa occupied Spain for over seven hundred years. They introduced Eastern spices, new foods, and advanced irrigation techniques that the Spanish Conquistadors brought to the New Worlds in North and South America. Israel is a land of a thousand flavors brought from immigrating Jews from all over the world. Italy is a land of loosely united kingdoms with intense regional pride. Everyone believes their culinary heritage is the best.

The origins of Mediterranean dishes are inherent in the peasantry and indigenous people of each land who lived through the triumphs and sorrows of past wars, famines, and celebrations. They continue to respond to life passionately, welcoming all of us to join in the dance of milk and honey.

Everything

is good in

its season.

—Italian proverb

~

Harmony through Opposites

Ancient and modern Oriental and Far Eastern cuisine blend opposite flavors, textures, and colors to create harmony. Sweet and sour dishes reflect the ancient belief of balancing the two opposing forces governing creation. It is through alchemy that these opposites blend into a new dimension of flavor. Like flowering plants, opposing tastes bloom through stress to express a higher form of creation.

❧ *Sweet and Sour Leeks* ❧

This sweet and sour sauce can be enjoyed on any vegetable. The Mediterraneans love to blend it with a strong-tasting vegetable.

- 2 pounds leeks
- 4 tablespoons safflower or walnut oil
- 3 crushed garlic cloves
- 1 tablespoon plus 1 teaspoon sugar
  juice of 2 lemons
- 1 tablespoon lemon zest

Wash and trim leeks, taking off older leaves and leaving the bulb and inner leaves. Cut lengthwise. Heat oil until it sizzles. Add garlic and 1 tablespoon of sugar. Cook until the sugar begins to caramelize, then add the leeks, coating all sides with oil. Squeeze out the juice of 2 lemons onto the leeks. Cover and cook over low heat 10 minutes. Sprinkle with lemon zest mixed with 1 teaspoon of sugar before serving.

The Grand Saffron Festival

Saffron is an ancient herb of Middle Eastern civilization. It has colored the robes of royalty and flavored the cuisine of every civilization of antiquity.

In Consuegra, central Spain, there is an annual contest for the honor of being chosen the Saffron Queen. She must prove her talent for picking the most stamens from fields of purple saffron blooms.

Spain has been the greatest source of saffron for centuries, although it originated in the Middle East. Saffron is partial to sunshine and known as the herb of cheerfulness. Ancients dyed their sheets with saffron to improve lovemaking and fertility.

The crocus can be grown in many locations in North America, set in the fall or spring in moist, rich soil. The corolla spike beautiful purple and red flowers every fall. They make a striking border or mass planting in a rock garden. Plant them in well-drained soil to enjoy sun or light shade. Separate them by six inches. Plant three to four inches deep and divide in the summer.

∾ *Saffron Rice* ∾

The Spaniards serve saffron rice with stewed chicken, vegetables, and the following almond sauce.

- 4　tablespoons sesame oil
- 2　cups rice, uncooked
- ½　teaspoon powdered saffron

Heat oil and add uncooked rice. Allow it to coat and cook for a few minutes. Shake in saffron. Slowly add 4 cups of water, bring to a boil and reduce heat. Simmer, covered, for 20 minutes or until small holes appear on the surface. Do not stir while cooking. Remove from heat and let stand uncovered for 10 minutes before serving. Serves 6.

∾ *Almond Sauce* ∾

Almonds are enjoyed as a meat substitute.

- ½　cup ground almonds
- 2　cups chicken or vegetable stock
- 1　crushed garlic clove
- ½　teaspoon sugar
   juice of 1 lemon or lime
- 2　tablespoons fresh, chopped parsley

Bring almonds in chicken or vegetable stock to a boil. Add garlic, sugar, lemon or lime juice, and parsley. Reduce heat and simmer 5–20 minutes until the sauce thickens. Serves 6 with saffron rice.

The Greek Goddess of Good Eating, Adephaghia

Greek cuisine is over twenty-five centuries old. Culinary tastes interested the Greeks before the Europeans and Turks knew much more than how to roast meat. Poets, philosophers, priests, and peasants were all enthusiastic authorities on gastronomical delights. Many of their original written work was lost in seventh century A.D. during a fire that destroyed the Library of Alexandria.

Professional cooks appeared during the time of Alexander the Great and made cooking an art. The first culinary schools were established in Athens to teach the art of cooking to free men whose reputations were held in high esteem. The student would be schooled for two years before achieving recognition as a chef. Chefs were held in such high esteem that they were often referred to as wise men. Aghis of Rhodes was the first chef recorded. He was known for flavoring fish with aromatic herbs.

The Roman conquest of Greece led to radical changes in their cuisine. Every known Greek cook and apprentice slave was brought to Rome to flavor the elaborate, exotic, imported foods from every conquered country. The Greek cooks not only taught the Romans how to cook, but also invented utensils so they did not have to eat with their hands.

During the next few centuries, Italian city-states ruled by wealthy merchants conquered the entire Greek empire. They learned from their Grecian ancestors that love and good food are synonymous. As previous conquerors of Sicily, the Greeks had proclaimed the love of good food and festivity by dedicating a temple to the Greek goddess of good eating and merriment, Adephaghia. Now a part of Italy, Adephaghia still stands to honor the Greek culinary proverb, "cook and taste often."

> *Cook and taste often.*
>
> —Greek proverb

❧ *Garlic Sauce: A Greek Pesto* ❧

Here is a versatile sauce created to enhance vegetables, salads, and meats. Use the variations to change the flavor and create a new dish. The breadcrumbs will absorb the acidity of the vinegar, leaving only the aromatic flavor of the herbs.

- 4 garlic cloves
- 3 tablespoons white wine vinegar
- 1 cup soft bread crumbs
- ½ cup water
- 5 tablespoons extra virgin, cold pressed olive oil

Combine and blend until smooth.

Variations: Add ½ cup almonds, piñon nuts or walnuts; 1 teaspoon thyme, lemon thyme and ½ teaspoon rosemary; 1 teaspoon Greek oregano; or 1 teaspoon vegetable no-salt herbal blend (page 287).

ᕉ *Rigani Dressing* ᕇ

In May, the mountains of Greece are dotted with flowering wild marjoram *(Origanum dictamnus)*. The Greeks harvest the herb to flavor meat dishes. Mediterranean marjoram is much sharper in flavor than domestic marjorams or oreganos. It is marketed in other countries as "Spanish hops" because it was used to brew a fine ale. Here is a salad dressing to enjoy with fresh greens.

    ½ cup extra virgin cold pressed olive oil
       juice of 1 large lemon*
    ½ teaspoon rigani (wild marjoram), or dried oregano as a substitute
    1 teaspoon fresh mint, finely minced
    1 tablespoon chopped onion or garlic chives
    1 tablespoon cilantro or parsley
    1 teaspoon fresh cinnamon basil, finely minced
    ½ teaspoon lemon thyme

Combine, bottle and refrigerate for a few hours before serving on a dinner salad. Serves 4.

*To extract the juice, pour a cup of boiling water over the lemon and allow to cool a few minutes before squeezing it.

Arabic Herbal Remedies: "Toward the One"

The intent of the Arabic herbalist is to avoid disease and avert illness; as written in the Rig Veda, "Where the herbs are gathered together like kings in an assembly, there the doctor is called a Sage, who destroys evil and averts disease." The following herbs have their Arabic names in parentheses.

ANISE SEED *(anisun)*. Simmer 1 teaspoon of crushed seeds in 1 cup of water for 10 minutes. Strain and drink as the tea cools. This tea made of crushed anise seeds is used for the following conditions: promote milk flow, increase menstrual flow, soothe intestinal colic, promote digestion, strengthen eyesight, increase male potency.

APPLES *(tuffah)*. Sour apples and their seeds are eaten to strengthen the heart.

BARLEY *(sha'ir)*. Soak 1 tablespoon of barley in 1 cup of water for 30 minutes. Strain and drink the juice to alleviate a sore throat. Cook the remaining grain and ingest to reduce fever.

BASIL *(rayhan)*. The aroma of basil is used to increase intelligence and strengthen the heart. Basil soaked in water is sprinkled on the head and forehead to promote peaceful sleep.

BUTTER *(zubdah)*. Butter is mixed with dates and honey to abate food cravings of pregnant and menstruating women. Combine 1 tablespoon of unsalted butter with 2 tablespoons of honey and 2 tablespoons of chopped dates.

CARROTS *(jazar)*. The root and tops are eaten cooked to promote sexuality and to increase urination and menstrual flow for women.

CHAMOMILE *(babunaj)*. Chamomile tea is the first drink given to babies no longer nursing. For women, the tea is given to promote menstruation and increase urine flow. Steep 1 teaspoon of flowers in 1 cup of water for 5 minutes. Strain and drink sweetened with honey.

COCONUT *(narjil darjai)*. Coconut meat and juice were used to increase fertility.

COFFEE BEAN *(qahwah)*. Drink an infusion of freshly crushed coffee beans to alleviate dysentery and small amounts to increase intelligence.

CORIANDER *(habb al suda)*. The seeds are crushed and made into a tea to alleviate colds and fevers and to increase venous circulation. Coriander oil was rubbed on the scalp to promote hair growth and heal scalp conditions. The seeds were also burned to repel insects. Coriander is believed to cure every disease but aging. To make coriander tea, simmer 1 teaspoon of crushed seeds in 1 cup of water for 10 minutes before straining. To make coriander oil, slowly simmer 1 tablespoon of crushed seeds in 1 cup of oil for 5 minutes. Steep until cooled; strain and bottle before refrigerating. Apply warm.

CINNAMON *(darchini)*. Cinnamon is used as a culinary spice to improve digestion and circulation.

CITRON *(utrujj)*. Citron is eaten after meals as an after-dinner digestant and to promote a feeling of satisfaction after eating. It is believed to lift depression and is rubbed on the skin to remove freckles.

CUMIN *(kammun)*. Soak cumin seeds in boiled water and drink the tea to alleviate indigestion and flatulence. Soak 1½ teaspoons of crushed seeds in 1 cup of boiled water for 10 minutes before straining and drinking.

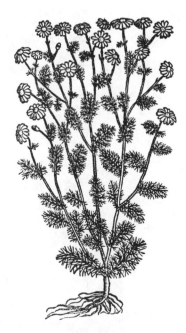

CHAMOMILE

FENUGREEK *(hulbah)*. Fenugreek is believed to strengthen the heart, reduce excess mucous, and increase male potency. The seeds and sprouts are eaten as food.

GARLIC *(thawm)*. Garlic is cooked with vegetables to expel afterbirth and warm those suffering from cold.

GHEE *(samn)*. Ghee (clarified butter) is mixed with honey to antidote toxins.

GINGER *(zanjabil)*. Ginger is cooked with foods to increase digestion and circulation and improve sexuality.

HONEY *('asal)*. Honey was diluted in warm water and drunk on an empty stomach every morning by the prophet Mohammed. Small amounts of honey may be eaten daily to abate the onset of disease.

There is no healing but Yours.

—Mohammed

MARJORAM *(marzanjush)*. Marjoram is especially eaten by those who have sinusitis and have lost the ability to smell.

MINT *(na'na')*. Mint leaves are steeped in milk to prevent curdling. The leaves are chewed to alleviate hiccups. Mint tea is drunk to promote digestion. Lemon balm tea is drunk to make the heart merry.

OLIVE OIL *(zaytun)*. Cooking with olive oil is believed to delay aging. The leaves are chewed and applied to inflamed skin and hives.

ONION *(basal)*. Cooked onions are used to reduce mucous. Eat them or wear them as a compress.

PARSLEY *(karafs)*. Parsley is eaten to correct bad breath and increase sexuality.

POMEGRANATE *(rumman)*. The fresh juice is used as a cough suppressant.

SAFFRON *(za 'faran)*. Saffron is cooked with grains to build blood and reduce joint pain. It is believed to increase male potency.

SALT *(milh)*. A pinch of salt before and after eating is believed to reduce bowel complaints.

SENNA *(sana)*. Senna tea is used as a purgative. The leaves are steeped with raisins and violets to produce peristalsis.

SPINACH *(asfanakh)*. Spinach is cooked with yogurt to cleanse the bowel.

THYME *(sa 'tar)*. Thyme is cooked with meats to increase digestion and is drunk as an infusion to remove tapeworms.

VINEGAR *(khall)*. Vinegar is combined with equal amounts of rose water and is drunk to relieve headaches. It was also applied as a compress remedy for toothaches.

Arabic Cuisine

The Arabic people utilize simple foods to correct imbalances that create diseases of the mind and body. Their meals balance the temperament of the four essences, or humors, of the body. They enhance digestion, assimilation, and bile and blood formation. Before each simple meal they pray to allow this food to uplift themselves and all of humanity. The following table contains the Arabic and English name of the herb and its uses in Arabic cuisine.

Herbs in Arabic Cuisine

ARABIC	ENGLISH	USES IN ARABIC CUISINE
Bagdownis	Parsley	Salads, soups, stews
Baqli	Purslane	Leaves and flowers in salads
Bhar hub wa na'im	Allspice (pimento tree berry)	Baked goods, meat pastries
Hub al hal	Cardamom	Ground in Turkish coffee
Hub et il baraky	Caraway seed	Tea to relieve colic, seeds in Syrian bread
Gunzabeel	Ginger plant and root	Used as a tonic in tea
Kamoun	Cumin seed	Add 1 teaspoon to glass of water for indigestion; added to egg dishes
Kizbara	Cilantro leaf and coriander seed	Cooked with fava beans, meats, and vegetables
Mohleb	Black cherry kernels	Ground in Syrian and Anise bread
Marda Koosh	Marjoram	Flavors soup, salad, meats
Ma war id	Rose water, orange water	Flavors, baklava syrup, pudding, pastries, cakes
Na'na	Spearmint, mint	Teas, soups, salads, lamb
Num name	Sweet basil*	Filling in lamb, rolls; pestos, salads

* The Orthodox church uses basil as an altar plant during Easter. During a pilgrimage, Constantine's mother is believed to have found basil growing under the cross where Jesus was crucified.

Continued on next page

Arabic	English	Uses in Arabic Cuisine
Simsum	Sesame seeds	Tahini oil and butter, Turkish candy
Thume	Garlic	Flavors meat and salads
Waraq al gar	Bay	Tea used as an antiseptic externally and to clean clothes; whole leaf used to flavor soups, stews, meats
Yansoon	Anise seed	Anise tea for digestion, anise bread
Za'tar	Thyme	Powdered and blended with sumac; also flavors meat, poultry

Dandelion Leaves: Hindee Mut-bookh

Dandelion greens are cooked as bitters to promote detoxification of the intestinal tract.

    1 small, minced onion
    1 minced garlic clove
    1 tablespoon cold pressed olive oil
    2 cups dandelion leaves
    1 tablespoon fresh lemon thyme, chopped
      lemon slices

Brown onion and garlic in olive oil. Add leaves and thyme and coat them with the oil. Cover and steam 5 minutes. Serve with lemon slices. Serves 4.

Sesame Garlic Dressing

Sesame and garlic stimulate metabolism and enhance digestion.

    ¼ cup sesame oil
    1 garlic clove
    2 tablespoons lemon juice
    1 tablespoon tahini (ground sesame seed)
    2 tablespoons water
    ½ teaspoon oregano
    ½ teaspoon parsley or cilantro

Blend and serve on vegetables or salads.

❧ *Qroon Cakes* ❧

These cakes, an easy version of baklava, are served during Lent.

> 3 cups flour
> ⅔ cup vegetable oil
> ½ cup sugar
> 1 teaspoon anise
> ½ cup warm water

Filling:
> 2 cups ground nuts
> 1 tablespoon orange water
> ¼ cup sugar

Syrup:
> 3 cups sugar
> 2 cups water
> 2 tablespoons strong lemon verbena tea or juice of 1 lemon
> 1 teaspoon orange blossom water or orange mint tea

Combine and knead first 5 ingredients to form a dough. Cut into small pieces and flatten to 2½ inches in the palm of your hand. Add filling and fold over edges into a crescent. Bake at 350 degrees until the bottoms begin to brown. Cool and dip into syrup, made by bringing to a boil 3 cups of sugar and 2 cups of water. Add lemon verbena tea and cook for 15 minutes. Add orange blossom water. Yields 40–50 qroons.

❧ *Turkish Coffee: Qahweh* ❧

Mohammed named this drink Qahweh, "the wine of Araby," after prohibiting the use of wine. It is cooked in brass coffee pots and served in demitasse cups. The coffee beans are first roasted until almost burned and then crushed or ground. Turkish coffee beans are commercially available in specialty stores.

> 1 teaspoon sugar
> 2 tablespoons Turkish coffee
> 2 cardamom pods

Boil 2 cups of water in a brass coffee pot. Add sugar. Sprinkle in coffee. Stir and allow to boil and become frothy. Add cardamom pods and remove from heat. When the froth subsides, return to the fire and boil again. Repeat 3 more times, removing the coffee before it can boil over. The froth can be spooned into demitasse cups before pouring the coffee.

Mediterranean Herbal Vegetarian Pleasures

Mediterraneans enjoy a variety of fresh herbs and vegetables throughout the year. They have created a sauce to complement each vegetable as a main dish and accompany it with fresh bread or pasta. Like the Mediterraneans, learn to eat light and live longer.

∾ *Artichokes: Carciofi con Basilico* ∾

Artichokes open obstructions in the kidneys and ease childbirth.

    12 small artichokes
     1 tablespoon lemon juice
     6 tablespoons cold pressed virgin olive oil
     1 crushed garlic clove
     1 cup dry white wine
    ¼ cup chopped, fresh garden basil
     1 teaspoon minced, fresh lemon thyme
        cayenne pepper to taste
    ¼ teaspoon vegetable no-salt blend, optional (page 287)

Prepare artichokes by removing any tough outer leaves and the stem. Rub the bottom with lemon juice. Snip the tips of the leaves with scissors. Slice lengthwise about ¼-inch thick and soak in 4 cups of water with lemon juice for 1 hour. Drain on paper towels. Only cook artichokes in glass or enamel to avoid discoloration. Heat olive oil in a skillet with garlic, the artichoke slices, white wine, basil, lemon thyme, and a sprinkle of cayenne pepper. Add vegetable no-salt blend, optional, for seasoning. Cover and simmer 20 minutes, uncover, and allow the liquid to reduce by half. Serve on garlic toast. Serves 6.

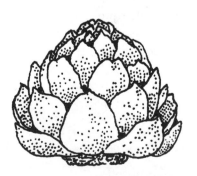

ARTICHOKE

❧ *Beets: Barbabietole con Erbe* ❧

Beets are baked in Mediterranean countries, rather than boiled.

    2   pounds beets, skinned and sliced
    ½   cup butter
    1   mashed garlic clove
    ½   cup fresh herbs, minced: marjoram, basil,
        chervil, parsley, cilantro, or mints

Bake skinned and sliced beets at 350 degrees until tender. Cook garlic in butter until the mixture turns golden and add to beets. Garnish with fresh herbs. Cook for 1 minute longer to blend flavors. Serves 6.

❧ *Asparagus: Asparagi Italiana* ❧

Italians cook white asparagus, but green will do. Asparagi is served as a main course.

    ½   cup butter or ghee
    2   tablespoons ground hazelnuts
    2   pounds asparagus
    ½   cup freshly grated romano and parmesan cheese
    ¼   cup fresh, chopped parsley, basil, and thyme or lemon thyme

Heat butter or ghee until it turns golden. Remove from heat and blend with 2 tablespoons of hazelnuts. Cook asparagus in non-aluminum pot 12–17 minutes. Drain, sprinkle herbs and cheese on top of asparagus and spoon the hazelnut butter over them. Serves 6.

❧ *Fennel Sauce: Arancia e Creama di Finoccio* ❧

Fennel has an anise flavor enhanced by the tangy taste of orange juice.

    1   pound fennel
    3   tablespoons extra virgin olive oil
    ½   cup orange juice (the juice of 1 large orange)

Remove the outer stalks of fennel and cut into 2-inch sections. Simmer in boiling water until tender. Drain well. Whip olive oil and orange juice until it makes a cream. Pour over freshly cooked fennel and garnish with the feathery fennel tops.

⚬ *Broccoli: Broccoletti e Olive* ⚬

Broccoli is often cooked in wine with garlic and, of course, olive oil.

    1 mashed garlic clove
    ½ cup virgin cold pressed olive oil
    2 pounds broccoli, cut lengthwise
    1 cup black olives, pitted and diced
    1 teaspoon lemon thyme
    ½ cup provolone cheese, grated
    2 cups red wine
    1 cup croutons

Cook the garlic in olive oil until it sizzles. In a heavy casserole, pour the oil on top of the broccoli spears. Sprinkle the olives, thyme, and cheese on top of them. Pour the wine over the casserole. Cover and cook 20 minutes over medium-low heat. Serve sprinkled with croutons. Serves 6.

⚬ *Cardoons: Cardi* ⚬

Related to thistles, cardoons are an artichoke served as an entrée. Like celery, the stalks of the inner leaves are eaten. Immediately rub them with lemon juice to prevent discoloration.

    2 bunches cardoons
    ½ cup butter or ghee
    1 tablespoon fresh parsley
    1 tablespoon mint
    1 tablespoon thyme
    2 tablespoons freshly squeezed orange juice
    ⅓ cup parmesan bread crumbs

Cook cardoons and drain. Heat butter or ghee with parsley, mint, and thyme. Add orange juice and pour on top of the cardoons. Sprinkle with parmesan bread crumbs. Serves 6.

❧ *Peas: Piselli alla Menta* ❧

Here's a chance to use some of the mint taking over your yard.

2 pounds fresh, shelled tiny peas
4 tablespoons butter or ghee
3 tablespoons freshly minced mint leaves
2 sage leaves
　pinch of sugar

Cook peas in water until tender. Timing depends on the size and maturity of the peas, about 3–5 minutes. Drain. Heat the ghee and herbs in a frying pan for 3 minutes. Add the peas and pinch of sugar. Serves 6.

❧ *Eggplant: Melanzane Napoletana* ❧

Eggplant originated in India. The Italians first imported it and began cultivating eggplant by the seventeenth century.

2 eggplants, sliced ½ inch thick, sprinkled on both sides with salt
½ cup flour
½ cup virgin cold pressed olive oil
3 cups tomato sauce
4 tablespoons fresh, chopped basil
½ pound provolone cheese, thinly sliced
　fresh thyme to taste

Drain eggplant on paper towels for 1 hour to reduce the water content. Rinse off the salt before cooking and dust with flour. Heat olive oil in a frying pan and brown each side of the slices. Arrange layers in a greased casserole, covered with tomato sauce, basil, provolone, and a sprinkle of fresh thyme. Bake at 450 degrees for 10 minutes and serve hot. Serves 6.

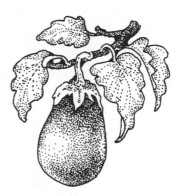

EGGPLANT

❧ *Peppers: Peperoni* ❧

Peppers are a tropical American plant. They are grown in southern Mediterranean countries with longer growing seasons. They are served as an entrée, over rice, or in casseroles.

- 4 large green, red, or yellow peperonis
- ¼ cup cold pressed extra virgin olive oil
- 1 medium sweet red onion, chopped
- 1 mashed garlic clove
- 2 tomatoes, chopped
- 2 cups bread crumbs
- 1 tablespoon basil, chopped
- 1 tablespoon parsley, chopped
- ½ cup pecorino cheese, grated*
- ¾ cup ricotta cheese*
- 1 egg
- 10 black olives, chopped

To remove the peperonis' skin, char over a flame and rinse under cold water. Core and remove seeds. Make sure the hole is large enough to stuff. Heat olive oil in a skillet. Sauté onion and garlic. Heat for 3 minutes, then add tomatoes, bread crumbs, basil, parsley, pecorino, ricotta, egg, and black olives. Blend and stuff peppers. Stand upright in a baking dish close together. Bake at 375 degrees for 1 hour, basting with juices several times. Serves 4.

*Pecorino is a sharp-tasting cheese made from sheep's milk. The cheese is popular with the Romans and Genovese. Ricotta is a fresh cheese with a smooth texture and bland taste. It is used to make lasagna and for stuffing macaroni and peppers.

❧ *String Green Beans: Fagiolini Verdi* ❧

My mom would often serve string beans as a cold summer salad.

- 1 pound string beans
  garlic to taste
- ⅓ cup wine vinegar
- ⅔ cup cold pressed extra virgin olive oil
- 1 teaspoon each fresh basil and thyme
- ½ teaspoon savory

Steam beans until tender, about 7–10 minutes, and drain. Rub a large wooden salad bowl with fresh garlic. Combine wine vinegar, olive oil, basil, thyme, and savory. Toss with the green beans. Refrigerate 3–4 hours before serving.

❧ *Zucchini: Zucchini con Erbe* ❧

A versatile vegetable, zucchini absorbs the flavor of these seasonings.

    1 pound zucchini, sliced ½-inch thick
    ½ cup flour
    ¼ teaspoon pepper
    4 tablespoons olive oil or ghee (page 183)
       dried parsley, basil, or oregano to garnish
       parmesan to taste

Wash, cut off the ends of zucchini and slice ½-inch thick. Dredge in flour and pepper mixture. Fry in olive oil or ghee. Drain, garnish with dried parsley, basil, or oregano and parmesan. Serves 4, immediately (zucchini gets soggy after cooking).

❧ *Squash Blossoms: Fiori di Zucca* ❧

Squash blossoms are eaten to reduce anxiety and balance the emotions. Male squash blossoms are stuffed and fried in early spring.

    ½   cup bread crumbs
    ¼   cup parmesan, grated
    1   tablespoon combined chopped parsley, basil, thyme
    ⅔   cup grated mozzarella
    ¼–⅓ cup olive oil, enough to hold the stuffing together
    1   pound squash blossoms, washed and dried
    ¾   cup flour
    1   egg yolk
    ⅓   cup water
    1–2 cups olive oil for frying

Combine bread crumbs, parmesan, herbs, mozzarella, and olive oil. Stuff and close each flower. Dip the stuffed blossoms in a batter of flour, egg yolk, and water that has been beaten and allowed to rest at least 20 minutes. Deep-fry in hot olive oil. Serves 6.

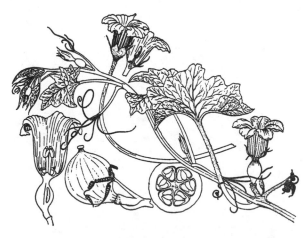

SQUASH

❧ *Tomatoes: Sughi di Pomodori* ❧

Cook a teaspoon of sugar with tomatoes to reduce the acidic content.

- 2 pounds fresh tomatoes, peeled, seeded, drained, and chopped or 2 pounds of canned Italian plum tomatoes
- 1 bay leaf
- ¼ teaspoon cayenne
- ½ teaspoon each thyme, parsley, marjoram, and oregano, fresh or dried
- 2 teaspoons fresh basil, chopped
- 2 mashed garlic cloves
- 1 teaspoon vegetable no-salt herbal blend (page 287)
- ½ cup fresh parmesan, grated

Combine in a large pot and cook 30–45 minutes over low heat. Serve on pasta. Serves 6.

❧ *Spinach: Spinaci* ❧

Spinach is cooked with olive oil and raisins to keep the bowels regular.

- 2 pounds spinach
- 1 garlic clove
- ½ cup ghee or cold pressed virgin olive oil
- 2 tablespoons pignoli or pecans
- 3 tablespoons raisins, soaked in water to cover for 1 hour and drained

Rinse spinach leaves thoroughly; cut off stems on older leaves and cook in non-aluminum cookware. Steam spinach; drain, cool and squeeze dry. Simmer garlic in olive oil or ghee for 2 minutes, then remove. Add spinach, pignoli or pecans, and soaked raisins. Cook 5 minutes. Serves 4.

∾ *Pesto Genovese* ∾

This is an excellent sauce for potatoes, rice, or pasta.

- 1 cup fresh basil leaves
- 4 spinach leaves
- 1 teaspoon fresh marjoram
- 2 teaspoons fresh parsley
- 3 garlic cloves
- ⅓ cup parmesan cheese, grated
- ⅓ cup pecorino cheese, grated
- 1 cup cold pressed extra virgin olive oil
- ½ cup pignoli or other nuts, optional

Blend to a smooth paste. Yields 1½ cups.

∾ *Mushrooms: Funghi* ∾

Mediterranean country folks gathered edible mushrooms for a variety of dishes. Store-bought will do.

- 4 tablespoons cold pressed virgin olive oil
- 3 garlic cloves, mashed
- 1 pound mushrooms, sliced*
- 3 tablespoons freshly chopped Greek oregano, or
  mixture of tarragon, marjoram, and savory
  cayenne or nutmeg to taste

Heat oil and garlic in a frying pan. Adding a few mushrooms at a time, quickly brown them and remove with slotted spoon. When all are cooked, reduce heat, add the oregano or tarragon, marjoram, and savory, and cook 1 minute before returning all the mushrooms. Cook 3 more minutes. Season with a dash of cayenne or nutmeg. Serves 4.

Variation: Substitute onion *(cipolle)* for mushrooms.

GARLIC

∾ *Beans: Fagioli* ∾

Dried beans were often served on Fridays and during the Lenten season, often with pasta (pasta fagioli).

- 1 pound dried white, black, or red beans.
   herbal bouquet of thyme, bay, cilantro, or epazote
- ½ cup cold pressed virgin olive oil
- 12 fresh sage leaves
- 3 tomatoes, chopped and seeded
- 1 teaspoon vegetable no-salt herbal blend (page 287)

Soak dried beans overnight in twice as much water. Discard any beans that float to the top of the water. Cook the beans in two quarts of water with an herbal bouquet such as thyme, bay, cilantro, or epazote for 1½–2½ hours. When the outer skins peel off easily, the beans are done. Heat olive oil and sage until the leaves sizzle. Add the beans and stir for 5 minutes, coating them well. Add tomatoes. Allow to simmer 10 more minutes, adding the vegetable no-salt herbal blend. Serves 6–8.

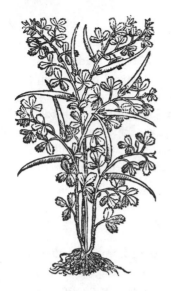

8

Ancient Healing of the Mystics

Health is self-affirming. As we maintain it, we have its reward.
We create health and through our efforts we are validated.

Ayurvedic healing is recorded in the ancient Sanskrit texts of India. It is known as the "science of life," a healing system practiced in India for over five thousand years. The teachings are recorded in the world's oldest literature, the Vedas. Ayurveda is the healing gift of the ancient sages of Vedic culture (originated by 5000 B.C.) and culminated in the age of Krishna (about 1500 B.C.). Ayurvedic practices have been incorporated by Tibetan, Chinese, and southeast Asian Buddhist cultures. The Greeks and later European cultures also referred to the Vedas. Today, Ayurveda is part of a newly emerging global culture revolutionizing the concept of healing. The nature of Ayurvedic medicine is an integration of the mind, body, and soul. Ayurveda relates to Shakti, the divine nurturing principle in Mother Nature's bounty.

Healing begins with self-awareness and ends with a union with the beloved soul. As we recognize oneness, we can expand into cosmic consciousness (the Tao in Chinese philosophy, and the Brahman in the Vedic cultures).

Eastern health practices are subjective, derived from observation and insight by rishis, ancient seers and spiritual leaders. The system of

Ayurvedic medicine is an integration of the mind, body, and soul.

~

Ayurvedic medicine is individualized, whereas Western medicine is objective, based on analysis and deduction from the general population. The only norm in Eastern medicine is creative growth encouraged by self-healing. Each individual is taught to achieve longevity through balancing the physical, emotional, and mental processes, achieving self-harmony. One not only recovers, but also achieves self-realization and liberation from attitudes that hold back our greatest achievements. In Eastern terminology, we unfold like the thousand petals of the lotus flower.

An East Indian Herbal

Herbs and spices are at the heart of East Indian home remedies. Various blends are used in seasonings and teas to encourage, balance, and harmonize us. Mental, emotional, and physical well-being are balanced through proper diet, exercise, and lifestyle habits. The addition of appropriate herbs and spices is determined by the individual needs of each personality.

ANISE SEED *(Pimpinella anisum)* is roasted and chewed after meals as a digestant. Roast one cup in an ungreased pan for 30 minutes at 300 degrees.

ASAFOETIDA *(Ferula),* "hingu" in ancient Sanskrit texts, is a hot, pungent gum extract from the tree root of the ferula asafoetida used to relieve spasms, rheumatic pain, and earaches. More pungent than garlic, asafoetida is also high in sulfur-bearing amino acids that promote digestion and may be used as a parasiticide. As a digestant, add a pinch to a pot of beans as they cook. For spasms or rheumatism, make a paste with ¼ teaspoon asafoetida to 1 tablespoon water, honey, or ghee, and apply externally to unbroken skin. For earaches, saturate a cotton ball with ⅛ teaspoon asafoetida in 1 teaspoon olive oil. Place loosely in the affected ear. It is not recommended for inflammatory disease.

AJOWAN *(Trachyspermum copticum)* is a relative of caraway native to southern India. It tastes like thyme and has similar antiseptic properties. The seeds are eaten to relieve indigestion or crushed and cooked in a tea for colic, bowel complaints, or chronic asthma. Crush 1 teaspoon of ajowan seeds and simmer in 1 cup of water for 3 minutes. Strain, add honey, and sip to relieve digestive disorders or asthmatic complaints.

CARDAMOM *(Elettaria cardamomum)*, "ela" in Sanskrit, is an ancient East Indian breath freshener and digestant. Bedouins added the seeds to a strong brew of coffee to detoxify the caffeine. Cooked in milk, the East Indians believe the refreshing taste stimulates joy in the heart. Cardamom is often baked with fruit.

CLOVES *(Caryophyllus aromaticum)*, "lavanga," are native to the Indonesian Spice Islands. Cloves are best known for their analgesic properties. Saturate a cotton ball with clove oil and apply to a toothache, enlarged lymph node, or earache. Inhale clove oil as a decongestant to clear the lungs. Cook clove buds as a tea or in milk as a warming digestant.

CUMIN *(Cuminum cyminum)*, "jeera," is a stimulating digestant and anti-spasmodic. It is used as a digestant for those who bloat after eating. It is powdered and roasted and added to soups, stews, and pulses (beans and peas). It is not recommended for inflammatory conditions.

EAST INDIAN DILL SEED *(Anethum)*, "sowa," is made into a tea to improve digestion and increase breast milk. Steep ½ teaspoon of crushed seeds in 1 cup of water for 5 minutes. Strain and add honey.

FENUGREEK *(Trigonella foenum-graecum)*, "menthi," is a home remedy for diabetes, impotence, congestion, hair growth, and increasing breast milk. The seeds are soaked overnight in water and the liquid is drunk as a remedy. The seeds may then be sprouted for salads and stir-fries.

GOTU KOLA *(Hydrocotyle asiatica)*, "brahmi," is one of the famous Ayurvedic rejuvenating tonic herbs for nerves and brain tissue. A cup of gotu kola tea is drunk before meditation as gotu kola has mildly narcotic properties that quiet and soothe the nerves. It is believed to increase memory and intelligence, reducing the effects of aging. As a blood cleanser, gotu kola is used for chronic skin diseases as a tea or salve. It especially aids red and itching skin. As a liver tonic, gotu kola clears heat and harmonizes organ function, similar to Chinese bupleurum and American goldenseal. Gotu kola bolts easily from seed and may be grown in the shade and as a container plant.

ANISE

GALANGAL *(Alpinia galanga)* is a member of the ginger family with bright green sword-like leaves and white flowers with pink veins. The rhizome is used medicinally for upper respiratory congestion and indigestion. Galangal may be purchased at Oriental grocery stores. It is used extensively in Thai and southeast Asian cuisine in curries and stir fries for its spicy/sour taste. The rhizome can be grown like ginger, using containers and greenhouses during the winter. Galangal respiratory tonic and digestant is made by grating 1 teaspoon of galangal and combining with the juice of 1 fresh lime and ½ cup of boiled water. Steep for 5 minutes and strain before drinking.

Ginger is known in India as "vishwabhesaj," a universal medicine.

∼

GINGER *(Zingiber officinale)* is known in India as "vishwabhesaj," a universal medicine. Fresh ginger juice is added to the powdered root to make a thick jam and rolled into pills. It is taken with honey to relieve congestive illness, with rock candy to relieve inflammatory and febrile disease, and with rock salt to relieve flatulence, arthritis, and constipation. The energy of ginger is warm and dispersing. It is used as a diaphoretic to drive out colds, flu, and nausea. It is also helpful in reducing hypertension. Ginger tea is made by simmering 1 teaspoon of grated fresh ginger or ¼ teaspoon of dried ginger in 1 cup of water for 10 minutes. Strain and add a few drops of honey to relieve nausea at the onset of a cold or virus. It is not recommended for inflammatory diseases. Although ginger has been helpful in healing gastric ulcers, it can also encourage ulcers and inflammatory "non-ulcerous" disease. It can be used cautiously in a diluted form with honey and discontinued if any burning or discomfort occurs.

GARLIC *(Allium sativum)*, "rashona," is a tonic for digestive, respiratory, reproductive, and circulatory systems. In Sanskrit, rashona means "lacking one taste" (garlic only lacks the sour taste). The root is hot and pungent, high in sulphur-bearing amino acids for detoxification. The stem is astringent, facilitating digestion. Garlic leaves are bitter, pulling toxins out of the reproductive system. The seed is sweet, which is nutritive. Research has been on the raw clove. Two or three raw cloves eaten daily had these effects: garlic thins the blood, promotes circulation, and cleanses fungus and some bacteria from the skin and intestines. It expels mucus from the lungs and can reduce blood pressure for some hypertensives. Garlic is a hot, stimulating herb that is not recommended for those with inflammatory conditions, fevers, and thin blood.

HONEY is used by East Indians in tonics and medical preparations as a carrier. Honey moves the nutritional and medicinal properties of an herbal combination to bodily fluids and tissues for assimilation. Externally, honey is used as an antiseptic to heal wounds.

JASMINE FLOWERS *(Jasminum grandiflorum),* "jati," are used to increase love and compassion. They are a cooling blood purifier and excellent female tonic to prevent breast cancer and eradicate uterine bleeding. They have also been used by yogis to alleviate lymphatic congestion and lymphatic cancer. Combined with sandalwood, jasmine flowers reduce fever and increase mental clarity. Jasmine flowers can be added to any tea or soaked in 1 cup of water overnight to drink as a flower water tonic. Since jasmine essential oil is rare and expensive, jasmine flowers can be simmered in oil or ghee to reduce fever and enlarged lymph nodes. Homemade jasmine oil is made by soaking 12 flowers with each ounce of heated ghee or sesame oil until cool. One tablespoon of gotu kola leaves and sandalwood chips may be added for further soothing properties. Strain and apply the oil locally to lumps, cysts, or on each side of the temples.

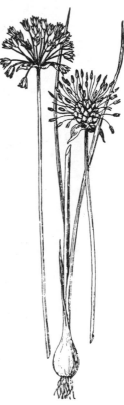

GARLIC

LEMON GRASS *(Cymbopogon citratus)* as a tea is a digestant that reduces fever. The essential oil is used for commercial flavoring and citronella insect repellent. Lemon grass tea is made by steeping 1 tablespoon of leaves or 1 teaspoon of the bulb in boiled water for 10 minutes. Strain and drink warm as a digestant or cold to reduce fever.

LOTUS SEED *(Nelumbium nuciferae),* "padma," is India's sacred herb. The seeds open the heart and calm the mind and spirit to improve speech and communication skills. They can be added to rice dishes as a nutritive herb or cooked in a tea to quiet restlessness and unsettling dreams. A tea is made by simmering 6 lotus seeds in 1 cup of water for 20 minutes. Strain and drink or add to heated milk. Lotus seed tea combines well with chamomile and skullcap tea. Lotus root is a nutritive, starchy herb cooked in milk for chronic or debilitating conditions. It is used for hemorrhoids and diarrhea as an astringent demulcent. The root or powdered root may be added to soups, stews, or rice dishes. Lotus root tonic is made by simmering 2 tablespoons of lotus root powder in 1 cup of milk or soymilk for 10 minutes, stirring to prevent sticking. Flavor with cinnamon, spices, and honey to taste, and enjoy.

NEEM *(Azadiracta indica)*, "nimba," is a cooling blood purifier used topically for inflammatory skin diseases. An infusion of the bark and leaves is made into a medicated oil or ghee. Steep 1 tablespoon of ground neem in 3 ounces of heated coconut oil or ghee for 15 minutes. Apply to ringworm, eczema, or hives. Neem is a powerful insecticide effective for over 160 pests. In India, a tea has been used to treat malaria during intermittent spells of fever.

NUTGRASS *(Cyperus rotundas)*, "musta," is a common weed used to alleviate menstrual disorders and irregularity. It is not recommended if constipation simultaneously occurs. To make a tea, steep 1 teaspoon of dried and powdered nutgrass in half a cup of boiled water for 10 minutes before drinking. It may be repeated 1 or 2 times daily until menstrual pain abates. Then, discontinue.

PEPPER *(Piper longum)*, "pipali," is related to black pepper. It is prepared in milk to relieve bronchial congestion and asthma. Pepper is used as an appetite metabolic stimulant, analgesic for back pain, and an aphrodisiac. It has a very powerful taste. Pipali is combined with freshly ground black pepper and dry ginger powder to make a famous Indian digestant called trikatu (page 183).

SAFFRON *(Crocus sativus)*, "nagakeeshara," is used as a tonic to increase circulation, tone the female reproductive organs, and reduce cystitis. Simmer a pinch of saffron in milk, ghee, or with an herbal combination to improve potency. Safflower is often used as a less expensive substitute.

SALT is a bitter antiseptic used externally to cleanse and relieve swelling. It can be heated in a dry pan and applied locally to painful areas by wrapping it in a clean cloth. As an addition to food, take a pinch of salt before meals to stimulate digestion and promote proper assimilation. To make a salt pack for pain, heat 1 pound of salt in a dry frying pan for 10 minutes, stirring to heat evenly. Pour into a clean towel or cloth and apply locally to a painful or swollen area.

SANDALWOOD *(Santalum album)*, "chandana," cools the body, mind, and emotions, relieving fever, thirst, and pain associated with inflammation. It can be applied externally to infected sores or ulcers, or used as an essential oil to open the heart. A homemade sandalwood oil is made by simmering 8 tablespoons of sandalwood powder in 2 cups of sesame oil or ghee for 15 minutes. Do not boil. Apply warm. Sandalwood powder may be added to an herbal tea as a remedy for acute and inflammatory conditions. The East Indians use it externally on the feet more often than internally.

SESAME *(Sesamum indicum)*, "tila," is fifty percent oil, similar to olive oil. It is a healthy oil because it withstands heat without turning rancid. The East Indians use it to reduce nervous conditions and build strong bones, gums, teeth, and platelets. They believe the black seeds are best. The oil can be heated with any combination of herbs to prepare a medicated oil that can also open and purify the heart (see jasmine, page 179).

SUMAC *(Rhus coriaria)* is an astringent red berry that is dried and added to lentils and yogurt for a sour, fruity taste. Cooked in a tea, it is used to alleviate bloating and stomachaches caused by indigestion and too much food. The tea is made by cooking 5 dried berries or ½ teaspoon of powder in 1 cup of water for 10 minutes. Strain and sip.

TAMARIND *(Tamarindus indica)* is the seed pod of a flowering legume. It is known as the East Indian date. The slightly narcotic effect sedates the bowels in a traditional treatment for dysentery in India. The sour taste sedates and cleanses the liver. Tamarind is added in small amounts to Asian fish and poultry entrées for its rich source of vitamins and trace minerals. For some, tamarind works as a laxative.

TURMERIC *(Curcumae longa)*, "haridra," is a natural antibiotic that can also be used to strengthen ligaments and muscles. In India, it is associated with prosperity. In a milk-based drink, turmeric improves digestion, increases intestinal flora, and purifies the blood. It is not recommended during pregnancy or for those with inflammatory diseases.

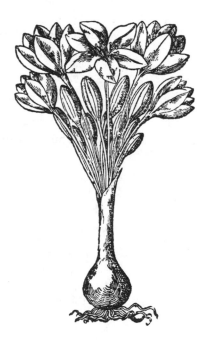

SAFFRON

Traditional Ayurvedic Remedies

My study with an Ayurvedic Brahman encouraged healing the body with many different topical applications. The following recipes help promote health through stress relief.

～ *Brahmi Oil* ～

Brahmi oil is considered the most healing tonic for the skin and nervous system. Apply to relieve stress and anxiety. This also promotes a deep sleep. East Indians also apply brahmi oil to the feet and abdomen to sedate and nurture nervous or hyperactive individuals.

2–3 tablespoons dried gotu kola leaves
1 quart sesame oil

Simmer dried gotu kola leaves in sesame oil for at least 10 minutes. Strain. Apply warmed to the feet or locally to any body part, and relax.

～ *Insomnia Tea* ～

This tea will reduce stress, promote mental clarity, and provide a good night's sleep.

1 tablespoon gotu kola, fresh or dried
1 tablespoon milk, cooked (optional)

Steep gotu kola in 1 cup of boiled water for 20 minutes. Strain and add cooked milk if desired.

～ *Healing Touch Skin Cream* ～

This can be used to soothe eczema, chronic skin conditions, and varicose veins.

1 tablespoon gotu kola leaves, fresh or dried
4 ounces coconut oil, ghee (page 183), or sesame oil, warmed

Steep gotu kola in warm coconut oil, ghee, or sesame oil for 30 minutes. Strain and apply locally 2–3 times daily to alleviate itching and rashes.

☙ *Fever Buster Tea* ❧

Drink this tea or use it as a compress to produce sweat and reduce fever.

- 1 cup gotu kola tea (see recipe for insomnia tea, page 182)
- ⅛ teaspoon black pepper
- 1 teaspoon basil, fresh

Steep gotu kola tea, prepared as above, with black pepper and fresh basil.

☙ *Ginger Soak* ❧

For aches and pains, this is a stimulating, dispersing, and circulating soak. It is a great way to warm up in the winter too!

2–3 tablespoons fresh ginger, grated

Cook grated ginger in 4 cups of water for 10 minutes. Add water and ginger root to your bath or footbath. Relax in warm water for 30 minutes.

☙ *Ghee* ❧

Ghee is eaten as a nerve and brain tonic and also builds strong bones.

- 1 pound unsalted butter
- 1 tablespoon fresh or dried gotu kola, licorice root, basil, ginger, or sandalwood chips, optional

Melt butter over low heat. Add herbs when melted, optional. Bottle and refrigerate overnight in a glass or plastic container with a wide mouth. As the mixture solidifies, scrape off the white milk fat on the top and discard. Eat the yellow ghee and discard any white milk fat that settles at the bottom.

☙ *Trikatu* ❧

A digestant and metabolic stimulant.

- 1 teaspoon long pepper
- 1 teaspoon black peppercorns
- 1 teaspoon dried ginger
- 1 teaspoon fresh ginger juice
- 1 teaspoon honey

Grind equal parts of long pepper, black peppercorns, and dried ginger into a powder. Mix well and add fresh ginger juice to form a paste. Roll in honey and form pills, placing on waxed paper to set. Makes 12 pills. Take 1 before meals. **Note:** Pepper and dried ginger are not recommended for inflammatory conditions.

∾ *Pipali (Pepper) Tonic* ∾

A bronchial congestion tonic.

- 3 peppercorns
- 1 cup milk
- ½ teaspoon honey

Simmer peppercorns in milk for 10 minutes. Strain, add honey, and sip.

∾ *Pipali (Pepper) Plaster* ∾

For sciatica, arthritis, and back pain.

- 10 peppercorns
- 2 cups sesame oil or ghee (page 183)

Simmer peppercorns in sesame oil or ghee for 15 minutes. Strain and apply locally, warm. Avoid broken skin.

∾ *Turmeric Tonic* ∾

Haridra (turmeric) stimulates digestion, increases menstrual flow, and dissolves gallstones.

- ¼ teaspoon turmeric
- 1 cup milk
  honey to taste

Simmer turmeric in milk for 5 minutes. Honey may be added to temper the warmth.

∾ *Turmeric Ghee* ∾

For sprains and bruises.

- ½ teaspoon turmeric
- ½ cup ghee (page 183)

Simmer turmeric in ghee for 5 minutes. Allow it to steep 10 more minutes before applying locally.

Traditional Ayurvedic Recipes

*S*ince East Indian cuisine evolved from a combination of several races, religions, and climates, there are an infinite variety of roasted and ground spices, roots, and berries that make East Indian cuisine unique. In India, cooks take pride in homemade, authentic dishes. Chutney is spicy and adds flavor to vegetarian menus. The spicy, hot chutney takes the place of a meat in the energy it releases without taxing the digestive system like a heavy meat. A yogurt dish with two vegetables is added to a main lentil and grain dish. The spices selected are seasonal, like cinnamon in the winter and tamarind in the summer. Fresh, whole spices are roasted and ground in a mortar or electric coffee grinder to be served on rice and vegetable dishes. The following are a few homemade spice mixtures you can make and store for up to three months in a tin. **Note:** Traditional East Indian recipes are too spicy for those who have inflammatory intestinal history.

The intelligence of pure feeling is contained in the expressions of Nature.

—The Rig Veda

 Sambhar Masala

From Southern India, sambhar masala is used to flavor lentil and bean dishes and is a sauce for stewed vegetarian dishes.

- 1½ teaspoons cumin seeds
- 1½ teaspoons whole black peppercorns
- 1½ teaspoons fenugreek seeds
- 4 tablespoons coriander seeds
- 12 whole dried red chilies
- 1½ teaspoons whole split beans
- 1½ teaspoons yellow mung beans
- 1½ teaspoons yellow split peas

In a heavy frying pan, dry-roast the cumin seeds, whole black peppercorns, fenugreek seeds (in East Indian or health food stores), coriander seeds, and red chilies, stirring constantly for five minutes. Remove from heat and cool while you dry-roast the whole split beans (urad dal), yellow mung beans (moong dal), and yellow split peas (channa dal) for 10 minutes. Allow all ingredients to thoroughly cool, then grind in an electric coffee grinder. Store in an airtight tin for up to three months.

❧ *Garam Masala* ❧

There are many varieties of garam masala, this one from Northern India. Add sparingly to pilafs, meat, and poultry dishes.

- 1 tablespoon green cardamom seed pods
- 1 (3-inch) stick of cinnamon
- ½ tablespoon whole cloves
- 1 teaspoon black peppercorns
- 2 tablespoons cumin seeds
- 2 tablespoons coriander seeds

In a heavy frying pan, dry-roast all of the above ingredients until brown, shaking and stirring to avoid burning. Cool thoroughly; grind and store in an airtight tin for up to three months.

❧ *Mint Chutney: Pudina Ki Chatni* ❧

Serve this delightful chutney as a relish with a rice dish or on pita bread.

- 2 cups fresh mint, coriander, or spearmint leaves
- 1 small white onion
- 1 fresh green chili (seeded for a milder flavor)
- 2 fresh garlic cloves
- 1 tablespoon lemon or lime juice
- 1 teaspoon cayenne
- 1 teaspoon vegetable no-salt herbal blend (page 287)
- ½ cup water

Blend or process all of the above ingredients into a thick paste. Cover and refrigerate 2–3 hours before serving. This relish can be prepared a day before serving and chilled overnight.

❧ *Indian Cheese: Paneer* ❧

Paneer can be stir-fried and added to spicy vegetable dishes.

- 2 quarts (8 cups) milk
- 4 tablespoons lemon juice

Heat milk, stirring to avoid skin on top. As it begins to boil, stir in the lemon juice and remove from heat. The milk curdles instantly. Pour it through a cheesecloth-lined strainer placed over a bowl so the whey drains out. Let it set 1 hour or longer. Gather the curd in the cheesecloth and put on a large plate with a heavy lid or weight on top. Leave it several hours. Cut into cubes. Refrigerated, it will keep at least two days.

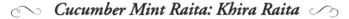

Cucumber Mint Raita: Khira Raita

Serve this as a vegetable relish with chappati bread to balance a very spicy dish. Substitute spinach for cucumber, if desired.

     1 large cucumber
        pinch salt
     2 scallions
     1 green chili, seeded for milder flavor
    10 ounces (1¼ cup) plain yogurt
     1 tablespoon fresh lemon juice
     1 teaspoon ground cumin
     2 tablespoons fresh mint, finely chopped
        mint leaves to garnish

Shred the large cucumber, sprinkle with salt, and refrigerate for 1 hour. Puree the scallions, green chili, yogurt, lemon juice, and cumin in a blender. Pour on top of the cucumber, adding fresh mint. Garnish with mint leaves.

Paneer Makhani

The East Indians eat hot, spicy vegetarian entrées to cleanse the blood by increasing perspiration and promoting proper digestion.

     1 cup paneer cubes (page 186)
     ¼ cup plain yogurt
     2 onions, chopped
     1 tablespoon sesame oil, vegetable oil, or ghee (page 183)
     1 teaspoon ground cumin
     1 teaspoon coriander
     1 teaspoon turmeric
     1 teaspoon garam masala (page 186)
    1½ cups tomatoes, peeled and chopped
     2 teaspoons cayenne
     1 tablespoon water
     ½ cup plus 1 tablespoon cream
     1 tablespoon fennel seeds, dry-roasted
        cilantro leaves to garnish

Deep-fry paneer cubes until golden. Drain, place in a bowl with yogurt. Stir-fry onions in sesame oil, vegetable oil, or ghee. Stir in ground cumin, coriander, turmeric, and garam masala, and heat for a minute. Add tomatoes, cayenne, and water; simmer 10 minutes. Add cream and heat through, being careful not to boil. Spoon in paneer and yogurt mixture and garnish with cilantro leaves and fennel seeds.

Hummus

Hummus is served with pita bread as a light lunch or appetizer before dinner.

    2   tablespoons olive oil
        juice of 1 lemon
    2   teaspoons curry leaves, finely chopped
    1   garlic clove
    ¼   cup tahini
    1   (17-ounce) jar or can of garbanzo beans, drained

Place all of the above ingredients in a blender and blend until smooth.

Chappatis

The East Indian War of Independence in 1857 was heralded by passing chappatis to each house.

    2   cups whole wheat cake flour
    ½   teaspoon salt
        up to 2 cups water
    1   tablespoon oil

Any of the following optional herbs:
    1   teaspoon combined ground thyme,
        lemon thyme, and lemon verbena
    1   teaspoon combined rosemary and lemon thyme
    1   teaspoon garam masala (page 186)
    1   teaspoon ground ginger
    1   teaspoon cinnamon basil, finely chopped
    1   teaspoon ground anise, fennel, or coriander seed

Sift flour and discard bran. Work in water a little at a time to make a firm dough. Knead and allow the dough to rest, covered with a damp cloth, for 1 hour. Divide into 6 pieces, roll flat to ⅛-inch rounds. Rest the dough, covered with a damp cloth, for 30 minutes. Heat 1 tablespoon of oil in a frying pan until it sizzles. Fry one chappati at a time until it bubbles. Turn over as brown spots appear. Add oil if necessary. Fry all. Serves 6.

❧ *Homemade Curry* ❧

In India, these spices are bought whole, toasted, and ground with a mortar and pestle. Store any remaining blend in an airtight container or tin.

- 2 teaspoons ground cumin
- 2 teaspoons ground coriander
- 2 teaspoons ground turmeric
- 1 teaspoon nutmeg
- ½ teaspoon cinnamon
- ¼ teaspoon cayenne
- ¼ teaspoon black pepper, freshly ground
- 1 teaspoon salt, optional

Combine and mix thoroughly.

❧ *Tahini: Ground Sesame Butter* ❧

Tahini can be used as a peanut butter substitute and in any nut butter recipe. Combined with rice, it makes an excellent complement and easy complete protein. Tahini contains vitamin T, an excellent blood builder that may enhance platelets.

- 3½ cups (1 pound) white sesame seeds, hulled

Spread onto an ungreased cookie sheet. Toast at 325 degrees for 8–10 minutes, occasionally stirring to toast the seeds evenly. Remove the seeds when they turn a pale straw color. Browning seeds will cause them to taste bitter. Blend at high speed to form a paste.

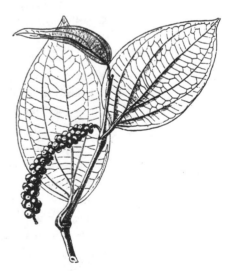

BLACK PEPPER

Lamb on Rose Petals: Yakhni

Kashmir, the "Indian jewel of the east," is surrounded by the Himalayas and emerald green lakes. In Srinagar, the capital, the Moguls built ingenious floating vegetable gardens complemented by floating lotus blossoms and electric kingfish. The gardens are arranged in quadrants with a shallow water channel running down the middle. Shalimar Bagh, the Garden of Love, is terraced with four flower beds rising above one another. The top terrace was reserved for Queen Nur Jahan's royal women. In elegant seclusion, a black marble pavilion opens up to the stars and the progression of the moon against the night sky. It is here that the women would feast on a national dish of lamb and curry, nestled on a bed of rose petals.

The Kashmir serve this dish on a bed of fresh red rose petals and edible silver foil, available at East Indian markets. The use of milk, fruits, and nuts give Kashmir curries a sweet, nurturing essence. This recipe was adapted from *A World of Curries* by Dave DeWitt and Arthur Pais (NY: Little, Brown and Co., 1994).

  1 teaspoon saffron
  ¼ cup milk, hot
  2 onions, chopped
  2 tablespoons fresh ginger
  6 garlic cloves
  ½ cup milk, cold
  1 cup plain yogurt
  6 tomatoes, chopped
  2 pounds fresh lamb, chopped
  ¼ cup ghee (page 183)
  1 teaspoon ground cumin
  1 chopped chili pepper (seeded to reduce heat)
  1 teaspoon ground coriander
  ¼ teaspoon cardamom
  ¼ teaspoon cloves
  ¼ teaspoon nutmeg
  ¼ cup almonds, chopped
  ¼ cup raisins, chopped
    red rose petals (optional)
    edible silver foil (optional)

Soak saffron in hot milk for 5 minutes. In another bowl, blend onions, fresh ginger, and garlic cloves into a paste. Combine cold milk and plain yogurt in another bowl. Cook tomatoes and lamb in a frying pan over medium heat for 20 minutes. Heat ghee in a small dish, add the onion paste, and cook over high heat until it turns a golden color. Add ground cumin, chili pepper, ground coriander, cardamom, clove, and nutmeg, and heat for 2 minutes. Add to the lamb and mix well. Add saffron milk, the milk and yogurt, and chopped almonds and raisins. Cook for 10 minutes to blend flavors and make a gravy.

East Indian Beverages: Thanda Garam

East Indians enjoy a variety of refreshing beverages and herbal teas made with aromatic leaves, fruits, and wood chips. They are served at many festive and religious occasions and holidays. The most common time to enjoy a drink is at noon or with afternoon snacks.

〜 *Homemade Yogi Tea* 〜

An excellent stimulant to promote well-being, Yogi tea is often drunk to enhance digestion.

- 2 teaspoons ginger, freshly grated
- 4 cardamom seeds
- 8 cloves
- 1 cinnamon stick
- 2 tablespoons milk

Add ginger, cardamom seeds, cloves, and cinnamon stick to 8 cups water. Cook to reduce the liquid by half. Strain and add milk.

〜 *Ginger Lemonade: Shikanjee* 〜

Ginger elevates lemonade to the height of taste. It can be used to abate nausea and stimulate bile flow.

- 1 cup sugar
- ½ cup fresh lemon or lime juice
- 1 tablespoon ginger juice
  candied ginger to garnish

Boil sugar in 2 cups of water for 1 minute. Cool and add lemon or lime juice, ginger juice, and 2 cups of cold water. Garnish with candied ginger. Makes 8 servings. Serve over ice.

Cumin Tea: Jal Jerra

A digestant tea served before dinner with a sweet-sour taste.

- 1 cup water, boiled
- 3 teaspoons tamarind
- 1 tablespoon mango powder
- 1 tablespoon cumin seeds, ground and roasted
- 2 tablespoons brown sugar
- 1 cup fresh mint
- 1 (½-inch) slice fresh ginger
- ½ teaspoon chat masala (East Indian black salt)

Soak tamarind in 1 cup of boiled water overnight in a glass or porcelain dish. Mash and squeeze out all of the juice. Add 2 more cups of water to the tamarind and squeeze out the juice. Add water to make 6½ cups. Discard the tamarind. Stir in mango powder, cumin seeds, and brown sugar.

Blend mint, ginger, and half a cup of water. Add the tamarind water. Stir in chat masala (do not substitute white salt). Allow the tea to steep 1 hour before serving 8.

Variations: Substitute for mint leaves and cumin: ½ teaspoon of cardamom, ¼ teaspoon of fennel seeds, ground. Add ½ cup of brown sugar and ⅓ cup of fresh lime juice.

Aam Lassi

This is the national favorite of East Indians, served a little differently in each region. Mango, an East Indian fruit, is served to guests and on special occasions in a variety of ways. There are over 1,000 varieties of mangoes cultivated in India.

- 1 cup plain yogurt
- ½ teaspoon fresh lemon juice
- ½ cup fresh mango
  dash of cinnamon powder
- 4 tablespoons honey
- ⅓ cup cold water
- 1 tray ice cubes

In a blender, blend all the ingredients, adding the ice cubes last. Serves 4.

✌ *Holy Basil Tea: Tulsi Ki Chah* ✌

Tulsi tea is given to abate illness and ensure recuperation.

- ½ cup holy (tulsi) basil leaves
- 2 cups water, boiled
- 1 slice ginger, grated or 2 pieces ginger candy, finely chopped
- 1 tablespoon honey

Steep basil leaves in boiled water for 5 minutes in a covered glass or porcelain pot. Add ginger or ginger candy and honey. Brew 3 more minutes before serving.

✌ *Fennel Tea: Saunf Ki Chah* ✌

Fennel tea is given to strengthen eyesight and promote cheerfulness.

- 1 teaspoon fennel seeds
- 4 cups water
- ½ cup fresh rose petals
- 1 tablespoon lemon peel, grated
- 1 tablespoon honey

Simmer fennel seeds in water for 5 minutes. Add rose petals (gulab) and lemon peel. Brew for 3 minutes. Add honey and serve over ice.

The Curry Connection

Curry is an ancient culinary and medicinal mixture of ancient spice blends. Traces of curry blends have been found in excavations of the Indus Valley (in what is presently Pakistan) dated 2500 B.C. This culture, known as the Harappa, used curries to flavor their food and to keep themselves healthy.

Curry spices are high in vitamins A and C as well as trace minerals deficient in western soil, like chromium and zinc. The hot chili peppers contain niacin, which converts to tryptophan and then serotonin in the brain, causing a relaxing endorphin release. Many of the present-day antidepressants are computer engineered to maintain serotonin levels in the brain. The ancients used chilies to maintain proper neurochemical, or brain, function.

The ancient East Indians blended curry because they immediately noticed beneficial results. The hot spices encourage proper digestion, preserve food from rancidity, destroy parasites, and reduce flatulence.

The resulting perspiration cleanses bodies of toxins, acting like an extra kidney and causing a cool-down, even in the intense heat.

East Indians use curry to treat a variety of ailments. The hottest spices—cinnamon, long pepper, cumin, and ginger—are combined to treat asthma, anemia, jaundice, and constipation, which is a serious condition in Ayurvedic medicine. Grated nutmeg, cloves, and long pepper are blended with camphor for an aphrodisiac and rejuvenating tonic for men. Turmeric is used to treat leprosy and less serious skin diseases, while an oil of nutmeg is used to abate insomnia.

Curry encourages proper digestion, preserves food from rancidity, destroys parasites, and reduces flatulence.

～

The East Indian system of medicine is based on prevention. They flavor their food with curry every day, using this and other food combinations to promote health and well-being on a daily basis. Spices are often dry-roasted before grinding to bring out their flavor, and can be stored in a tin up to three months. Dried ginger and turmeric must be crushed with a mortar and pestle before grinding them in an electric spice mill or coffee grinder. Curry must be freshly prepared to release digestive and tonic properties. It can be added to fruits, vegetables, stews, meat, and rice dishes.

Curry is believed to have originated on the Malabar coast of Southern India where pepper, cinnamon, ginger, cardamom, and turmeric grow wild. The seafaring Phoenicians and Arabs began buying them around 500 B.C. and sold them in Alexandria. From Egypt they were sent to the Mediterranean, where the profit increased manyfold. The Arabs concealed their source of spices as long as possible. Payment for spices was made in gold, silver, coral, cloth, and sometimes wine. The demand for spices became so great in Rome that the government, paying so much for spices, could not pay the army. Outposts were soon raided by barbarians and Moguls, and the Roman empire toppled for the love of curry.

Portuguese trade, which began in 1498, soon changed the nature of curry by adding the fiery chili pepper. They created a world market for spices and chilies. Each land added their special flavor and ingredients to create new regional curry dishes.

The Mogul conquerors encouraged cultivation of spices throughout India. Their rule began in 1526 and ended when the British moved in on the politically unstable conditions in 1757 to "civilize India." During British rule, India became the largest chili and spice producer in the world. The British initiated clove plantations and made English teas a national beverage before they left the country in 1947.

Curry is popular in Africa as well. Africa's cuisine was influenced by eight European countries who began colonizing in the 1600s (Belgium, England, France, Germany, Italy, the Netherlands, Portugal, and Spain). Malay slaves introduced exotic dishes from the Spice Islands made with anise seed, fennel, ginger, coriander, garlic, mustard, tamarind, cardamom, cumin, and turmeric imported for the Malay cooks. Chilies were introduced by Portuguese traders and naturalized by local birds, now known as African bird peppers. Curries called "kerrie-kerries" were cooked with seafood and meat, locally grown tomatoes and onions, and seasoned with a variety of spices. Curries were served with rice and roti bread, eaten only with the fingers. The popularity of curries throughout Africa crosses all cultural barriers and has been adapted to a variety of other foods, such as kidney beans, fruit, and even butter.

Eastern Africa

Ethiopia is an independent nation on the east coast of central Africa whose cuisine has remained independent of European influence. They enjoy a year-round growing season on the farmlands of their plateaus. Coffee plants grow wild and remain the largest cash crop. Other crops include millet, sorghum, peanuts, plantains, sugar cane, potatoes, barley, wheat, corn, and peas.

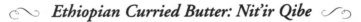

Ethiopian Curried Butter: Nit'ir Qibe

Ethiopians flavor their food with this delicious curried butter.

- 2 ounces fresh ginger root
- ½ cup onion, minced
- 1 garlic clove, minced
- 2 pounds butter
- 2 cloves
- 1 teaspoon whole cardamom seeds
- 1 (2-inch) piece cinnamon
- 1 tablespoon fresh Greek oregano leaves
- 1 tablespoon fresh lemon or cinnamon basil leaves
- 2 teaspoons whole cumin seeds
- ½ teaspoon turmeric

Combine ginger root, onion, and garlic clove. Pound into a paste with large mortar and pestle. Melt butter over low heat, skimming off all foam as it rises (or melt 2 pounds of clarified butter, already prepared). Add to the butter the paste, cloves, cardamom seeds, cinnamon, oregano leaves, lemon or cinnamon basil leaves, cumin seeds, and turmeric, cooking over a low heat for 20 minutes to blend the flavors. Strain and refrigerate. Remove white milk solid after it hardens and discard. Yields 2 cups.

Variation: ½ teaspoon cayenne or 1 chopped, seeded chili pepper can be added.

Western Africa

Guinea is a humid, tropical land divided into four regions: coastal, savanna, southeastern forest, and Fouta Jallon mountainous region. They receive up to 169 inches of rain annually, making rice their subsistence crop. Most Guineans are involved in agriculture and are semi-nomadic herders raising livestock. Cassavas, rice, millet, peanuts, corn, and sweet potatoes are grown to feed families. Coffee, bananas, peanuts, citrus, and pineapples are grown for trade.

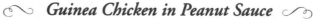

❧ *Guinea Chicken in Peanut Sauce* ❧

Serve on plain rice with sliced onions sprinkled with sugar and vinegar.

- 2 cups ground peanuts
- 1 cup coconut milk
- 2 tablespoons ghee
- ¼ teaspoon curry
- 4 cups chicken pieces, cubed
- 1 onion, finely chopped
- 3 tomatoes, chopped and skinned
- 1 garlic clove
- 1 tablespoon ghee, optional (page 183)

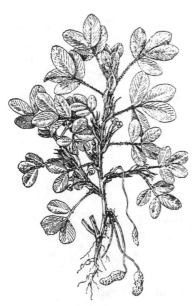

Cook ground peanuts in 2 cups of boiling water for 5 minutes until mixture thickens. Add coconut milk and set aside. Heat ghee and curry in a skillet and cook chicken pieces until golden. Remove from pan. Cook chopped onion, tomatoes, and garlic for 3 minutes, adding ghee, if desired. Add peanut sauce and chicken. Simmer 30 minutes.

PEANUT

South Africa

Cape Malays, descendants of seventeenth-century Malaysian slaves, developed South African cuisine. They incorporated Dutch and English ingredients into their special curries; one of them, Pinang Kerrie, a famous national dish of South Africa. The Dutch and English colonized South Africa to resupply their trade ships. They organized and stocked farms to feed their sailors and introduced many new foods to South Africa. Over twenty herbs and spices were available for culinary pleasure.

∾ *Pinang Kerrie* ∾

Do not suppose that pinang is just another curry.
—C. L. Leipoldt

    2 teaspoons Cape Curry (page 198)
    4 garlic cloves
    1 teaspoon turmeric
    2 bay leaves
    1 ounce ginger, minced
    2 tablespoons apple cider vinegar
    1 teaspoon tamarind paste
    1 teaspoon sugar
    1 pound lamb, cubed
    2 tablespoons sesame oil
    4 onion chive bulbs, chopped
       applemint and green onion chive leaves to garnish

Combine all of the spices. Add cubed lamb and coat well. Refrigerate 2 hours or overnight. Heat sesame oil in a skillet and sauté onion chive bulbs until brown. Add 1 cup of water, lamb, and marinade. Cook 45–50 minutes. Remove bay leaves. Serve on rice with a garnish of applemint and green onion chive leaves.

❧ *Cape Curry* ❧

This is the hottest curry I have ever tasted. Use it sparingly, and beware!

- 1 tablespoon whole cloves
- 2 tablespoons black peppercorns
- 3 tablespoons cumin seeds
- ½ cup coriander seeds
- 1 tablespoon fennel seeds
- 1 tablespoon mustard seeds
- 1 tablespoon ground ginger
- ¼ cup ground cardamom
- ¼ cup turmeric
- 3 small, hot, red chilies, stems and seeds removed

Roast all of the above ingredients in a dry skillet. Grind in a spice mill until well blended. Store in an airtight jar.

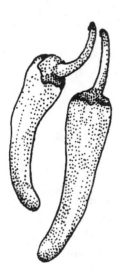

CHILIES

North Africa

Morocco is an Arab country in northwest Africa. Its location, bordered by the Atlantic Ocean and Mediterranean Sea, allows trade traffickers to enjoy a variety of cuisine and renowned hospitality. They are unique in being self-sufficient for agricultural and meat requirements. Their most favored dish is called tagines, a slowly cooked, fragrant meat stew (page 200). Meals are served on the floor and are eaten with their fingers.

Algeria is a former French colony located on the Mediterranean coast of North Africa. Along the fertile coastland dates, figs, olives, grains, grapes, and fruit trees are cultivated. The interior nomads raise livestock. Algerians are Sunni Muslims who ingest no pork or alcohol. They enjoy mint tea and strong coffee.

Tunisia is only eighty-six miles across the Mediterranean from the boot of Sicily. Tunisian cuisine reflects the Mediterranean cultures as well as the Islamic traditions of no pork or alcohol. Their food is served from one common bowl from where everyone eats with their fingers.

❧ *Harissa Chili Curry* ❧

This hot sauce is served in Morocco, Tunisia, and Algiers. It should be served with a hankie to catch the tears running down the face of any newcomer trying it. Harissa can be cooked in stews, served as a side dish for dipping breads, or as a relish. Curries can be served with yogurt and mint dishes to cool down the dinner.

- 12 dried pequin, serrano, or jalapeño chilies, seeded and deveined
- 1 teaspoon ground cardamom
- 1 tablespoon cumin
- 1 teaspoon ground cinnamon stick
- 1 teaspoon ground coriander seeds
- 1 tablespoon fresh mint
- 2 tablespoons virgin olive oil
- 5 garlic cloves

Reconstitute the chilies by soaking them in water until softened. Pan-roast cardamom and cumin seeds a few minutes in a frying pan over medium heat before grinding. Blend all ingredients to form a paste. Add an additional 1 or 2 teaspoons of water or olive oil if the mixture needs moisture. Yields 1–1½ cups.

∾ *Tagines Meat Stew: Flower Curry* ∾

This Moroccan curry is unusual in that it uses lavender and rosebuds to temper the hot flavor. Try it with rice dishes or couscous. This should clean out your spice cabinet!

- 2 tablespoons crushed, dried rose buds
- 2 tablespoons crushed, dried lavender leaves or flowers
- 1 tablespoon ground cardamom
- 1 tablespoon mace
- 1 tablespoon dried ginger
- 1 teaspoon red (cayenne) pepper
- 2 teaspoons dried, ground galangal, from an oriental food market
- 1 teaspoon ground cloves
- 1 tablespoon ground turmeric
- 1 teaspoon cinnamon
- 1 teaspoon ground fennel seeds
- 2 tablespoons freshly ground pepper
- 1 teaspoon nutmeg

Combine the ingredients in a spice mill and powder. Yields ¾ cup.

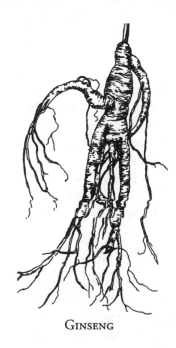

9

Oriental Secrets of Longevity

When the root is deep, there is no reason to fear the wind.

—Chinese proverb

hinese herbalism has been developed for over four thousand years and is actively practiced by the Chinese, Taiwanese, Indonesians, Koreans, Japanese, Malaysians, Vietnamese, Filipinos, and Thai. Today there are over one thousand prescriptions of herbal combinations in use to address an imbalance or disharmony in the physical, psychological, or spiritual nature of an individual. In a combination, the ruling herbs address the main symptom, while supporting herbs enhance the function. Assisting herbs drive and enhance the effect of the combination. Conducting herbs often enhance the assimilation and utilization of the herbal combination to assure success. Herbs are cooked twice to extract all the nutritive and therapeutic benefits. Chinese herbs are best cooked in glass or porcelain containers, or ginseng cookers. A ginseng cooker is a specially designed ceramic bowl with a fitted, flat lip and a dome lid that fits on top. Chinese herbs are cooked in water inside the ginseng cooker, which sits inside another pan of steaming water, like a double boiler. A Crock-Pot may be used as a substitute for a ginseng cooker, or when large quantities of herbs are cooked.

Herbal tonics are special brews meant to be used over a long period of time to promote "radiant health." They are not used for acute conditions.

Herbs are cooked twice to extract all the nutritive and therapeutic benefits.

~

Tonics provide nutrients that enhance the natural process of organic function. The body does not know age or order of difficulty, but it does know how to maintain health and can produce a radiant glow when provided with herbs and foods that promote health. The Chinese developed herbal tonics to promote longevity and fertility and to enhance the blessings of the spirit. These tonics are most beneficial when combined with a balanced diet, exercise, and harmonious lifestyle. Our bodies, like seeds, will be constantly renewed by Mother Nature to bloom again.

Inner Alchemy

*O*nce people connect to their inner strength, there is no end to the world of travel.

—Ding Ming Dao

∾

*C*hinese herbalists treat the individual rather than the disease. Oriental medicine looks for an underlying cause for a disease as it relates to the entire body. This describes what the Chinese call a "pattern of disharmony," which may cause psychological or physiological illness. The origin of an identical disease and its subsequent cure may be totally different in two individuals. Chinese herbs affect the personality's fears, behavior, and social reality, as well as the spiritual flowering. They also address environmental causes of disharmony. External influences are eliminated, like a viral or bacterial invasion, or an inability to adjust to the weather and its many changes. If humidity, rain, or a seasonal change adversely affects an individual, certain herbs are combined to counteract any detrimental effects.

Harmony includes being comfortable in one's environment. To the Oriental people, this includes a profound respect for Mother Nature. Orientals see humanity as part of nature, rooted like the trees, blooming under stress, and silent like the mountains. Their intent in combining herbs is to promote an easy flow and transformation in their environment, making life a safe place to creatively express themselves. We are here to contribute to the loveliness of nature, not to take away from it.

In the body, tonic herbs balance the organs, whose energy systems harmonize like an orchestra with the meridians, the channels and the pathways of energy, blood, and qí (chí). The interior of the body connects us with our environment, community, and fellow herbalists of every culture and color all over the world.

Chinese herbal treatments are often combined with acupuncture. Acupuncture is an Oriental system of relieving pain and inducing anesthesia by inserting thin needles into the body at specific points. Oriental medicine also uses acupuncture to enhance organ function, circulation, and strengthen the vitality of the recipient by increasing immune function. Herbal therapy is considered the nurturing, or yin, part of organ meridian therapy. Chinese tonic herbs are taken on a daily or long-term basis, alone or with other modalities. Chinese tonics release their rejuvenating energy through the process of cooking. Cooking will nullify any sulphur dioxide or preservatives. Grinding the herbs and putting them in capsules is not effective or recommended. Properly prepared tonics establish a deep connection to one's vital energy and initiates an appreciation of the anatomy, allowing every part to fulfill its ultimate potential. To be successful, we must pay attention to the mundane and little things in life. To be healthy, we must build strength, stamina, and a gentle spirit on a daily basis from the pure energy inherent in tonic herbs. Possibly the most popular Chinese herb used for health purposes is ginseng. The shape of the root indicates it is a whole body tonic. Among ginseng's greatest virtues is its ability to reduce stress while increasing energy.

Grades of Ginseng

These are the three categories of ginseng roots, called grades. Heaven grade is the best. Earth grade is made acceptable. Man grade is inferior.

WILD MANCHURIAN: Tung pei is the best. It may be up to two hundred years old and grows in slightly radioactive soil. This root is known to have the most pronounced effect on spiritual perception and is available in tiny amounts. Wild Korean ginseng is considered similar in excellence.

YI SUN is the next highest grade. It is grown commercially and sun dried.

SHIU CHU is commercially grown and harvested after six years. The roots are prepared by steaming and soaking them in date sugar. This variety is known to sedate the undesirable effects of ginseng, such as headaches, shoulder tension, and anger that would back down a tiger.

KIRIN is commercially available and the least expensive of the highest quality ginsengs.

KOREAN WHITE is peeled and preserved by sun drying. It is used as a light tonic and an energy booster, but is not therapeutic. Its benefit is short-term.

JAPANESE GINSENG lacks quality and has little of the earthy ginseng taste. It looks similar to higher quality ginsengs and is often sold to unsuspecting ginseng enthusiasts at a bargain price.

Heaven grade is the best; Earth grade is made acceptable; and Man grade is inferior.

AMERICAN GINSENG is very mild, but highly esteemed by the Chinese. George Washington had a successful ginseng business with the Chinese (Americans learned about the energizing properties of ginseng from the Native Americans).

POWDERED GINSENGS are often low grade and may contain lactose.

How to Cook Ginseng and Tang Kuei Roots

Ginseng root *(Panax renshen)* is cooked and eaten to raise the chí, or vitality, of an individual. Tang kuei *(Angelica sinensis)* can be cooked and eaten to build the vitality through the blood, hormones, and bodily fluids. Ginseng is often cooked for men, while women use tang kuei instead. Tang kuei is called the "female ginseng" and helps build the blood. Combined, they benefit the stamina and nurturing essence of an individual. However, neither ginseng nor tang kuei should be used when estrogen blockers have been prescribed.

Ginseng and tang kuei roots can be purchased and cooked, separately or together, in a ginseng cooker. Purchase a ginseng cooker in Oriental stores or substitute a double boiler. Bring one ounce of roots to a boil in two cups of distilled water. Allow to cook for one hour. Sip half a cup of tea once or twice daily for stamina.

To reboil the roots, add one cup of water for each ounce of herbs and boil for one hour. The Orientals believe the second cooking yields the finest tea. They often cook their roots three times before composting them.

If you choose to eat the root, do so after the first cooking as the nutrient energy is abundant (eating the root after the second cooking does not have this). Try eating only a small piece and wait an hour before eating any more. Those who are new to Oriental herbs should slowly increase, ingesting no more than an ounce daily to assure proper assimilation and metabolism of a new food. Chinese herbs are very potent and have an unusual, earthy flavor quite different from Western cuisine. Many of the roots have a heating property that could increase blood pressure or cause nausea and diarrhea in an enthusiastic novice.

To make an extract, place one ounce of roots in four ounces of brandy. Add a slice of Chinese licorice or two jujube red dates. A flavored brandy or vodka can be used. Use a glass jar with a secure lid. Steep at least three weeks before tasting. Begin ingesting by diluting one teaspoon in warm water up to three times daily. Dilute in at least one tablespoon of water.

If you let other people shape you, then you will never know independence.

—Ding Ming Dao,
36 Tao Daily Meditations

When the extraction is down to one half, add two more ounces of alcohol and steep three more weeks to keep a continuous supply of extraction.

When drinking ginseng teas and extracts be sure to notice any signs of "empty yang" symptoms. These would include headaches, hypertension, shoulder tension, irritability, or excessive sexual desires. Any of these symptoms occurring thirty minutes to one hour after ingesting suggest that the heat, or energy, is not being utilized properly. This indicates a need to reduce or avoid ginseng roots, or to combine the roots with other herbs to allow the energy to flow unhindered into the channels or pathways of the central nervous system.

Herbs that combine well with ginseng or tang kuei are:

> Chuan xiong, Chinese lovage *(Ligusticum wallichi)*
> Ho shou wu root *(Polygonum multiflorum)*
> Huang chí *(Astragalus membranicus)*
> Kan tsao, Chinese licorice root *(Glycyrrhiza uralensis)*
> Pai shao, white peony root *(Paeonia alba)*
> Shih hu (Chinese *dendrobium* orchid)
> Ta tsao, Jujube red dates *(Zizyphus jujube)*
> Tang shen *(Codonopsitis radix)*
> Ti huang, Chinese foxglove *(Rehmannia glutinosa)*

A Chinese Herbal

The following Chinese herbal determines which herbs are best for you. Add half of the amount of ginseng or tang kuei to any combination of these herbs in your cooker. Be sure to cook them twice. **Note:** Ginseng and tang kuei should not be used by women on estrogen blockers without the consent of their physician.

CHAI HU *(Bupleurum chinense)*. Bupleurum is a famous liver tonic with similar properties as gotu kola. The Chinese use it to bring out strong emotions of sadness or anger. Bupleurum is indicated for chronic disease and prolapsed organs, hypertension, and ulcers. It has anti-inflammatory and sedative effects useful in female, cardiovascular, and liver tonics.

FU LING *(Poria cocos)*. Fu ling is an excellent yin, or fluid, tonic. It has diuretic properties that may strengthen the urinary system, and sedative properties to soothe the heart and lungs. Fu ling is used as an assisting herb. The fungi should be white and firm. It is often sold as shavings, which cook faster. It can be used alone or with Western herbs that are diuretic, such as uva ursi, parsley, and dandelion leaves.

GINGER ROOT *(Zingiber officinale)*. Dried ginger root warms the stomach and tones the spleen and pancreas, enhancing digestion and assimilation. As a tonic, it relieves nausea, vomiting, and cramps. It is not recommended for gastritis or heavy menses. The Orientals use it as a driving, warming, and dispersing herb.

GINSENG *(Panax renshen)*. Ginseng is a warming energy tonic with a bittersweet, earthy taste. There are several grades, and the cost often indicates the therapeutic qualities. Ginseng is known as an adaptagen, containing stress-reducing, adrenal cortical-like hormones promoting longevity and increasing the quality of life. Wild Manchurian, tung pei and yi sun, heaven grade, also enhance spiritual perception. Ginseng is not recommended if inflammatory conditions exist and is best combined with herbs that help move the energy and sedate side effects. Ginsengs are used in many male longevity tonics that build chí, or vitality. The Orientals know that it is the cooking process that releases the therapeutic essence of ginseng.

HUANG CHI *(Astragalus membranicus)*, or Astragalus root. Huang chi is renowned as an immune and energy tonic herb. It is believed to strengthen the outer limbs, especially the legs. Athletes enjoy better respiratory function and endurance. As an immune enhancer, astragalus stimulates white cells, modifies T helper cells, and reduces T suppressor cells. It is also used to reduce fluid retention in the lower body. The best roots are large, straight, and yellow. This herb should be cooked up to sixty minutes to release its therapeutic qualities. Ground and powdered varieties have little or no benefit. One or two slices cooked in one cup of distilled water will benefit those who are convalescing or who want to improve their immune function. Since huang chi has very little taste, it is often combined with licorice root, ginger root, or other herbs that benefit the immune system.

HO SHOU WU *(Polygonum multiflora)*. Ho shou wu is the most famous longevity herb, enhancing chí, vitality, and sexual vigor. Its energy is warm and bittersweet, opening the heart in spiritual bliss. As a rejuvenating tonic, ho shou wu clears vision, increases fertility, and may return hair to its original color over a period of years. Cook large, dark slices in combination with tang kuei, ti huang, jujube red dates, or lycii berries for a powerful tonic.

KAN TSAO *(Glycyrrhiza uralensis),* or Chinese licorice root. Kan tsao is known as the "great harmonizer." The Chinese believe it revitalizes the center, digestive organs, and encourages a balance between the liver, spleen, pancreas, and stomach by detoxifying over twelve hundred toxins. They use kan tsao in combinations to eliminate side effects of other herbs. It is sedative and gently laxative. As a tonic, it regulates blood sugar, helping anorexia and addictive tendencies. **Note:** It is not recommended for hypertensive individuals and those who retain fluids. Check with your physician before ingesting.

Glycyrrhiza is similar to adrenal cortical stress hormones. The Orientals combine it with ginseng for a smooth release of boundless energy. The sweetest, yellow roots release fifty molecules of easily assimilated sugar during stress, enabling an individual to maintain vitality and clarity. Cook one or two licorice roots with each ginseng root. **Note:** Oriental licorice is a different variety than the licorice grown in the West and cannot be substituted with the same effect.

Kan tsao is known as the "great harmonizer."

~

KOU CHI TZA *(Lycii fructus),* or Matrimony vine berries. Kou chi tza are bright, red berries that promote cheerfulness, improve night vision, and enhance energy. The Chinese eat them to balance blood sugar, open the heart, and promote longevity. It is one of the few Chinese herbs with a pleasant taste. Lycii berries are believed to build the three Vital Treasures: jing, chí, and shen. Jing represents the source of vitality stored in the deepest organs: the "Sea of Energy." Chí is a life-activating energy derived from light, air, and food: "Where chí flows, blood follows." Shen is developed through compassion and experienced as unconditional love: the "light of chí." Cook the berries and eat them in cereal, bread, or combined with other herbs as a tea.

KUEI PI *(Cinnamon cassia).* Chinese cinnamon is very hot and spicy. It is a powerful assisting herb in energy and heart tonics benefiting circulation and reducing coldness. Small amounts can be chewed to abate flu and cold symptoms. Cinnamon becomes bitter when boiled. Simmer small amounts with jujube red dates to disperse its warming energy. Cinnamon is known to contain chromium, a blood-sugar regulating mineral deficient in Western soil.

LIGUSTICUM *(Chinese lovage).* Ligusticum is a female and blood tonic, increasing circulation, detoxifying the liver, and removing excess heat. It combines well with tang kuei, paeonia, ginger, or licorice root.

PAI SHAO *(Paeonia albaflora)*, or peony root. Peony root is an antispasmodic tonic that raises the threshold of pain and balances female hormones. It is used to abate dysmenorrhea, pain, and insomnia. Peony
restores the balance of the liver energy. Select pure white slices with a
hint of pink.

PAI SHU *(Atractylodes ovata)*. Pai shu is a mild energy tonic with a bittersweet taste known to regulate appetite and control weight. One or
two teaspoons of powdered pai shu taken daily as a tea is used to aid
weight regulation. All grades are acceptable. It is commercially available in pieces that look like wooden chips.

*Tang shen
is used as
a ginseng
substitute.*

SHIH HU *(Dendrobium hancockii)*. Shih hu is the Chinese dendrobium
orchid, a famous chí tonic of the sages. It is cooling and mildly sweet
and salty, restoring bodily fluids and alleviating fatigue. Large golden
stems are dried and simmered with licorice or ginger to restore sexual vigor. This Chinese kidney yin tonic affects the lower back, knees,
and sexual vigor. To the Chinese, the kidneys rule the bone, bone
marrow, memory, hearing, and brain function. The kidneys store
ancestral chí and heredity, as well as having both yin and yang properties, restoring fluids and enhancing vitality.

TANG KUEI or DONG QUAI *(Angelicae sinensis)*. The energy of tang kuei is
warming, and its flavor is sweet and pungent. Tang kuei is a sedative
hematonic used by the Orientals as a blood builder and female
tonic. The cooked root benefits the female endocrine system.
Benefits may include improved circulation, lower blood pressure,
more energy, and less constipation. It reduces PMS, menstrual irregularity, and menopausal symptoms. The Orientals use tang kuei as a
female longevity herb. Traditionally, the Orientals cook a large tang
kuei root with a spring chicken as a blood-cleansing spring tonic.
Tang kuei also can be very relaxing. Large roots are best. They are
available in thin slices.

TANG SHEN *(Codonopsitis radix)*. Tang shen is a mild energy tonic also
used as lung tonic. It has a neutral energy and is used as a ginseng
substitute. Since it is not heating, tang shen is safe for those who
cannot handle ginseng. The long, straight roots can be used for any
immune deficiency or weather sensitivity. The Orientals believe the
lung rules the wei chí, or first line of immune defense. Nursing

mothers use tang shen to increase their milk. It combines well with astragalus and licorice as an immune or children's tonic. Follow the directions and cook like ginseng.

TA TSAO *(Zizyphus jujube),* or jujube red dates. Jujube red dates are delicious and nourishing assistants. They disperse the energy of other herbs throughout the twelve acupuncture meridians. Jujubes promote smooth flow of circulation, aid in digestion, and relax abdominal muscles. The smallest dates are best. Remove pits after cooking. Jujube shrubs are native to Texas and grow in many southwestern climates in North America.

TI HUANG *(Rehmannia glutinosa).* Ti huang is prominent in female and blood tonics. It is the bittersweet root of the Chinese foxglove plant. The Orientals use the prepared root as a kidney tonic in cold weather and the raw root as a blood detoxifier in the summer. Steaming the root changes its property totally. The steamed root is sliced thinly, tastes sweet, and looks like tar. It builds and nourishes the blood. The Orientals consider blood tonics excellent for producing, storing, directing, and circulating bodily fluids, including hormones. Fertility may also be enhanced by blood tonics. In the summer, raw ti huang is taken to cool the blood, reduce blood pressure and anxiety, and aid in rehydrating body tissues.

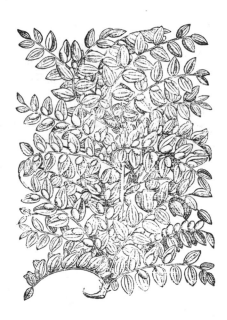

WU WEI TZA *(Schizandra fructus).* Schizandra berries contain all five flavors representing the five Chinese elements: wood, fire, metal, earth, and water. It is a yin fluid and yang vitality tonic, alleviating fatigue and driving out tension. The berries are high in tannic acid and must be soaked overnight before draining and cooking in a tonic.

ZIZYPHUS JUJUBE

Chinese Remedies

𝒯he following tonics are a few of my favorites. They are mild and effective, soothing the mind and body while harmonizing the spirit.

❧ *Shoulder and Neck Relaxing Tonic* ❧

This tonic will ease tension and anxiety and take the edge off a bad day. I use it as a sleep tonic.

- 3 cups distilled water
- 2 small tang kuei roots (or 1 large slice)
- 2 jujube red dates
- 4 (2-inch) slices white peony root *(Paeonia alba)*
- 1 slice fresh ginger or 1 dried Chinese licorice root

In distilled water, simmer the above ingredients. A ginseng cooker or porcelain pot and lid make the best cooking utensils. Simmer for 1 hour, without lifting the lid. Strain and drink ½–1 cup to relieve tension.

❧ *Clear Skin Tonic* ❧

Schizandra was popular with the wealthy Chinese and royalty as a radiant skin tonic. It protects the skin from sun and wind exposure, and is used in many aphrodisiac tonics. It is also known to be mildly sedative.

- ½ cup schizandra berries
- ½ cup jujube red dates
- 1 piece licorice or ginger root

Soak schizandra berries immersed in water overnight; drain and combine with 4 cups of fresh water, jujube red dates, and licorice or ginger root. Simmer, covered 15–20 minutes. Sip one cup daily.

∾ *Chinese Nightcap* ∾

The Chinese believe that women who drink peony root tea will become as beautiful as the peony flower.

   3 slices white peony root *(Paeonia alba)*
   1 licorice root
6–8 Chinese chrysanthemum or chamomile flowers

Simmer peony slices and licorice root in 2 cups of water for 15 minutes. Add Chinese chrysanthemum or chamomile flowers and steep 5 minutes before straining and nodding off . . . .

∾ *Female Tonic* ∾

This tonic builds vitality, beautiful skin, and regulates the female reproductive system. It is mildly sedative and beneficial for women of all ages.

  1 small root, 1 ounce, or 1 thin slice tang kuei
  2 slices white peony root
     (Paeonia alba)
  3 pieces bupleurum
  2 jujube red dates
  1 piece licorice or ginger root

In 2–3 cups of water, simmer herbs for 1 hour. Strain and drink up to 1 cup daily. (I use 2 cups of water to produce a stronger estrogenic brew.) **Note:** Omit tang kuei if estrogen blockers have been prescribed or consult your physician first.

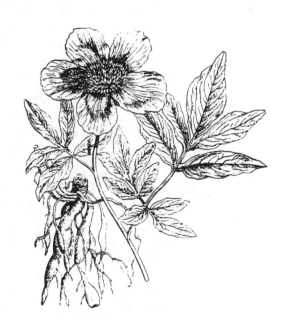

PEONY FLOWER AND ROOT

Chinese Cuisine

*A*dversity, imagination, and an ever-growing population encouraged the Chinese to master the art of cooking. The Chinese were one of the first civilizations to discover fire and learn to cook food. Famines, floods, and the lack of fuel changed their cuisine into an economical art form. They learned to cook quickly, steaming rice instead of baking bread and farming grains instead of grazing cattle. The only cattle they raised were for working the land. They raised pigs and chickens for food because they required minimal care and did not interfere with their farming. The sea offered a variety of fish and sea vegetation, which they learned to dry and preserve indefinitely. They combed the land and sea for new and unusual sources of food. Like the Native Americans on the other side of the world, Chinese survival depended on a harmonious relationship with Mother Nature and ingenuity in living off the land.

Hasten slowly and you shall arrive.

—Chinese proverb

∾

Today, we admire Chinese cuisine because it is predominantly vegetarian, low fat, low calorie, and nondairy. To the Chinese, their cuisine offers a relaxed, social pleasantry that contributes to a peaceful coexistence. Although they do not designate one main dish, each serving has a fragrance, texture, and color that is balanced with a delicacy and flavor meant to please all the senses. Their sauces turn an ordinary dish into a gastronomic pleasure, retaining simplicity and individuality.

Availability of fresh food determines what combination of entrées will appear on the table. Chinese never shop with a grocery list. First, they search the market for ingredients. Then they match the cooking method with the food to preserve the flavor and enhance the nutritious qualities of the meal. Fish is steamed, duck is simmered, vegetables are stir-fried; a delicate blend of seasonings penetrates every part of the food.

What is unique about Chinese cuisine? Only the cook cuts and seasons the food. Knives are considered barbaric and kept in the kitchen, away from the children. Preparation time is much longer than cooking time and salt shakers are scarce. The meals are so satisfying that desserts are unnecessary to silence a growling stomach. The Chinese know greatness is achieved in little things; to them, ruling a country is like cooking a small fish, as every detail is given great concern.

Canton: Gateway to the West

Canton was the first seaport open to the West. The Cantonese soon immigrated to open the first Chinese restaurants in Europe and America. Their cuisine is original and versatile, displaying a vast variety of local produce. They season with soy sauce, ginger root, and sherry, often using a light chicken stock as a base. Their chefs originally came from Peking. They are renowned for stir-fries, fried rice, and delicacies such as Bird's Nest Soup and Shark Fin Soup.

Canton is the capital of Kwangtung province in the southeastern region of China. It was populated with a large wealthy class who moved south from Peking when the Ming Dynasty was overthrown in the seventeenth century. They brought with them a wealth of culture and cuisine, including their chefs, who were delighted to live in a land so rich in natural resources. They developed a cuisine with light sauces to blend with the natural flavor of each ingredient. Originating from Peking, Canton cuisine is a true art form, contrasting color and texture in a variety of ways.

Peking Cuisine

Peking, the capital city of China, and the province of Shantung developed simultaneously. Peking was the cultural center and intellectual hub in the Imperial Palace. Great banquets continued for days, as chefs from Peking and Shantung combined their talents to create elegant meals. They accented their dishes with garlic, leeks, and chives, and created spring rolls wrapped in rice papers. Culinary students were given a one-year course on raising, slaughtering, dressing, and cooking the famous Imperial Peking Duck.

North of Peking lies the vast outposts of Manchuria and Mongolia. These people were nomadic. They herded goats and ate a variety of lamb and mutton "firepot" dishes. An entire group would sit around a common large pot of simmering soup stock, immerse each bite of vegetable or lamb in the pot and dip the cooked food into an individual bowl of spices and condiments. The condiment bowl was often laced with chrysanthemum blossoms.

❧ *Plum Sauce* ❧

Plum sauce is a blend of sweet and sour tastes. It is used to stimulate digestion and often is served with chicken.

- ½ cup chutney, any flavor
- 1 cup plum jelly
- 1 tablespoon brown sugar
- 1 teaspoon rice vinegar

Chop chutney and cook with plum jelly, sugar, and vinegar. Stir and heat thoroughly. Add water to thin. Bottle and cap in a sterile glass jar.

⟋⟍ *Peking Spring Rolls* ⟋⟍

Egg rolls are served to relatives and special friends after the Chinese New Year. They became known as spring rolls due to the season they were served. This recipe is by Fran Goreham.

  2 tablespoons peanut oil
  4 carrots, grated or shredded
  1 small head of cabbage, thinly sliced
  1 onion, minced
  1 bunch of green onions, sliced
  1 can bamboo shoots, cut into ½-inch pieces
6–7 mushrooms, diced
  ½ cup soy sauce
  ¼ teaspoon pepper, optional
  ½ teaspoon vegetable salt, optional, or
    vegetable no-salt herbal blend (page 287)
  1 package firm tofu, well-drained and diced
  1 package egg roll wrappers
  1 cup hot vegetable oil for frying

Heat 2 tablespoons of oil in a large skillet. Combine ingredients (except egg roll wrappers) in order listed. Cook about 20 minutes. Remove to large

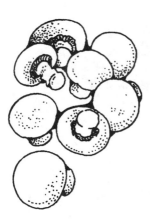

bowl, draining any remaining liquids. Begin heating frying oil in a large Dutch oven or deep fryer. Following directions on the wrapper package, put about ¼–⅓ cup of filling in the center of wrapper and seal edges with water. Cook in hot oil until golden, turning with tongs to cook both sides. Remove with tongs to drain on several layers of paper towels. Serve with hot mustard, sweet and sour sauce, or plain. Makes about 20 egg rolls. Leftover filling can be frozen.

MUSHROOMS

Hunan Cuisine

Hunan follows the Yellow River in the central area of China, where carp are abundant. Their cuisine is not only famous for a variety of carp delicacies, but also sweet and sour sauces.

❧ *Vegetables with Sweet and Sour Sauce* ❧

The Chinese often balance their meals by combining opposites.

For each ½ cup of thinly sliced vegetables, prepare:

    1 garlic clove, minced
    2 tablespoons peanut or vegetable oil
    ½ cup sugar
    ½ cup rice vinegar
    ½ cup water
    2 tablespoons soy sauce
  1½ tablespoons cornstarch or arrowroot starch
    ½ cup water

Sauté garlic in hot oil. Add vegetables and cook three minutes or until softened. Add sugar, vinegar, water, and soy sauce. Stir and cook until dissolved. In a separate bowl, blend cornstarch and water to form a paste. Add to stir-fry and allow it to thicken the mixture. Pour over steamed rice. Serves 2.

Suggested vegetables: carrots, snow peas, bean sprouts, bamboo shoots, water chestnuts, green peas, bell pepper, ginger root, onion, mushrooms, coconut and pineapple pieces.

Fukien Cuisine

In Fukien, the eastern region of China, chefs created egg rolls and clear soups. Many of their dishes are seafood, but they are also renowned for cooking pork two and three times. Early in Chinese culinary history, the chefs learned to cook pork and chicken with ginger root to destroy salmonella and other unwanted animal organisms.

✺ *Mustard Dressing Sauce* ✺

This Fukien recipe is served with egg rolls.

- 1 tablespoon powdered mustard
- ½ teaspoon sesame oil
- 2 tablespoons soy sauce
- 2 tablespoons rice vinegar
- 1 teaspoon brown sugar

Combine all ingredients. Put in a clean glass jar and refrigerate to blend the flavors.

✺ *Matrimony Vine Soup* ✺

The berries of this vine are believed to increase fertility. This soup is often served to a newly wedded couple to wish them a happy family.

- 6 cups vegetable or chicken stock
- 1 cup chopped lean pork
- 6 bunches matrimony vine (*Lycium chinensis*, Chinese Wolfberry vine), chopped, with stems discarded
- 1 teaspoon sea salt or a no-salt herbal blend (page 287)
- 2 eggs, beaten

Boil stock and pork for 15 minutes. Add matrimony vine and salt. Cook 5 minutes. Slowly pour in eggs and remove from heat. Matrimony vine is slightly bitter and detoxifying. Serves 4.

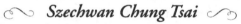 *Lotus Root Soup*

Lotus root is a very nourishing, starchy food eaten to relieve stress and promote health for elderly and convalescent family members.

> 1 pound fresh lotus root, peeled and cut into ¼-inch pieces (from Oriental market)
> 6 jujube red dates
> 2 slices ginger root
> 6 cups water or soup stock
> 1 tablespoon soy sauce
> 1 teaspoon salt or a no-salt herbal blend (page 287)

Cook lotus root, red dates and ginger in water or soup stock for 30 minutes. Add soy sauce and salt before serving. Serves 4.

Szechwan Cuisine

The far opposite western province of China is Szechwan. Their cuisine is well known for hot, spicy dishes laden with dried peppers and cooked in hot oil. Szechwanese enjoy deep-fried foods prepared with a variety of local mushrooms. Their climate is quite warm and their people more assertive than other Chinese.

Szechwan Chung Tsai

The Szechwanese use mustard green hearts in this spicy appetizer as an aid to digestion.

> 1 tablespoon peanut oil
> ½ teaspoon whole anise
> 1 tablespoon chopped onion chives
> 1 teaspoon chopped ginger
> 1 teaspoon chopped garlic
> 1 pound mustard green hearts

Heat oil, add anise and allow to brown. Remove anise from the oil. Stir-fry chives, ginger, and garlic, then add mustard green hearts. Cook 1 minute. Remove, place greens in a dish, and press down. Cover with a tight lid. Refrigerate 5 days before serving as an appetizer. Serves 4.

Hot Pepper Oil

The Szechwanese eat chilies as a vegetable to stimulate digestion and improve cardiovascular circulation.

1½ tablespoons peanut oil
3   dried red chilies, whole

Heat peanut oil and add dried red chilies. Cook until it turns red. Strain.

Soy Milk

Soybeans are known as the "Chinese cow." They are a nutritious, complete protein and nondairy substitute.

1 cup soybeans
   vanilla extract
   cocoa powder or ¼ cup orange juice

Soak soybeans overnight in cold water. Wash and drain well the following day. Place ¼ cup of beans in a blender with 1 cup of water. Blend at high speed for 1 minute, then add 1 more cup of water and blend again. Continue until all beans are blended. Strain the liquid through a cheesecloth, squeezing out as much liquid as possible. Flavor the soy milk with vanilla extract and cocoa powder or orange juice. Refrigerate.

Cook the remaining bean mixture over medium heat until it simmers. Remove from heat and serve as a breakfast cereal. Serves 4.

Soy Milk Gelatin

The Chinese blend the bite of ginger with the crunch of coconut to produce a delicious dessert with a light, creamy texture.

2 packages unflavored gelatin
5 cups soy milk
   preserved ginger to garnish
   coconut flakes to garnish

Dissolve gelatin in soy milk over low heat. Cool and refrigerate until it sets. Cut into servings and serve with preserved ginger and coconut flakes.

❧ *Warming Winter Congee* ❧

In the Orient, this soup would be served to build strength and immunity for the winter. I often prepare it for my students who study herbs at my home.

- 2 tablespoons astragalus root
- ¾ cup millet, toasted
- 12 black or red dates, soaked and pitted
- 2 carrots, cut and peeled (or use sweet potatoes)
- 1 inch fresh ginger plus ½ teaspoon powdered ginger
- 1 teaspoon cardamom seed, crushed or powdered ·
- 8 cups vegetable stock or coconut milk
- 2 tablespoons ghee
- 2 teaspoons cinnamon powder or 1 stick cinnamon
   maple or brown sugar to taste

Tie astragalus root in a muslin bag and simmer with millet, dates, carrots, ginger, and cardamom in 8 cups of stock or coconut milk for 1½ hours. Remove astragalus and season with ghee, cinnamon, and maple or brown sugar. Soy sauce and sesame oil may also be used for seasoning. Rice or barley may be substituted for the millet.

Optional additions for winter congee: Cilantro (Chinese parsley) is a great addition to any soup. It may be served raw as a side dish too. Dice lemon grass roots and add to season stock, stir-fry, and soups. Lotus seeds can be cooked in soups and tonics to "strengthen the heart and calm the spirit," and can be purchased in small cellophane bags at your local Oriental food market.

How to Brew Tea

Tea has been cultivated in China since A.D. 500. Today, there are over two hundred varieties made from green or black tea. Green tea is unfermented. Tender green leaves are picked from the top of the bush and dried. Black tea, allowed to dry on the bush, is gathered, dried, and fermented. The flavor is strong and full. The Chinese refer to it as red tea because it looks red after it is brewed. Oolong tea is only partly dried and fermented, producing a rich pungent tea and served after dinner. Only the Cantonese serve tea during meals. Scented teas are balanced with flowers. They are served between meals and at special occasions. The most popular flowers are jasmine, rose petal, and Chinese chrysanthemum. The tea plant itself is a species of the camellia family.

Flowers beyond reach are sacred to God.

—Chinese proverb

~

Freshly brewed tea is clear and has a fragrant bouquet. Brew tea in porcelain or glass, as metal containers change the flavor. Always boil the water, then pour it over the tea leaves and allow it to steep up to 5 minutes in a covered teapot. For each cup of water, add ½ teaspoon of tea leaves. A second infusion can be brewed from Chinese teas (the Chinese believe the second infusion is the best). The benefits of tea drinking are perhaps best said in this traditional Chinese tea drinking song:

> Tea in the morning stimulates thinking, revives one's spirit.
> Tea after meals clears the throat, helps digestion.
> Tea during the day quenches thirst, does away with frustration.
> Tea after work soothes the muscles, melts away fatigue.

Several fresh herbs combine well with Chinese teas to produce a unique flavor. Here are a few of Mother Nature's blends.

Mother Nature's Chinese Tea Blends

- Add 1 teaspoon of chopped lemon grass for every cup of Chinese tea.

- Add 1 teaspoon of spearmint or peppermint for every cup of Chinese tea. Chocolate mint combines very well with Chinese black teas.

- Add ½ teaspoon of dried lemon verbena leaves
  to every cup of green tea.

- Add ½ teaspoon of fresh honeysuckle flowers
  to every cup of green tea.

- Add ½ teaspoon of fresh or dried chamomile flowers
  to every cup of green tea.

- Add ½ teaspoon of chopped lavender flowers
  to every cup of green or black tea.

Chinese Flower Teas

The Chinese use flowers to correct emotional as well as physical imbalances, perceiving both as an expression of energy.

CHINESE CHRYSANTHEMUM is a nervine used to improve mental clarity. It is the tea to drink after long hours of study and mental gymnastics. The Chinese use it like westerners use chamomile flowers.

GARDENIA is anti-inflammatory and is known as the happiness herb. It is believed to relieve "liver congestion" and blocked emotions. It calms the heart and reduces heat.

HONEYSUCKLE FLOWERS reduce fever and thirst.

MAGNOLIA BUDS correct imbalanced energy. The Chinese use it to reduce facial swelling and as an expectorant and hair tonic. The energy becomes more cooling as the bud opens, enhancing bodily fluids.

ROSE PETALS are an emmenagogue for PMS and amenorrhea. They relieve a heavy feeling in the chest and tummy. Pick young flowers.

YARROW FLOWERS reduce fever.

The Blessings of a Chinese New Year, Tuan Nien

Preparing for the Chinese New Year is a joyous exercise in imagination and creativity. Along with family traditions and exceptional food, honorable deeds and kindness are practiced during the celebration. It is a time to affirm both spiritual and material blessings. Spiritual blessings include longevity, radiant health, love, and happiness. Material blessings include good food and wealth to enjoy all the personal comforts life offers. Specific Chinese calligraphy characters are displayed on walls, pictures, and scrolls during the celebration. *Fu:* Blessed are those who find happiness in their food. *Lu:* Blessed are those who enjoy health and can afford comfortable clothes. *So:* Blessed are those who enjoy inner peace and relaxing sleep for they will enjoy long life.

Everyone stays awake on New Year's Eve, celebrating "Shou Swei," bringing long life to the parents of each family who "guide the year out." The New Year begins with the dragon dance amidst cymbals, gongs, and the explosion of firecrackers. Red is the color symbolizing the New Year. The Chinese wear it and serve red food during the celebration.

Various foods representing the best wishes of the New Year are served. The seeds and fruit of the red

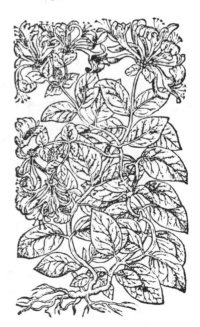

HONEYSUCKLE

pomegranate represent the blessing of fertility. The golden tangerine brings prosperity. An evergreen twig pushed into a tangerine and set in a bowl of uncooked rice stands for ten thousand years of food, "wan nien liang." Sugar cane is displayed to assure ongoing success, while chunks of lotus root symbolize longevity and a harmonious family. Watermelon seeds may be sprinkled by each plate, wishing each person this blessing: "may what you think and what you say always be pleasant." A special New Year cake is served to assure a year filled with sweetness. Other sweets include candied water chestnuts, lotus roots, red dates, and tea sweetened with preserved fruit.

Often these delicacies are served at "dim sum." Dim sum is a progression of soups, dumplings, meats, custards, preserved fruits, and a variety of snacks served in bite-sized portions. The Chinese enjoy tasting many foods as they gather for social and family occasions. Dim sum means "your heart's desire," referring to the different tastes, textures, and fragrances of these foods. The chefs often stay up all night preparing an infinite variety of menus representing the blessings of the spirit and desires of the heart.

⌒ *Ginger Zucchini Carrot Cake* ⌒

This Chinese New Year specialty assures a year filled with sweetness and the blessings of the New Year: health, happiness, and inner peace.

    3 cups flour (unbleached is best)
    2 cups sugar
 1½ cups grated carrots
    1 teaspoon baking soda
 1½ cups grated zucchini
    3 eggs
    2 teaspoons cinnamon
    1 cup safflower oil
    1 teaspoon finely shredded ginger root

Beat eggs, adding oil and sugar. Blend carrots, zucchini, spices and soda into mixture. Then slowly add flour, half a cup at a time. Pour into a greased tube pan. Bake at 350 degrees for 1 hour. Cool 15 minutes and remove cake from pan. Serve with ginger cream sauce.

∾ *Ginger Cream Sauce* ∾

Enjoy this crunchy sauce as an icing or as a dip for fresh vegetables.

    1 cup sour cream or yogurt
    2 teaspoons minced candied ginger

Blend sour cream or yogurt with minced candied ginger. Allow the flavor to blend a few hours or overnight before enjoying. Serves 8.

∾ *Herbal Fortune Cookies* ∾

Every herb has its fortune . . . and so does every herbalist! Recipe and the following herbal fortunes by Fran Goreham.

    2½ dozen paper fortunes (2½ inches x ½ inch wide)
     ½ cup all-purpose flour
     ¼ cup sugar
     1 tablespoon cornstarch
        dash of salt
     ¼ cup vegetable oil
     1 teaspoon almond extract
     2 egg whites
     1 tablespoon dry or fresh chopped herbs of choice: mints (such as
        apple mint, spearmint, peppermint, chocolate mint), scented
        geraniums, rosemary, lavender, lemon verbena, lemon balm.
        Try whatever herbs you would like—be creative.

Prepare paper fortunes.* Heat oven to 300 degrees. Mix flour, sugar, cornstarch, and salt. Beat in remaining ingredients until smooth. For each cookie, spoon 1 heaping teaspoon of batter onto well-greased cookie sheet; spread into 3½-inch circle with back of spoon. Bake only 4 cookies at a time; cool cookie sheet and grease well each time. Bake until golden brown, about 10 minutes.

Working quickly, remove 1 cookie at a time with a wide spatula; flip into protected hand (leave remaining cookies in oven). Place paper fortune on center of cookie; fold cookie in half. Holding points of folded cookie with both hands, place center of fold over the edge of bowl and pull points downward to make a crease across the center. Place cookie in ungreased muffin cup so it will hold its shape while cooling. If cookie cools before it is formed, heat in oven about 1 minute. Store in tightly covered container. Makes about 2 dozen.

*For fortunes, quote herbal lore (see page 224) or Chinese myths. Or, instead of the paper fortune, add a small sprig or leaf or two of a fresh herb before folding the cookie. This is fun for gardening or herbal groups.

Herbal Fortunes

Aloe	Through patience comes wisdom.
Basil	Romance your soul and be one.
Bay Laurel	Greatness is achieved, honor restored.
Betony Lamb's Ears	Negative thoughts are gone.
Borage	You have the courage of your convictions.
Chamomile	Relax and join nature.
Curry	Hidden worth is easily brought forth.
Dill	The "evil eye" of one close to you will not work.
Dittany	Passion has many forms, look closer.
Fennel	See all around. Believe half.
Garlic	Magic is afoot.
Horehound	You can break the spell.
Lemon Balm	Sympathy is needed for someone close.
Parsley	Have a party.
Pot Marigold	Joyfully play with the fairies.
Rosemary	Remember the good times.
Rue	The state of grace knows no boundaries.
Santolina	Trust your instincts; proceed cautiously.
Savory	Visualize your expectations.
Thyme	Join the nature beings.
Violet	Modesty has its rewards.

SECTION II

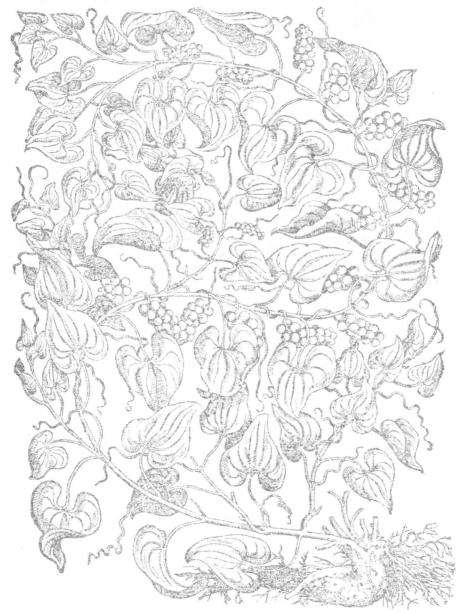

Grow and Use
Your Own Herbs

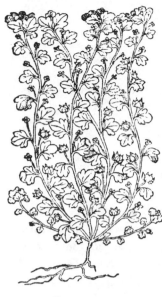

10

How to Organically Grow Herbs

SPEEDWELL

A good gardener is a man who cultivates the soil.

—Karel Capec

The study of herbs heralds a return to a more natural way of life from our preindustrial heritage. In studying herbs, we look at their usefulness to humanity and our environment. Herbs are intricately linked with our scientific, economic, and belief systems. Herbs are coming back into vogue as culinaries, medicinals, cosmetics, and insect repellents.

By 2700 B.C., the Chinese had begun cultivating herbs for medicinal teas on a scientific premise. It is believed they learned much of their knowledge from the Tibetans, who farmed state-owned medicinal gardens. The Persians planted the first herb gardens, accenting aromatic, scented plants that attract bees. Municipal gardens were available for popular use in Nineveh. In European herbals and pharmacopoeias, the Greeks and Romans provide references to herbs useful to this day.

Herbs lost popularity during the industrial age. The medical profession has now returned to the study of herbs to free us from the undesirable side effects of many chemically produced drugs. Herbs are marketed for profit with little regard for old-fashioned herbalism, where our hands are in the soil and our hearts are enjoined with the miracles of Nature.

Herbs are intricately linked with our scientific, economic, and belief systems.

~

However, the individual continues to search for simple, inexpensive, and safe ways to enrich vitality.

Organically grown herbs create an ecologically balanced and unpolluted environment. They are attractive, easy to grow and maintain, and supply vitamins and minerals for a wide variety of homemade products. Enjoy!

Amend the Soil

Herbs thrive in a soil pH of 6.5 to 7.0, which is considered neutral. Soil pH is a value that measures the acidity or alkalinity of soil. Measurement begins at 0 and ends at 14. Below 7.0 is acidic; above 7.0 is alkaline. Acidic soil is sandy; alkaline soil is clay, chalky, or rocky. Correcting soil pH will assure proper absorption of nutrients from the soil. If you have acidic soil, add woodashes, eggshells, limestone, or dolomite. Alkaline soil can be corrected with sand, leaf mold, and pine needles. To prepare leaf mold, rake your leaves in the fall, wet them with tap water, and allow them to decompose. Work amendments into the soil until it crumbles easily. Amendments, such as dolomite and limestone, have suggested amounts listed on the packaging. The soil should remain dark in color after the final amendments, a sign of high nutrient content.

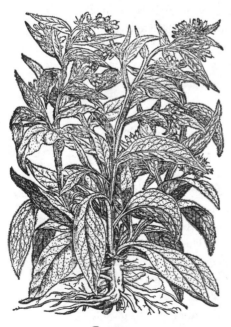

COMFREY

Soil pH can be tested by your local county extension service or local nursery. Samples from several areas should be gathered and sent to a lab in a packaged container obtained from the agent. An analysis will be mailed with suggestions that will balance the acidity and provide missing nutrients, such as nitrogen, calcium, magnesium, zinc, and iron. The cost is usually under ten dollars.

To improve texture, drainage, and aeration, combine well-drained loamy soil, humus, compost, and organic matter. Dig sand into clay soils. Add bone meal, lime, and eggshells to increase alkalinity for plants such as rosemary, thyme, sage, and rue. Use compost to replace commercial fertilizers. Seaweed may be used to fertilize container plants. Add earthworms and earthworm castings to aerate garden soil. Amendments are usually done twice a year, before spring and fall planting.

Deeply rooted herbs can be grown to break up dense and poorly drained soils. Some examples are comfrey, elecampane, echinacea, evening primrose, french sorrel, and valerian.

Herbs that tolerate clay soil include bee balm, dandelion, sweet annie, burdock, yellowdock, perilla, artemesia, and several of the hardiest mints (applemint, spearmint, blackstem peppermint, and lemon balm).

Herbs that thrive in sandy soil include borage, roman chamomile, lavender, fennel, tarragon, wild carrot, and winter savory.

The Fine Art of Sowing Seed

Many gardeners enjoy growing herbs from seed. It is certainly less expensive and many herbs bolt easily from seed, like garden sage and salad burnet. Purchase seeds that are organic and untreated with fungicide and chemicals. Seeds may be started inside in late winter and late summer for spring and fall gardens. Begin six to eight weeks prior to the beginning of the season. Lightly press seeds into well-composted soil ⅛-inch apart. Use a seed tray or a shallow, rectangular planter. The diameter of the seed determines the depth of planting. Sow the tiniest seed on the surface, otherwise plant seeds three times deeper than their diameter. Directly sow the largest seeds, such as garden sage, borage, and salad burnet, into a prepared garden in early spring. Sow chervil and coriander outside in autumn and they will flourish until the following summer. Mark the area by inserting a stick through the label and planting it nearby. Use a scarecrow to deter birds from feasting on the seedlings. To ensure germination, keep the soil moist by watering daily with a fine spray to avoid disturbing the seeds.

Fine seed can be sown by shaking it from a can with tiny holes poked into the bottom. I save a juice can, poke holes in it with a knife, and use it as a seed shaker. Be sure to use soil that is of light texture and easy to crumble. This ensures that adequate light will penetrate the seeds for germination. Inside gardeners should place seed trays in a warm, sunny window or suspend grow lights three to four feet above the seed trays (grow lights may be purchased at hardware stores and require 150-watt bulbs). Fluorescent lights may be used as an alternate light source, also suspended three to four feet from the seed trays. Choose a grow light source that is compatible with you. Many gardeners are sensitive to fluorescent lights and notice a drain in their energy. I find that grow lights work better for me by increasing energy during the winter months and reducing depression. Full spectrum lights may be the best source for you and your plants; check for a local source in the phone directory.

If the seeds are sown in a flat, water it from below. Place the flat in a pan of water and allow it to soak up the moisture for several hours. Conserve moisture by covering the seed flat with black-and-white newspaper, plastic, or by slipping a plastic bag over the flat. The best temperature for seeds is 70–80 degrees. Check the seeds daily for a whitish mold, which indicates poor circulation. If this occurs, place the seeds in front of a low-speed fan until the mold disappears. Also, remember to check daily for proper moisture and always water the flat from below.

When the seeds sprout, remove them from the plastic. Continue to water from below. Seaweed can be diluted in water in a 1 to 20 proportion to facilitate germination and growth. Adding a little seaweed to water helps to produce plants with a better immune system. Spray weekly with chamomile tea to prevent damping off, which is a disease that affects waterlogged seedling roots. Without warning, the seedlings shrivel and fall over, indicating the roots are dead. If this occurs, do not use the soil, compost it; sterilize the container and begin anew with a fresh soil medium. Transplant the seedlings into bigger pots when they are 1½ inches tall. Moisten the soil before transferring the seedlings.

Check the Roots

When purchasing plants from the nursery, take a close look at the roots. Slip the plant out of the container by tapping gently on one side. Tip the plant so the soil and roots can be inspected. First, make sure there are roots: young, tender to the touch, and white. Old roots that are tough, fibrous, and discolored may be growing out of the bottom of the pot. These can be snipped off before transplanting. Established plants should have root growth to match the height of the plant. Herbs with puny roots may have been forced with chemical fertilizers and go into shock and die shortly after transplanting, or succumb to disease easily.

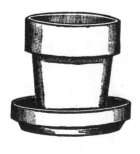

To test a good root system, roll a piece of exposed root between the index and thumb fingers. If it breaks easily, the plant will easily weaken and be unable to draw sustenance from the soil. Find herbs with a good, strong root system. Then inspect the foliage to make sure it is free from mold, rust, or insect invasion.

Begin Planting

Clean and soak all new pots you purchase. The clay pots will rob the potting soil of moisture unless soaked before using. Soak new pots two to three hours before planting. The water will saturate the pot and prevent it from absorbing moisture from the soil after the herb has been potted. Old pots can be reused if sterilized properly. Wash plastic containers with soap and water very thoroughly. Another cleaning in the dishwasher should make them safe. Clay pots or seed trays can be boiled for twenty minutes to disinfect them. Clay pots coated with hard water salts or chemical fertilizers are best discarded.

Harden off the seedlings in a cold frame or shady area before exposing them to outdoor conditions. Three days is necessary for transplants that are four to six weeks old. Hardening off is a process that prepares seedlings to make a transition to the outside garden. To harden off seedlings, move them to a shady, protected area near the house, away from wind and harsh weather. A cold frame offers an excellent environment to harden the tissues of tender seedlings. It also reduces injury from sudden temperature changes and drying wind.

A cold frame is a box with a plastic top or hinged glass top. It is often made from sealed wood two inches thick. Cedar and redwood would provide a medium that does not require a sealant. Otherwise, buy wood sealant from the hardware store and paint it on the wood to prevent rotting. We paint sealers on twice, letting them dry overnight between coats to ensure saturation of the wood tissue. Never use creosote compounds to treat cold frame wood, as toxic fumes may injure or kill the plants. Cut the boards in equal lengths and hammer them together using aluminum nails (cedar and redwood contain corrosive compounds that eat regular nails).

After four to six weeks indoors, seedlings are ready to be hardened off, weather permitting. Keep them inside until all danger of frost has passed. Allow the seedlings three days to harden off before transplanting them into a prepared garden.

Plant seedlings on a cloudy day or after sundown. Water the seedlings before removing them from the pot. Keep the original soil around the roots. Dig a hole slightly larger and deeper for the transplant—space up to eighteen inches apart to allow room to grow. Remember herbs need free circulation of air to prevent fungal infestation and space to fill out. Choose a spot that ensures proper light requirements for each herb. Water the hole with diluted seaweed (10 to 1) and make sure the water drains quickly

Harden off the seedlings in a cold frame or shady area before exposing them to outdoor conditions.

~

before inserting the herb. Then fill the hole with loose, crumbly soil and pat firmly to secure the transplant in its new home. Pinch off the top, or terminal, stem with your fingertips, pinching to the next set of lateral leaves. This encourages bushier growth. Pinching can be repeated whenever the top growth becomes spindly. After firming the top soil surrounding the plant, water again with diluted seaweed water and bless the land.

Water weekly or as needed to prevent wilting. Use well-rotted organic matter to mulch. Herbs can be mulched four to six inches deep to protect the roots against summer heat and winter frost.

Mulching

*M*ulch is a protective covering such as shredded wheat straw or shredded redwood bark spread under plants to reduce water evaporation, control weeds, and protect the roots of herbs and trees. Mulching prevents erosion by breaking the force of driving rain and irrigation while at the same time encouraging water absorption. Mulching reduces the spread of viral and fungal diseases, which can be spread by splashing water.

Mulching reduces the spread of viral and fungal diseases.

~

Organic mulch is a natural way to reduce weeds and competitive plants. Herbicides are potentially damaging to all plants, and only work at certain times of the year. Some organic sources of mulch include pine needles, wheat straw, decomposed leaves, black and white newspaper, and compost.

Pine and redwood mulches can be attractive as well as functional. They are applied two to six inches deep. The courser the material, the deeper you mulch. I have used cocoa hulls as an attractive and fragrant mulch in show beds.

Trees and shrubs are mulched deeper than plants. Organic mulches are applied one to two times yearly. Probe deeply to check soil moisture before watering. Mulching will save you dollars in watering costs and improve drainage in heavy soils. Better aeration of soil improves root growth and activity.

Compost may be used as a source of mulch, or added to an existing mulch. The compost will improve soil texture as it decomposes, adding micronutrients and increasing the population of beneficial organisms preventing fungal and bacterial diseases. Use compost to mulch during spring and fall planting when you want the mulch to decompose rapidly and nourish the soil.

Sources of Organic Mulch

Blood Meal is an excellent source of available nitrogen, acidifying the soil and repelling rabbits from your garden.

Buckwheat Hulls are fine-textured and last longer than most mulches.

Comfrey Leaves, Foxglove Leaves, and Nettles are high in iron and minerals. They are best dried and shredded, then worked into soil, compost, or other mulches.

Cottonseed Hulls are fibrous and long-lasting, yet many are contaminated with herbicides or contain verticillus wilt spores.

Grass Clippings are best composted before seeds appear. It must be applied thin and used dry or it smells and gets slimy.

Greensand supplies potassium in a slow release form.

Hay is readily available and high in nitrogen. Leguminous hays decompose faster.

Hops are available from breweries or through growers. They are fire resistant and odorous until decomposed. Their light color may add variety to your gardens and beds.

Manure may burn plants unless very decomposed. Manure normally contains many salts, airborne insects, nematodes and diseases when fresh or moist.

Oak Leaf Mold is readily available and adds acidity to the soil. Remove any wood as it may contain oak root disease. Keep moist to stop it from blowing away. It is a short-lived mulch.

Peanut Hulls normally contain many chemicals. Check your sources.

Peat Moss dries out quickly, is costly, blows away, and is already decomposed, so it adds few nutrients to the soil.

Pine Needles acidify soil as they decompose, but can catch on fire if they dry out.

Pine and Redwood Bark are long-lasting and stay in place. Make sure these have not been treated with chemicals.

Rice Hulls repel water due to high silicates. They work well in rainy climates.

SEAWEEDS are nutrients, but are not attractive and may be contaminated from oil spills. Check your sources.

STRAW does not decompose, so add nitrogen. Chop for aesthetic value.

WHEAT STRAW is readily available. It is an excellent winter mulch, but may blow away if not secured.

WOOD CHIPS last longer than sawdust and cause less nitrogen deficiency. They do not easily blow away.

WOOD SHAVINGS may pull nitrogen from the soil. They blow away easily and are unattractive. Compost first.

Hints about Compost

Composting is the acceleration of the decaying of organic matter.

Composting is the acceleration of the decaying of organic matter. Compost is a natural amendment that improves all types of soil. It is the organic breakdown of leaves, grass, black-and-white newspaper, vegetable and plant debris, pine needles, and non-animal kitchen leftovers: coffee grounds, tea, eggshells, parings of vegetables, fruits, and whatever the pets won't eat. Animal fat, skins, or flesh foods are not for composting. Cat litter makes a dangerous byproduct and is not advised for composting. Other animal manure (cow, goat, rabbit, et cetera), as well as bone meal and blood meal, will hasten the breakdown of material. Before composting, shred all plant materials with a rotary mower or shredder. Water down the pile weekly and turn it with a pitch fork every two weeks. It will heat up in the center and break down seeds and weeds. The heat will eventually repel ants, but meanwhile you can spread red pepper flakes around the compost to deter them. Ants can be beneficial in breaking down compost and helping move the materials, which will aerate the compost. Use red pepper flakes and citronella sprays to prevent them from mounding near the pathway to your compost. A citronella spray can be made by diluting one teaspoon of orange or lemon essential oil in two cups of water. Use a hand sprayer to mist the area. Mist your legs, arms, and feet to help deter ants and mosquitoes during visits to the compost.

Composting can be done in a loose pile, a wired bin, a brick or stone structure, above or partially below ground. It can be fancy or plain. Many gardeners prepare three compost bins for different degrees of breakdown. The first pile is in the very initial stage of decomposing. In one to two months, it is moved to a second pile and more manure, blood meal, and actinomycete microorganisms are added. When the material begins looking like course dirt, it is moved to a third pile. It is spread thinner and watered to enhance the decomposition. Having a succession of compost bins will speed the processing time and ensure a ready supply of compost.

You can make an indoor compost to decompose non-animal leftovers in the kitchen. Use a plastic container, such as a margarine tub, and add one tablespoon of bloodmeal or nitrogen for every four cups of materials. Sprinkle eight tablespoons of dirt in the tub and cover it with the container lid. Keep it covered. Instead of adding water, I blend scraps with a cup or less of water, then add it to the container. The finished product is a crumbly, finely textured, almost silky soil.

Gardeners amend soil with compost and humus to loosen clay and thicken sandy soil. Humus is high in nitrogen and holds water and nutrients like a sponge. Composting can also be accelerated by commercial products that add microorganisms and bacteria, increasing decomposition. Compost that normally takes one year will be ready in three to four months without the addition of manure or nitrogen. Actinomycete microorganisms ensure a steady supply of nitrogen-producing microorganisms. They may be purchased at feed stores or through mail order businesses.

You can apply less textured, more fibrous compost to fallow soil and it will continue to break down until planting season. A moderate amendment of three inches of compost will balance the soil. The pH of compost is neutral. This allows plants to freely choose their nutrients.

Compost can be worked into the soil twelve to eighteen inches deep or used as a top dressing from a half inch to three inches. Half-rotted compost can be used as mulch for the winter and worked into the soil in the spring. Plants are enhanced by increased protein metabolism, transported like ions in a chemical reaction, thus experiencing better respiration, synthesis, and photosynthesis as a result.

If you have acidic soil it can be balanced with composted limestone, wood ashes, and eggshells. Alkaline soil benefits from leaf mold, sand, pine needles, and peat moss. Peat moss aerates the soil but does not contain nutrients. These can be amended directly into the soil or topically applied as mulch. Herbs have shallow roots requiring protection with summer and winter mulching.

Add compost to container herbs when they are repotted. Seedlings can be rooted in one-half cup compost to avoid damping off. Die back of new growth and root rot fungus is rare in composted mediums because the organisms produce antibiotics and antifungal agents that offer protection to herbs grown in it.

Tips on Watering

*H*erbs may require watering when the soil is dry one inch below the surface. Insert your finger to the first knuckle or a toothpick one inch into the soil. If the soil is dry or the toothpick comes out clean, it is time to water. With rosemary and lavender, wait until the tips of the top branch droop to water. Brown tips indicate overwatering.

When testing potted plants, tap the side of a terra cotta or clay pot with a hose or your finger. If a hollow sound occurs, it is time to water. A dull sound indicates adequate moisture. When using plastic or stone containers, test the first inch of soil for moisture content or water when the soil pulls away from the sides. Whiskey barrel containers can be tested similarly.

Be sure to plant herbs in well-drained soil so the water will not stagnate and cause root rot. Amend or change the soil every six months.

Water early in the morning to allow foliage to dry in the morning sun. Watering at night can invite fungal disease because the foliage remains damp. The combination of dampness and darkness promote fungal growth. Test the water temperature to make sure it is not unusually hot or cold. Herbs prefer water temperature to be 70 degrees. This temperature will feel tepid on the inside of your wrist. Flush the soil every few months to reduce salt buildup. This tends to be more of a problem when chemical fertilizers are used, but flushing is also a time-honored practice of organic gardeners. To flush the soil, run the water at full force on the soil, allowing the ground to be thoroughly rinsed of any debris or salts. Salt buildup can occur with alkaline water, yet flushing with the same source of water still seems to refresh the soil. Salt buildup on the soil has a layer of discoloration with a gray or off-white color.

Deep-watering may be necessary for large herbs and roses. Use soaker hoses or drip water from a single hose into the area. Deep-water trees where herb beds are located during the summer and before a freeze to reduce shock and encourage the plants to establish a deeper root system. Even plants that become dormant in the winter need occasional watering. The roots remain active and require water, proper drainage, and air circulation.

During the winter months, bring potted plants inside to protect them from exposure to wind and freezes. Test the soil for moisture content every four to five days. Pots dry out faster inside with a low humidity. Before you bring your potted plants inside, it's an excellent time to repot them. New soil will help retain a higher amount of moisture content and keep the herbs healthy during the winter.

Water early in the morning to allow foliage to dry in the morning sun.

Even perennial potted plants should be sheltered inside for the winter and watered regularly. Perennials are herbs that live from year to year. Many perennials die down to their roots during the winter months and releaf in the spring. Comfrey is an example of a perennial that dies back. Some perennial herbs are evergreen, such as yarrow and soapwort.

Root Division

Perennials are divided by their root stock and planted in the spring or fall. They grow very slowly from seed and may take as long as two years to produce. Herbalists take cuttings or root divisions to start perennials. They can be purchased as an established two-year plant in gallon containers from local nurseries. Perennials can be divided after completing two years of growth. Use a sharp shovel to dig up the rootstock, which will appear as a clump of dirt, rhizomes, and roots. Divide the rootstock vertically with the shovel to subdivide the clumps of rootstock. I divide perennials into two- or three-inch diameters of roots, but there is no set rule. Gather the divided perennial and place in an appropriately sized pot, two inches wider than the diameter of the plant, or relocate the plant to a new area in the garden. Since the root system is already developed, the plant will quickly begin to produce foliage and more root growth. To ensure successful growth and avoid any further shock to the plant, water after relocating with a ten-to-one seaweed solution. Repeat every week until new growth is evident.

If you are confused as to when a perennial is ready to be divided, the herb will become invasive or the center of the plant will die, leaving a circle of foliage around the bald spot. Dividing the perennial will regenerate the plant and cause it to begin multiplying again. Be sure to dig up and compost the woody center of the clump.

Cuttings

Many herbs can be propagated from stem cuttings: lavender, sage, thyme, rosemary, geraniums, curry, pineapple sage, mints, basil, oregano, and lemon verbena. If the herb has four inches of tender stem growth, you can root a cutting. It is the same process your grandmother called taking a "slip."

Choose a healthy plant to propagate cuttings. Dip a sharp pair of scissors in alcohol for sterilization and allow to air dry before cutting. Choose a tender, mature, nonwoody stem four inches in length. The item should bend easily and not be in bloom.

Strip the bottom third of leaves and dip the stem into a ten-to-one dilution of seaweed water. The exception is scented geranium cuttings, which are left to harden overnight in a cool, shady spot before planting in rooting soil. A good rooting medium is equal parts sharp sand (to facilitate drainage) and compost. A very finely textured organic potting soil will also work to root cuttings. Insert each cutting into damp, loose soil. I make a hole with my index finger or a small stick, then I place the cutting into the soil and push the soil together. This will ensure the cutting is not damaged by pushing it into the soil. Use a clean two-inch pot, container, or seed flat, washed thoroughly with warm, soapy water (dish soap will do). Be sure to rinse in warm tap water three or four times to complete the cleaning process.

After placing the cuttings in a container, water with seaweed solution and place the container in a loose plastic bag and secure with a twist tie. This will increase humidity and reduce moisture loss until the cuttings develop roots. Leave the cuttings away from direct sunlight for seven to ten days, then water with a ten-to-one solution of seaweed water. The cuttings have grown roots by the tenth day. When the tops show new growth of foliage, remove the plastic bag and water every other day with a ten-to-one seaweed solution. Keep the new plants in a warm spot to increase root development and prevent the rooting medium from waterlogging. To prevent the cuttings from drying out, open the plastic bag and mist the cutting without disturbing the soil every other day. Use room temperature tap water or the ten-to-one seaweed dilution. The cuttings can be moved into the next larger-sized pot within two weeks.

Check the roots by turning the plant on its side and tapping lightly to dislodge the plant. The roots should fill the container before transplanting and may already be growing out of the bottom of the container. Trim off any roots that are not tender and white with a pair of sterilized scissors. Sterilize scissors by dipping them in alcohol and allowing them to air dry.

Occasionally I have neglected my transplants until they have become rootbound. The roots have tightly wound around the inside edges of the pot looking for a way out. Before transplanting into a larger container, I cut an X across opposite sides to cut through any dead roots and stimulate new growth (use your fingernails or a scissors to cut an X in the roots). Loosen the soil to allow the roots adequate growing space and compost any debris.

To transplant into the next larger container, fill the pot with the compost and potting soil in equal proportions. Water the medium with a ten to one seaweed water dilution and create a space in the soil for the transplant. Either spoon out the soil or scoop it out with your fingers. Place the transplant into the soil, remembering to loosen the soil around the roots. Pat the soil into place, adding extra soil if necessary until the soil is half an inch from the top of the container.

How to Feed Your Herbs

*U*nderfed plants are targets for predators. Insects often prefer diseased leaves and plants. They are Mother Nature's cleanup crew. The two main varieties are sucking and chewing insects. They can be repelled by a strong herb's immunity; sturdy stems, often turning woody, and high concentrations of volatile oils may be toxic to many insects. Plants protect themselves from insect invasion by sending repellent or toxic compounds to sucking or biting insects. They also pressurize their cells to make nibbling difficult. Puny plants are a direct result of deficient and imbalanced soil. Organic amendments will replace nutrition in the soil and encourage beneficial microorganisms and balance the pH.

Overfed plants can attract unwanted insects.

Overfed plants also can attract unwanted insects. Overfertilized plants are called "forced." They are fertilized every week, instead of every six to eight weeks, to produce lush foliage. A problem occurs because the herb has not had time to develop an equal amount of roots to support it. The plant produces weak stems and the plant falls prey to insect invasion. Organic growers use compost, mulch, and natural amendments that contain beneficial microorganisms to control bugs and promote natural growth patterns. We fertilize our herbs with fish emulsion and seaweed. Fish emulsion is a nitrogenous fertilizer made from discarded fish parts. It is a time-honored fertilizer used by the coastal Native Americans. It smells so bad, even deodorized, that it is hard to overdo it. I dilute a tablespoon in a gallon of water and spray the leaves of my herbs. This is known as foliar feeding. The nutrients go directly to the leaves and are quickly absorbed. I use a lawn sprayer, which can be purchased at a nursery or hardware store. The greatest effects of fertilizing are evident in three to four weeks.

In general, herbs require very little fertilization, just good drainage and amended soil. Your county extension service can test soil to determine soil requirements. If your herbs look pale and the leaves drop easily, consider adding nitrogen from fish emulsion, compost, or by planting legumes nearby. Earthworms and bug excretions add nitrogen to the soil (so does lightning, in case you have a lightning rod).

How to Feed the Bugs

There's another reason insects prefer overfed and puny plants. They need the high carbohydrates produced by chemically fed plants. High percentages of carbohydrates in a plant make it smell and taste sweeter to an insect. Plants that are not grown in an organic medium, or are chemically fertilized, produce a higher percentage of carbohydrates compared to protein and trace minerals (Rodale Press, Inc., *The Organic Way to Plant Protection*). This spells dinner to a host of preying insects.

The following is a list of organic fertilizers that will feed your herbs instead of the bugs.

BLOOD MEAL is derived from dried, ground blood collected at slaughter houses. It has a high percentage of nitrogen: 15 percent. Use it sparingly as a fertilizer. Dilute one teaspoon in a cup of water applied to each herb, especially blooming herbs.

LEAF MOLD is the product of rotting leaves. They contain five percent nitrogen and are excellent fertilizers for acid-loving plants, such as comfrey, foxglove, and roses.

DRIED MANURE of rabbits, sheep, goats, horses, and cows contains at least two percent nitrogen. Make a solution with one cup of manure to a gallon of water and apply to the soil.

COLLOIDAL PHOSPHATE is an excellent source of minerals for blooming herbs. Add a teaspoon to your herbs to encourage blooms.

SEAWEED is another excellent source of minerals. Dilute one tablespoon in a gallon of water and foliar feed your herbs.

Common Deficiencies: How to Spot the Problem

A sick herb tells us the soil medium is imbalanced.

~

A sick herb tells us the soil medium is imbalanced. Plants naturally absorb proper nutrients from organic soil. Commercial formulas add nitrogen, phosphorus, and potassium to the soil in formulated proportions, like 5–10–10. The problem is that plants cannot add and your soil may not need one of those nutrients. When a nutrient is deficient in the soil, or blocked from absorption, the plant finds a way of telling us. Here's a few examples of common deficiencies.

PHOSPHORUS DEFICIENCY. Slow leaf production and whitefly infestation may be a phosphorus deficiency. Bone meal, blood meal, and natural rock phosphate added to indoor and outdoor plants will help. Just work a few tablespoons into the soil of established herb beds or a teaspoon to the soil of a potted plant.

IRON DEFICIENCY. When leaves begin to yellow and the veins remain green, it is an iron deficiency. This is common in alkaline soil where the high calcium content blocks iron absorption. Foliar feed with one tablespoon of fish emulsion in one gallon of water. Acidify the soil with organic compost such as leaf mold. Powdered, chelated iron can be directly added to the soil. Follow the directions listed on the container. If iron deficiency occurs in potted plants, repot them with fresh, organic soil.

SULFUR DEFICIENCY. When new foliage begins to yellow, without the veining evident in iron deficiency, it indicates a sulfur deficiency. This is prevalent in alkaline soil. The deficiency will eventually affect young and mature foliage. Sulfur dust can be added to the soil. Follow the directions listed on the package.

MAGNESIUM DEFICIENCY. Yellowing of leaves may also indicate a magnesium deficiency. Leaves will then turn bronze or reddish in color. Mature foliage may drop off or the leaves may become thin, brittle, and infested with mites. Mites leave a silvery spider web on the back of leaves. To balance the soil, dilute one cup of Epsom salts in a gallon of water and add it to the soil. Then work in some organic compost and watch your herbs grow for it. Magnesium deficiencies can be caused by overuse of chemical fertilizers high in potassium. The high potassium content blocks magnesium uptake from the soil. It's very important to keep the soil balanced in mineral content by adding organic compost. The herbs know what minerals they need and work with Nature to remain in balance.

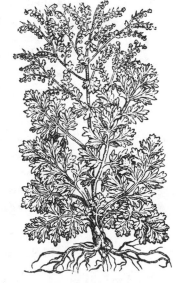

ZINC DEFICIENCY. Chemical superphosphate fertilizers can also cause zinc deficiencies, which is difficult to ascertain. The leaves may appear small or yellow between the veins. In Texas, zinc deficiencies are associated with puny pecans. Pecan growers spray a zinc amendment on their trees in March to ensure a good crop. Zinc sprays are easily absorbed by the plant and should be applied early in the day with minimum wind disturbance. Dilute three teaspoons in a gallon of water for foliar application. To prevent nutrient deficiencies in the future, add composted amendments rich in nutrients.

WORMWOOD

What Herbs to Grow: A Beginner's Herbal

As you meet these darlings of Mother Nature, choose ones suited to your soil and light requirements to grow in your kitchen garden.

ALOE *(Aloe* species, *liliacea).* I am a native of the African Congo and Mediterranean. My fresh gel is a home remedy for acne, burns, abrasions, and skin cancers. I prefer a sunny location with well-drained soil. Grow me as a container plant and propagate my pups. Protect me from winter freezes. Harvest my largest outer leaves by splitting them open and scraping out my gel.

ARTEMISIA *(Artemisia* species). I originated in the Mediterranean and now include over four hundred in my family. I love full sun and can grow in poor soil. I repel aphids and insects because my oil is toxic. I am grown as an ornamental. My Sweet Annie and wormwoods are also aromatic. I am safe to use externally as a pain reliever. I grow prolifically. I have naturalized in all temperate climates. I am especially liked because I repel mice.

BASIL *(Ocimum basilicum).* Because I am from the Mediterranean, I require several hours of sunlight and composted soil. I grow from seed and my cuttings root in water as an aromatic, culinary, medicinal, and cosmetic herb. My pesto makes a great meal out of the simplest pasta. Plant me near tomatoes, onions, and garlics and harvest me often.

BAY LAUREL *(Laurus nobilis).* I am a native of the Mediterranean grown as a tender perennial. I require protection from wind and cold winter freezes. I propagate from cuttings that take several months to root. My popularity comes as a culinary herb but my oil is also good for sprains. I used to adorn the heads of heroes, but now I am used in grains to keep weevils from hatching there.

BEE BALM *(Monarda didyma).* I am a mint with a delicious citrus flavor. My beautiful scarlet flowers attract pollinators and hummingbirds. My leaves are brewed into the Oswego tea that replaced English tea after the Boston Tea Party. I thrive in a wide variety of soils and light conditions. Leave me plenty of room to grow and I will make you a butterfly garden.

SALAD BURNET *(Poterium sanguisorba).* I am a member of the rose family with leaves that taste like cucumbers. I come from the Mediterranean and have naturalized in most soils and climates. I produce mounds of lacy green leaves and propagate easily from seeds. Enjoy me in salads and vinegars and allow me to mulch myself in the winter.

BETONY LAMB'S EARS *(Stachys officinalis)*. I am a perennial herb growing wild from Europe to Siberia. My soft leaves contain tannic acid and can be used as a natural band-aid. I propagate from seed and division in well-drained soil. Grow me as an ornamental or a pet.

BORAGE *(Borago officinalis)*. I am an annual native in many continents. I self-seed and need plenty of sun and room to sprawl in rich garden soil. My hairy leaves can be bruised to make a soothing compress and my beautiful blue flowers may help relieve a fever. Even my seeds are healing for the skin as a compress.

CATNIP *(Nepeta cataria)*. I am a native mint of Eurasia. Although cats get a little crazy by smelling me, people get calmer by drinking my tea. I am safe for children and combine well with other herbs to relieve colds and fevers. I propagate from seed and division and grow well in light shade.

CHAMOMILE *(Chamaemelum nobile* or *matricaria recutita)*. I am a native to many continents, soothing people of many nations. I propagate from seed sown in the early spring in sandy, well-drained soil in filtered light. My nobile variety is a perennial called Roman chamomile, a sweet-smelling lawn cover. The matricaria variety is the erect annual known as German chamomile. I can help in many ways, from soothing a baby's colic to keeping insects away. Try growing me in a fall garden when the heat is not so hard on me.

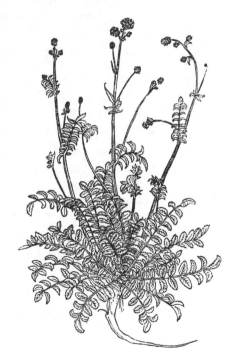

SALAD BURNET

CHIVES *(Allium* species). I am a native of the Mediterranean and Europe, a most ancient source of food and medicine. I love sunshine and propagate from seed and divisions, making an excellent border plant. Toss me in salads and dips, add my blossoms to soups, and allow my spicy flavor to season your food, lower your blood pressure, and repel insects in your garden. I give a lot and require only minimal care.

COMFREY *(Symphytum officinale)*. I originated in Eurasia as a great healer. I love rich, moist soil and filtered sunlight. I propagate easily from root division or seed. Externally, I can mend bones, regenerate skin, and heal a variety of skin ailments. Use me often or I will take over your garden.

CRETE DITTANY *(Dictamnus)*. I am a Mediterranean herb from the oregano family. I am an ornamental container plant with fuzzy, silvery leaves. Bring me inside for the winter and let the cats enjoy rubbing against me. I'm really cute.

Make an insect repellent from epazote leaves.

CURRY *(Helichrysum angustifolium)*. I am a tender perennial from the large compositae family. My silvery leaves love sunshine and repel aphids. I need winter protection and low humidity. My leaves taste like curry and my yellow button flowers are known as everlastings. Use me in dried fragrant herbal bouquets.

DANDELION *(Taraxacum officinale)*. I am a hardy perennial salad weed originating from Eurasia. Weed killers were invented for herbs like me. As a culinary herb, my leaves are an excellent blood tonic and diuretic. My roots can be roasted and brewed as coffee. Let me live near fruit trees and I will help them produce more fruit. Just don't pull me up—I'm a nonallergic lawn cover that blooms, perfect for xeriscaping.

DILL *(Anethum graveolens)*. I am an annual native of the Mediterranean. I grow easily from seed, but do not transplant me once I become established. I produce seeds and foliage for culinary pleasure in full sun and composted soil. Plant me away from fennel or you won't enjoy the flavor of either one of us.

ECHINACEA *(Echinacea pupura)*. I'm an all-American. I propagate easily from seed and root division in the spring and fall. Grow me in composted soil and watch for butterflies when I bloom. My 2½- to 3-year-old roots provide an antibiotic blood purifier and mild immune stimulant. My taste will make a lemon seem sweet.

EPAZOTE *(Chenopoduim ambrosiodides)*. I'm the Mexican and South American "bean plant." I make beans digestible. I grow anywhere and reseed for next year's crop. If you don't use me in beans, make an insect repellent from my leaves. Even grasshoppers stay away from me.

EUCALYPTUS species. I originate from Australia and Tasmania. The Aborigines discovered my antiseptic and germicidal properties. My essential oil is used in many commercial products. I am a very tender perennial that can be grown in a container or a greenhouse. I prefer sun, rich soil, and a good watering.

FENNEL *(Foeniculum vulgare)*. I am a native of the Mediterranean. I grow very large and reseed easily as an annual. My edible seeds and bulb are used as a digestant. I increase mother's milk and reduce colic in babies. My essential oil is soothing to the skin and eases rheumatic pain.

GARLIC *(Allium sativum)*. I am an herb of magical powers. My properties reduce infection, fungus, blood clots, worms, viruses, and blood pressure. My fresh bulbs are medicinal. I'm a companion with many plants and propagate easily from seed and root division. You can start me growing by putting my bulb in the soil. My summer blooms entice butterflies but my odor repels chewing insects. Plant me near roses to repel aphids.

HOREHOUND *(Marrubium vulgare)*. I originated in Eurasia and North Africa. I grow in dry, sandy soil where no one else thrives. I am renowned for breaking magical spells. My taste is very bitter, so the Shakers of colonial America created recipes adding sugar to my tea. Soon they learned to make cough drops to help people with colds and coughs. In England, I was once used to flavor ale and attract bees in gardens. Grow me in a sunny place with lots of space. When my blue-green leaves shimmer in the sunlight, I'm thought to be quite attractive.

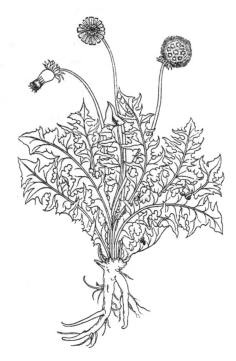

DANDELION

LAVENDER *(Lavendula* species). I am the herb of love and chastity. My aroma is calming and clean. Although my home is the Mediterranean, I've learned to live all over the world. Most of my species have crossed. My hybrid varieties yield the most oil. I can germinate from seed, but grow easily from cuttings. I must have well-drained soil and enjoy sunlight. I am an attractive container, garden, or edging plant. My French variety requires winter protection. English, Spike, and Munstead are more winter-hardy. I am a "must" for every gardener; I have a variety to suit every climate and every need.

LEMON BALM *(Melissa officinalis)*. I am a native of Southern Europe. My seeds are so vital, I have naturalized everywhere. I am a mounding mint with a reputation for lifting the spirits. My second birthday yields the most leaves for a refreshing tea. I enjoy sunlight and require well-drained soil. I look good in a container or a garden. Bees are especially attracted to me. I'm at my best growing wild on the hills of Greece, but I can adapt wherever you plant me.

LEMON GRASS *(Cymbopogon citratus)*. I'm a native of Southeastern Asia growing in tropical climates all over the world. From a distance, I may be mistaken as Johnson grass, but I'm really a very useful herb. I yield the finest commercial lemon oil and make the best culinary herb for lemon lovers. My bulb helps digest fatty meats and my leaves flavor teas, seafood, and vegetables. Grow me in full sun with lots of water. Propagate me from root division or buy a bulb at the Chinese vegetable market, root me in potting soil, and I'll be producing new leaves in three weeks.

LEMON VERBENA *(Aloysia triphylla)*. I am a native of South America. I am a deciduous lemony shrub that loses leaves every fall. Most people grow me in containers and cut me in half during the summer. I attract spider mites and white flies that suck the lemon right out of me. Check me often and spray a little pyrethrum and soapy water to kill the bugs, or plant marigolds to lure them away from me. Harvest my leaves for teas, cosmetics, and potpourris. Grow me in full sun and rich, light soil.

LIPPIA DULCE *(Stevia rebaudiana)*. I am the sweet herb of Paraguay, a cousin of kudzu. I am a newcomer to the herb market and am renowned as a sugar substitute. I grow well as a perennial ground cover in filtered light. Dry my harvested leaves before using me as a sweetener. I propagate easily from runners.

MINT *(Mentha* species). I am a native of most every continent. I once was a beautiful nymph until Persephone changed me into an herb. I've been around the world, renowned for being the most useful aromatic herb. I serve a million cups of tea daily and grow in most herb gardens as a perennial. I propagate easily from cuttings and can root in water. I like shade and moisture, but I can adapt to many conditions. Just don't plant me next to chamomile—I don't like the competition.

MARJORAM *(Origanum majorana)*. I come from North Africa and Asia and have done well in the Mediterranean countries. The Greeks know me as "the joy of the mountains," the herb of love, a favorite of Aphrodite herself. I am popular as a culinary, cosmetic, and strewing herb. Pro-pagate me from cuttings. Be patient if you sow my seeds. Plant me in a sunny, well-drained area or in a container. Protect me from winter freezes and I'll make you a wonderful butter.

MULLEIN *(Verbascum thapsus)*. I am a roadside weed grown in many countries as a biennial. My silvery-gray leaves and three-foot stalk of rosette flowers make an attractive container plant or background in the garden. I grow easily from seed every spring. My flowering stalk can be dipped in wax for a true herbal candle. My furry leaves make a fresh compress or a tea for sore throats and colds.

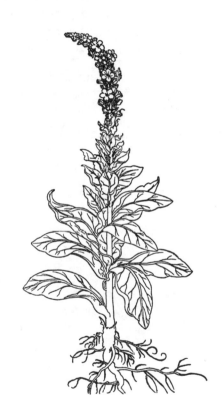

MULLEIN

OREGANO *(Oreganum)*. I am the jazzier cousin of marjoram, originating from the Mediterranean. I escaped in America and Europe to grow wild and free. Although my greatest fame has been culinary, my oil can be diluted to ease rheumatic and sprained joints. I grow in sunny, well-drained soil and can make an attractive hanging basket. I propagate easily from seed, root division, and cuttings. Keep me near the kitchen so you can enjoy me often.

Parsley is a culinary delight as well as a deodorant and diuretic.

~

PARSLEY *(Petroselinum crispum)*. I am a native Mediterranean culinary delight and a well-known deodorant and diuretic. I contain many vitamins and minerals when eaten fresh. Soak my seeds before sowing them into the soil. I germinate within six weeks. Although I am a biennial, I am often grown as an annual. My seed, leaves, and roots are all medicinal, especially when grown in moist, composted soil.

PERILLA *(Perilla frutescens)*. I am an Asian mint, known as "Japanese beefsteak." I have frilly purple leaves and I'm often mistaken for purple basil. I propagate from seed very easily and grow anywhere I land. My leaves make a beautiful, spicy, pink vinegar and my seed heads are quite attractive in dried arrangements. Wherever you plant me, you'll see me again next year.

ROSEMARY *(Rosemarinus* species). I'm the herb of remembrance, a perennial evergreen shrub from the Mediterranean. I grow in sunny places in well-drained alkaline soil. I propagate best from cuttings of soft, tender stems. Harvest me anytime you want to make an elegant chicken dish or an exquisite homemade hair rinse. My essential oil is a remedy for headaches, depression, and rheumatism.

RUE *(Ruta graveolens)*. I am a native European, the herb of grace. I like well-drained soil in a sunny, romantic garden. I can also be grown as an attractive container plant. My blue-green foliage looks great next to silvery herbs. I bloom bright yellow flowers all summer and propagate from seed, cuttings, and division. My volatile oil may cause photosensitivity and blistered skin, so plant me as a background plant.

SAGE *(Salvia officinalis)*. I am a native Mediterranean herb that has naturalized as far north as Canada. I'm a hardy perennial that requires little care. Because most people overwater me, I get root rot. I don't even like humidity. I bolt easily from seed and also propagate from cuttings. Gardeners use my tea as an insect repellent, cooks stuff their holiday turkeys with my leaves, and aromatherapists relax sore muscles with my essential oil. I'm a great herb for menopausal symptoms and a decongestant for sinus congestion. I'm reputed to be an excellent companion for longevity.

TANSY *(Tanacetum vulgare)*. I am a European weed, naturalized along roadsides in North America. I am a hardy perennial propagated easily from seed or division. I can repel ants and many insects, produce a yellow dye from my button flowers, and clear the skin of blemishes as a lotion. I enjoy full sun but can thrive in shade. Although my leaves are rather graceful, I've been accused of being invasive. I'm used to roaming freely along roadsides and still like to have my space.

THYME *(Thymus vulgare)*. I am the herb of courage, originating from the Mediterranean. I hid in the fleece of imported sheep and naturalized in North America. I'm a neat herb, requiring little space or care. I like sun, a well-drained, dry soil, and a small crevice to grow. My properties are antiseptic. I'm a real killer for colds. I enhance the flavor of many foods and taste good with many other herbs. I propagate easily from seed, cuttings, and division, growing as a perennial herb in a garden.

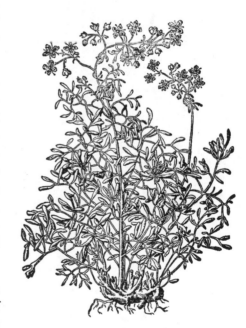

RUE

VIOLET *(Viola odorata)*. I am a Eurasian herb of innocence. I grow along shady, wooded areas and naturalize in limy soil. I propagate easily from division and self-sow by runners. I am a handsome addition to a rock garden or a border. My flowers can be candied and my leaves can be bruised and applied to wounds. My perfume is popular, but usually synthetic. I'm a favorite in nosegays and tussie mussies.

YARROW *(Achillea millefolium)*. I am a European weed named after the god of war, Achilles. My bruised leaves can stop bleeding and my flowers reduce fevers. The essential oil distilled from my flowers, azulene, is a powerful antiseptic. I grow in full sun and adapt to many soils. Propagate me by division or seed as a border plant or ground cover. I am an ancient healer who has been around since Neanderthal times.

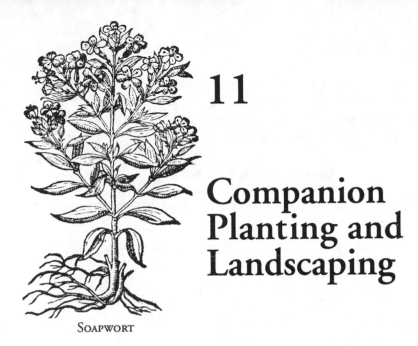

SOAPWORT

11

Companion Planting and Landscaping

Companion plants are friends and gardening
with them is like planning a party.

efore humanity can work with nature, we must first become a part of it. Herbs have become mediators between plants and humans, teaching us to utilize Nature's bounty to repel and attract pests and pollinators to harmonize with Mother Nature. An example of this is the concept of companion planting.

Companion planting is a practice organic gardeners use that demonstrates how certain plants are synergistic and aid one another by growing near each other. Edible companion plants also taste good together. For example, basil repels the tomato hookworm, thrives in similar light, soil, and water conditions as tomatoes, and tastes delicious when eaten together. Companion plants are friends. They have similar requirements, enjoy the same growing conditions, and ward off each other's predators. Chemical synergy will also encourage ripening.

Gardeners also use companion planting to reduce the need for insecticides and chemicals. Planting a variety of companion herbs in one area will lessen viral infestation and the need to compete for nutrients. The variety of scents, textures, and colors will confuse and repel pests and attract pollinators and beneficial insects. Beneficial insects, such as ladybugs, will eat aphids and harmful insects.

Before humanity can work with nature, we must first become a part of it.

～

Companion planting may enhance your garden by reducing the need for insecticides and chemicals. Interplanting will lessen viruses and competition for nutrients. The variety of colors, odors, and textures may confuse or repel pests, as well as attract pollinators and predator insects.

Advice on Pest Control

*H*ere's a better way to prevent insect invasion than choking your herbs with chemical sprays.

- Create a balanced, organic soil environment. Use organic compost and amendments.

- Adjust the soil pH to 7.0.

- Companion plant to reduce infestation. Plant chives or silvery herbs like silver king artemisia to reduce aphids.

- Vary the color, size, texture, and scent of plants to confuse insects.

- Rotate crops, amending the soil biannually, to reduce fungal and viral disease prone to one crop. Amend the soil to introduce microorganisms which will reduce nematode and fungal growth.

- Use plant traps, colors, and pheromones to lure insects away from your garden. Marigolds will lure spider mites away and yellow or sticky paper will attract whiteflies and catch them.

- Remove dead or diseased debris and weeds to prevent insects such as grasshoppers from hatching or overwintering in their protection.

- Row covers and netting deter chewing insects. They are available at feed stores and nurseries.

- Use biological insect control. Release ladybugs at night to reduce aphids. Dig earthworms into the soil to enhance aeration and reduce fungal disease. Use lizards and frogs to reduce the insect population. (They are obtainable from local nurseries, except for the frogs. Visit a nearby pond and catch a few. For advice, ask an eight-year-old.)

- Spray with soapy water and plant-derived insecticides only when necessary and after using biologicals, companion planting, and common sense. See recipes under Natural Insecticides, page 255.

What's Eating Your Herbs?

*A*lthough these insects are described in the singular, they may never appear in your herb beds alone!

APHID *(Aphidae* family). A pear-shaped, soft-bodied insect ⅒-inch long. There are over four thousand varieties of green, yellow, or black aphids. They suck the nutrient juices from the underside of new plant growth and excrete a sticky residue called honeydew. They are repelled by silvery plants such as silver king artemisia and curry.

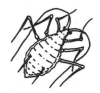

APHID

CARROT WEEVIL *(Listronotus oregonensis).* A long, brown, hard-shelled insect whose larva tunnel into the tops and roots of carrots, parsley, dill, and fennel plants.

CUTWORM *(Noctuidae* family). A ½-inch long chewing insect that characteristically curls up when disturbed. They come in a variety of colors and feed at night. Cutworms chew at the base of a plant, cutting it off at the stem. They lay dormant near the base of the plant during the day and can be removed easily.

IRIS BORER *(Papaipema nebris).* An inch-long caterpillar that burrows into the orris iris from the top down to the root, causing browning and rotting.

LEAF MINER *(Liriomyza* species). A ⅛-inch maggot that tunnels between the upper and lower leaf surfaces. They leave a white trail on the affected leaves and hatch into a small, black fly with yellow stripes, reproducing three to four times a year.

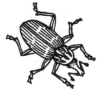

CARROT WEEVIL

MEALY BUG *(Pseudococcus adonidum).* A ¼-inch elliptical, short, spiny, sucking insect. The spine is white and waxy, allowing any eggs laid to stick to soft-stemmed plants for feeding. The honeydew secretions promote sooty mold visible on the plant's stem. They infect house and greenhouse plants.

MINT FLEA BEETLE *(Longitarsus menthaphagus).* A tiny, dark beetle that hops around like a flea. The mature adult eats holes in mint leaves, leaving them looking riddled. The larva is white and feeds on mint roots, often destroying the plant.

NEMATODE *(Meloidogyne).* A microscopic worm that feeds on the root of plants. The affected roots form galls, which appear as knots on the plant's roots. Galls prevent the uptake of water and soil nutrients resulting in stunted growth and eventual death to the affected plant.

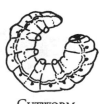

CUTWORM

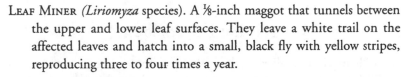

PARSLEY WORM *(Papilio polyxenes asterius)*. A 2-inch, bright green caterpillar with yellow and black stripes. They have a voracious appetite and feed on parsley, dill, fennel, and carrots before transforming into beautiful black swallowtail butterflies.

SCALE *(Coccidea* family). A sucking insect of various colors and shapes. The insect is 1 inch long and encased in a hard shell. Their secretions create honeydew and promote sooty mold. Affected plant leaves may become chlorosed, turning yellow with characteristic green veins.

SCALE

SLUGS AND SNAILS *(Mollusca* phylum). These are slimy, dark mollusks with prominent antennae. They can be ½–4 inches long. Their soft bodies leave a white trail on leaves. They feed at night on soft-stemmed plants and seek shelter in cool areas during the day.

SPIDERMITES *(Tetranychus urticae)*. A microscopic orange, brown, or green spider. Both adult and nymph suck on plant leaves until the leaves become speckled with silver spots and turn yellow. To test for spidermites, tap a plant sample over white paper. Spidermites will look like tiny red or black specks that move. They thrive in dry climates and often infest nurseries and green houses.

WHITEFLY *(Trialeurodes vaporariorum)*. A microscopic moth that sucks nutrients from the leaves, stems, and buds of a variety of plants.

Natural Insecticides

*M*illions of insects live off the herbal kingdom. They coexist in a way that has not deterred the natural balance and development of plants. However, there comes a time in every organic herbalist's life when an infestation occurs that requires an insecticide. My first choice is usually an herbal repellent (see next page). My next choice is a soapy water spray made from one tablespoon of insecticidal soap, or dish soap other than Ivory, to one gallon of water and spray it on my herbs. (A wise gardener once warned me not to use Ivory on plants because it would burn the leaves. Of course, then I had to try it . . . and he was right!) If soapy water does not work after four or five days, I get really serious and prepare a bug juice spray from the local population (see below). This usually does it, but if not, the following list of naturally derived insecticides will surely interest you.

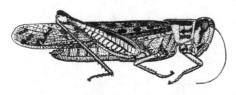

GRASSHOPPER

DIATOMACEOUS EARTH (dust) agricultural grade offends slugs, fleas, and chewing insects. D.E. kills ants and slugs. Follow the directions on the package. Dust affected plants only.

NEEM, from a tree sap in India, is nontoxic to mammals, fish, and our environment. More than one hundred sixty pests are offended by Neem. I have used Neem to kill wood borers when nothing natural worked. If you are in doubt about the nature of your pest, consider using Neem. Combine a squirt of dish soap into your solution and it will stay on the plants longer. For dilution proportions, check the label instructions.

SOAP AND/OR SOAPWORT SPRAYS are toxic to chewing insects: aphids, spider mites, mealybugs, whiteflies, stink bugs, thrips. The soap erodes the waxy outer coating of the insect's cuticle, destroying their watertight seal and causing dehydration and death. Dilute 1 tablespoon to 1 gallon of water for foliar sprays.

SULFUR DUST helps control fungal disease, although chamomile spray is safer and more effective. Soak dried chamomile flowers in cold water, covered, for several days. Strain and spray.

SALT WATER repels garden worms and spider mites. Dilute 1 tablespoon to 1 gallon water. Mist lightly.

∽ *The Ultimate Herbal Repellent* ∿

This repellent is my first choice for dealing with an infestation. Brew ½ cup each fresh thyme, sage, epazote, and garlic (use ¼ cup dried) in a quart of water for 30 minutes and strain it. Allow to cool before spraying it on the affected herbs.

∽ *Bug Juice Spray* ∿

Bugs won't land if they believe your plants are already occupied. The best part about bug juice is that it can be frozen and saved for next year. So, make some room in your freezer before the season begins! Catch several grasshoppers or crickets and put them in your blender. Blend ½ cup of bugs in 2 cups water or the above herbal repellant. Strain and spray on plants to repel infestation.

❧ *Tomato Leaf Spray* ❧

An old favorite of organic gardeners. Steep 1 quart of tomato leaves in 1 quart of boiled water for 1 hour. Strain and spray on plants to repel or confuse insects.

Herbs that Repel Insects

Insects use smell and taste to locate their dinner. These aromatic herbs may help to confuse or repel pests. **Note:** Occasionally herbs, such as cayenne and eucalyptus, can cause an allergic reaction after coming in contact with sensitive skin. Stay clear from the drift of the spray, wear long sleeves, and spray on days when only a mild breeze prevails. In case of irritation, wash thoroughly with mild soap (Ivory is fine) and cool water. Pat the skin dry.

BAY. Weevils do not easily hatch in grains when bay leaves are present.

CAYENNE. Brew 1 teaspoon in 2 cups of water for 5 minutes for a particularly offensive spray.

EUCALYPTUS OIL. Dilute 1 teaspoon in 2 cups of warm water. Rub onto skin of animals or people for insect repellent. Spray on plants.

FEVERFEW. Pyrethrum, the active component in feverfew, paralyzes many chewing insects. Commercial varieties of pyrethrum are isolated chemically and often added to other ingredients. To make your own brew, steep 1 cup of leaves in 2 cups of boiled water for 15 to 20 minutes. Strain and spray.

GARLIC. Companion plant near roses, fruit trees, or garden vegetables. Garlic spray may deter insects and animals. Add several grated cloves to one quart of boiled water. Strain and spray.

HOLY BASIL. Companion plant to confuse insects.

LAVENDER OIL. To repel moths, apply to a cotton ball and hang in the closet.

LEMON BALM. Steep 2 teaspoons in 1 cup of boiled water. Spray on greenhouse or house plants to repel insects and flies.

MARIGOLDS. Repels nematodes in the garden. For best results, plant them three months prior to planting vegetables. Gardeners till the marigolds into the soil just prior to planting.

OREGANO, WILD MARJORAM. Dry and steep 1 cup in 2 cups of boiled water. Spray to repel aphids and pests. Be sure to pick oregano that has flowered. It is much stronger.

PENNYROYAL OIL. Rub a dilution of 5 drops to 1 cup of water on skin to repel insects on animals or people. One cup of the leaves can be crushed and simmered in 2 cups of water or oil to make a home-made brew. Braid the plant around string to make a flea collar.

SAGE OIL. Repels flies, cabbage moths and aphids. Mix 1 teaspoon of sage oil in 2 cups of water or steep 1 cup of bruised leaves in 2 cups water. Strain and spray.

TANSY ROOT AND LEAVES. Strew or spray on plants to repel ants, beetles, worms, and squash bugs. Steep 1 cup in 2 cups of boiled water for 5 minutes. Strain.

THYME FLOWERS. Dry with fresh linen to repel moths and closet bugs.

THYME OIL. Dilute and spray on plants to repel and confuse aphids and pests: 1 teaspoon oil to 2 cups of water, or bruise 1 cup leaves and steep 15–20 minutes in 2 cups water. **Caution:** Thyme oil is a skin irritant.

WORMWOOD. The active ingredient is thujone, a poisonous narcotic and convulsant. Hang in closets or on wreaths to repel moths and insects.

Companion Herbs: Herbs that Grow Well Together

Here's a list of herbs and their companions. This year, plan to grow basil near your tomatoes to improve their flavor, and garlic chives near your roses to repel aphids.

BASIL: tomatoes, peppers, onions, chives, oreganos, salad burnet.

CHIVES: roses, carrots, leeks, comfrey, lavender.

CILANTRO: oregano, lemon balm, basils. Plant away from fennel and dill.

DILL: cabbage, cucumbers, basil, tomatoes. Plant away from fennel.

EPAZOTE: artemisias, lavender cotton.

FENNEL: tomatoes, flowering herbs, perilla. Fennel needs plenty of room and can be an attractive background plant.

LEMON BALM: parsley, fennel, tomatoes, onions.

LEMON VERBENA: attracts bees and butterflies. Plant near flowering herbs, bee balm, pineapple sage.

MARJORAM: thyme, lemon grass, oreganos, bee balm.

MEXICAN MARIGOLD MINT: sage, thyme, rosemary, winter savory, Mexican oregano.

MINTS: intermix basil and oregano, or holy basil and catmint.

OREGANO: thyme, lemon verbena, lemon balm, parsley, cilantro.

PARSLEY: tomatoes, roses, mints, oregano, thyme, chives, basil.

ROSEMARY: sage, dill, cabbage, lemon grass, thyme, soapwort, kale.

SAGE: rosemary, lavender, thyme, germander.

SALAD BURNET: thyme, mint, basil, oregano, tomatoes, chives, silvermound Artemisia.

SAVORY: beans, onion, tomatoes, chives, sorrel, basil.

SORREL: leeks, onions, chives, epazote, rosemary, savory, Mexican marigold mint.

How to Accent Your Landscape with Herbs

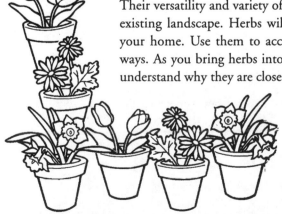

*H*erbs are a sensual and exciting addition to every landscape. Their delicate fragrances and colors appeal to the appetite, are visually attractive, and aromatically alluring. They touch every part of our senses. Their versatility and variety offer innumerable possibilities to enhance an existing landscape. Herbs will complement native plants and decorate your home. Use them to accent borders, pathways, patios, and entryways. As you bring herbs into your home and garden, you will begin to understand why they are close to Mother Nature's heart.

CONTAINER GARDENING plays a major role in design and landscaping. Containers may be made from urns, tubs, whiskey barrels, window boxes, hanging baskets, and raised beds. Terra-cotta, stone, clay, and wood are popular. Choose containers to suit your home or garden. Coordinate the colors with the surroundings. Consider seasonal and temporary plants for bedding and borders. Choose containers that are easy to move for tender shrubs, like bay and eucalyptus trees. Citrus trees and myrtles are fragrant and decorative on patios, foyers, and entrances. Look for places in and near the garden that will enhance the effect you are creating. Choose a dark green background or cluster several ornamental containers together near a walkway or brick wall. Patios are complemented by a cluster of container herbs with many colors. Cranesbill, purslane, periwinkle, butterfly, ginger, salvia, and curry plant add color and variety. A double wall is often used around a porch or patio. These ornamental stone walls look like narrow, raised beds. Rock garden herbs look good here, especially creeping thymes.

Herbs are a sensual and exciting addition to any landscape.

ORNAMENTALS, such as scented geraniums, pineapple sages, and old or miniature roses make a striking effect. Upright rosemary, lemon balm, lavender, and lemon verbenas make attractive focal-point herbs. Whenever possible, line containers with trailing rosemaries and thymes and surround the container with society garlic, yarrows, tansy, violets, ornamental sages, santolina lavender cotton, or salad burnets. Mints are appropriate when space is available.

FRAMING is another way to use containers to flank doorways. Clipped bay laurels and large topiaries of rosemaries are distinctive in pairs. Steps and sunken gardens and decks can be lined with a variety of fragrant and flowering herbs. Gates and archways can be framed with containers of miniature herb gardens, dye gardens, and "dry" flower pots. Make sure your container plants are in sufficiently deep containers and window boxes to avoid drying out easily. Mulch with an organic composted material to retain moisture.

HANGING BASKETS should be placed where they are easy to care for and are sheltered from the wind. Color and variety depends on the background. A plain wall looks good with multicolored herbs, such as variegated scented geraniums, tricolor sages, and lemon thyme, as well as trailing herbs, such as pennyroyal, prostrate rosemary, and catmint. Use lightly colored herbs against shady or dark walls. During the summer, hanging baskets may require daily watering. Buy large baskets with adequate depth to reduce withering. Wallpots of nasturtiums, calendulas, tansy, and trailing rosemary are quite attractive against brick or plain walls. Balcony containers are also attractive with trailing herbs and mints. Use lightweight containers and two inches of composted mulch.

BORDER HERBS in many varieties can be sprinkled on paths and walkways. Creeping thyme, woolly thyme, elfin thyme, and Roman chamomile can be walked on. Lamb's ears, old-fashioned stock, lemon balm, and foxglove add romance and color. Wildflower walkways may include nicotinia, evening primrose, bee balm, echinacea (purple coneflower), mullein, perilla, rose campion, and dandelion. Italian dandelions are best for their aesthetic quality.

Envision an herb garden that will harmonize with the style of your house. Formal knot gardens will enhance traditional architecture with neat rows of compact, intertwined thymes and santolinas, while modern-designed homes look better with a loosely flowing landscape of flowering perennial herbs of varying sizes, such as lavenders, rosemaries, sages, and yarrows. A kitchen herb garden can be planted outside the back door with a border of thyme and winter savory, a ground cover of oregano, and a background of rosemary, dill or fennel, sage, and lemon grass or lemon balm.

Envision a herb garden that will harmonize with the style of your house.

~

Outline the perimeters of the areas to be planted before planting. Use stakes and string to enclose the area, tapping the stakes into the corners with a hammer and stapling the string to each stake to enclose the garden. Look for areas with five to six hours of morning sun, sheltered from wind. An eastern and southern exposure is best for decorative and tender herbs, such as violets, calendulas, foxglove, tarragon, chamomile, and nasturtiums. For areas with afternoon or full sun, plant silvery herbs such as curries, sages, and artemisias, with annuals such as basil, borage, and epazote. In shady areas, catnip, mints, parsley, comfrey, and sweet woodruff will thrive.

Be sure to locate sprinklers, drip irrigation, and water sources near the herb gardens. Keep tall and drought-tolerant herbs, like lavender cotton, artemisias, sages, mullein, perilla, and lovage, as background plants against the house, wall, or fence. Annuals generally need greater watering requirements to complete their growing season. Consider planting summer savory, basil, borage, dill, chamomile, and watercress in well-watered areas.

Choose a ground cover to meet water and light requirements. Pennyroyal likes shade and water, oregano enjoys sun and rocky, dry soil. Woolly thyme and Roman chamomile are excellent choices for ground cover and thrive with minimal water and varying light requirements. These and other low-growing herbs, such as bouncing bet, violets, Corsican mint, and lamb's ears will soften every garden landscape. Plant ground cover on slopes and in cracks, corners, and rock gardens.

Fragrant herbs can be enjoyed when planted near doors, entryways, patios, and windows. Some of my favorites are antique roses, such as Champneys pink cluster, Louis Phillip, and Country Marilou. Lavenders, lemon verbenas, and rosemaries complement one another, as well as the antique roses. Scented geraniums, tangerine southernwoods, lemon balms, and pineapple sages are aromatic, low-maintenance herbs to accent entryways.

When planting herbs, give them plenty of space to grow up and out. Herbs require eighteen inches in diameter of growing space to ensure proper growth and air circulation. Be sure to balance the herb garden with a variety of tall, medium, and low-growing, colorful herbs. Choose a border of garlic chives, prostrate rosemary, salad burnet, marigolds, and winter savory to enclose the garden. Enclosure will magnify the effect of your garden. Color, varying height, and variety are appealing to the eye, appetite, and beneficial insects who will chomp diligently on invading pests. Choose native plants and varieties less likely to succumb to viral and fungal disease. Contact local herb growers, nurseries, and your county extension agent for information about the best native plants for your herb garden.

Planning the location, size, and variety of your herb garden is crucial for success. You will learn new ideas, techniques, and skills from every gardening experience, along with any mistakes. Your next design can only get better. Keep a sense of humor for the lessons Mother Nature will teach you on your path of herbal delights.

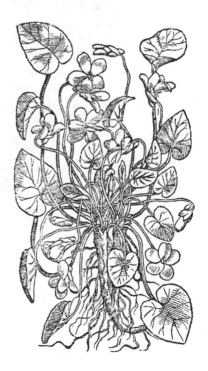

VIOLET

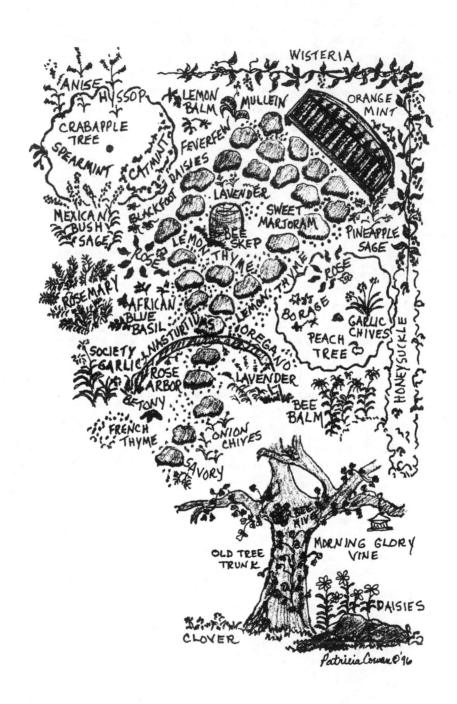

BEE GARDEN

Theme Gardens for Herbs

*N*ow that you have an idea of where your herbs are going to be growing, consider choosing a theme for your garden. Each theme will set a mood and evoke memories and feelings for every visitor walking the path leading into your special garden. Here are some suggestions to add to your own garden design.

Bee Garden

A bee garden will invite a variety of beneficial insects and hummingbirds to protect and pollinate your herbs. Bee gardens are enhanced by a sundial centerpiece or bay laurel tree as a focus. They are reminiscent of Mediterranean herbs, with a variety of scents, colors, and tastes to set the mood. Pick a sunny location with rich, well-drained soil. Select as many herbs from the following list as you can comfortably make space for in your garden design and get ready to make new friends.

Basils	Marjoram
Bee Balm	Mints
Betony	Mullein
Borage	Nasturtium
Bush Sage	Oregano
Catnip	Pineapple Sage
Egyptian Onions	Society Garlic Chives
Feverfew	Thyme
Lemon Balm	

Annual Culinary Garden

The following selection of herbs grow quickly and compete with one another to get to the dinner table. Remember to give these herbs adequate growing space, eighteen inches in diameter, and all enjoy full sun except parsley and watercress. Plant these in the shade of a taller annual like perilla or summer savory. Use the flowering annuals, marigolds, chamomile, and nasturtium, as an attractive border which will also attract pollinators and beneficial insects. Culinary herbs prefer rich, moist, well-drained soil and space to sow seeds for next year's dinner.

Basils	Marigold
Borage	Mustard (Fall planting)
Chamomile	Nasturtiums
Chervil	Parsley (Biennial)
Dandelion	Perilla
Dill	Summer Savory
Ginger	Watercress

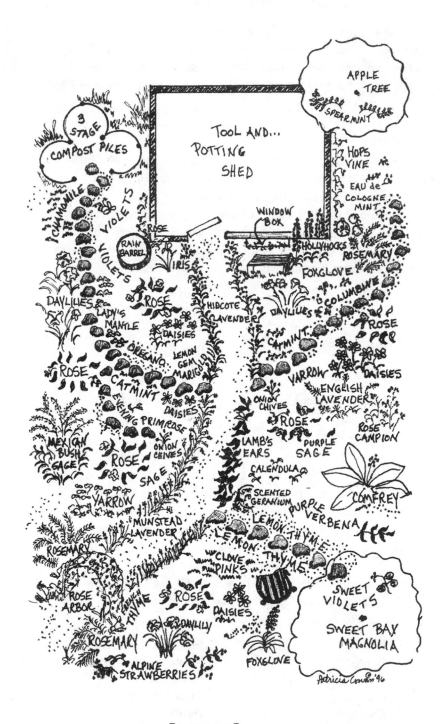

ROMANTIC GARDEN

Romantic Garden

Sunshine and waves of gentle colors greet the visitors of a romantic herb garden. Memories of medieval knights visiting young maidens with billowing skirts and garlands of daisies in their hair float through the imagination until the eyes focus on a marble statue surrounded by lilies, iris, and hollyhocks in full bloom. The following herbs enhance a romantic garden and may be interplanted in full or partial sun in sandy loam soil amended with compost and protected with an aromatic mulch, such as cocoa shells.

Columbine	Lilies
Comfrey	Marigolds
Daisies	Myrtle
Evening Primrose	Perennial Sage
Foxglove	Rose Campion
Hollyhocks	Rue
Iris	Violets
Lamb's Ears	Yarrow

Fragrant Garden

While you drift off into dreamtime in the peaceful embrace of the romantic garden, you might dream of a fragrant garden to plant nearby. The fresh scent of Sweet Annie, lavender, and rosemary under a trellis of climbing, fragrant roses, such as Lady Eubanksia, comes to mind. The nearby blossoms of wisteria and honeysuckle hanging on a nearby fence float by, while the scent of mints, violets, and sweet woodruff crushed underfoot rise to further stimulate the senses as you pass. Select a variety of scents from the following list to plant in a protected, morning sun location. Add well-composted organic amendments to the soil, such as alfalfa and horse, goat, or rabbit manure, and a few handfuls of earthworms to keep the soil aerated.

Bouncing Bet (Soapwort)	Roses
Curry	Scented Geraniums
Lavender	Southernwood
Lemon Verbena	Sweet Annie
Mints	Sweet Woodruff
Patchouli	Tansy
Pennyroyal	Violets
Rosemary	

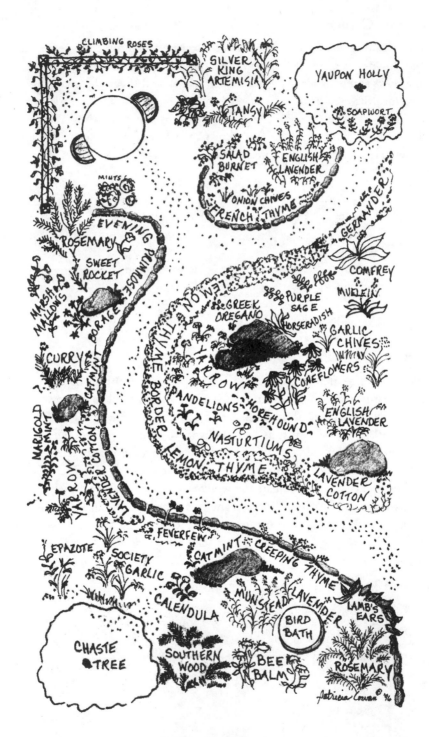

CLIMBING ROSES

SILVER KING ARTEMISIA

TANSY

YAUPON HOLLY

SOAPWORT

MINTS

SALAD BURNET

ENGLISH LAVENDER

ONION CHIVES

FRENCH THYME

GERMANDER

EVENING PRIMROSE

ROSEMARY

SWEET ROCKET

BORAGE

COMFREY

MARSH MALLOWS

CATMINT

CURRY

LAVENDER COTTON

MINT

MARIGOLD

YARROW

LAVENDER COTTON

LEMON THYME BORDER

GREEK OREGANO

PURPLE SAGE

MUELLEN

HORSERADISH

GARLIC CHIVES

YARROW

CONEFLOWERS

DANDELIONS

HOREHOUND

ENGLISH LAVENDER

NASTURTIUMS

LEMON THYME

LAVENDER COTTON

FEVERFEW

CATMINT CREEPING THYME

EPAZOTE

SOCIETY GARLIC

CALENDULA

MUNSTEAD LAVENDER

LAMB'S EARS

BIRD BATH

CHASTE TREE

SOUTHERN WOOD

BEE BALM

ROSEMARY

Patricia Cowan © '96

SURVIVOR'S GARDEN

Survivor's Garden (Tolerates Poor Soil)

For those whose yard suffers from well-drained soil deprivation, there is a survivor's herb garden. The following herbs tolerate poor, rocky soil and have been known to thrive just about anywhere. Once established in your garden, they will multiply quickly and compete for your attention by displaying unique beauty. They will bloom more when planted in areas with five to six hours of sunshine and prefer an area where they can grow uninhibited. Keep the tall plants in the background, namely bronze fennel, artemisias, epazote, evening primrose, and mullein. Use lamb's ears, chives, yarrow, thyme, germander, and salad burnet for borders. Fill in remaining space with any of the following herbs that are native in your area. Check with your local nursery or county extension agent for information on native plants.

Artemisia	Horehound
Bee Balm	Horseradish
Dwarf Borage	Lamb's Ears
Bouncing Bet (Soapwort)	Lavender Cotton
Chives	Marigold Mint
Curry	Mint
Dandelions	Mullein
Epazote	Munstead Lavender
Evening Primrose	Salad Burnet
Fennel	Tansy
Feverfew	Thyme
Geraniums	Yarrow
Germander	

Shade Garden

This garden provides a quiet, shady spot to rest. The refreshing, graceful herbs suggested here will prepare you for a quiet meditation under the outstretched arms of a shade tree. Choose an area with dappled sunshine or cool shade. The soil should be light, moist, and a little sandy with plenty of space for a comfortable chair.

Calendula	Parsley
Catnip	Pennyroyal
Foxglove	Pineapple Sage
Lemon Balm	Salad Burnet
Lovage	Tarragon
Mints	Violets

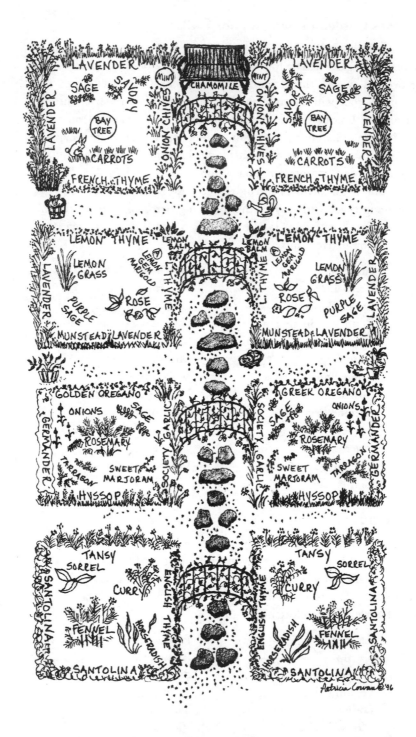

CULINARY PERENNIAL GARDEN

Culinary Perennial Garden

Culinary perennials belong near the kitchen, combined with the culinary annuals or separate if space allows. Perennial herbs die back during the winter and return in the spring. Gazing at a perennial culinary garden takes me back in time to Mexico, Central America, and South American travels. Their gardens become favorite community social areas where food is prepared nearby. That's my idea of garden fresh! In these cultures, the men grow and tend the gardens and the women cook and create new recipes of herbal delights. The following herbs enjoy growing in a culinary perennial garden in sunny, well-drained areas. Select the ones most likely to find their way into your kitchen cuisine and prepare for a bountiful harvest.

Bay	Marjoram
Carrots	Mints
Chives	Onions
Curry	Oregano
Epazote	Rosemary
Fennel	Sages
Horehound	Sorrel
Horseradish	Tarragon
Lemon Grass	Thymes
Lovage	Winter Savory

Choose edible borders of thyme, winter savory, chives, and purslane from the list of borders.

BORDERS:

Betony	Santolina
Germander	Society Garlic Chives
Hyssop	Tansy
Purslane	Thymes
Rosemary	Winter Savory

Biblical Garden

Herb gardens that tolerate poor soil bring to mind our humble roots. A biblical garden can be designed with herbs that remind you of a favorite Bible verse, holiday, or childhood memory. For example, costmary leaves were used to mark the Bibles during colonial times and angelica was so named because it bloomed on St. Michael's Day every spring. Rosemary was said to be used to lay Jesus' swaddling clothes to impart its evergreen fragrance and myrtles are mentioned numerous times in the Old Testament during Solomon's time. The following Biblical herbs enjoy partial shade and morning sun and thrive in rich, moist soil.

Aloe	Mullein
Angelica	Mustard
Comfrey	Myrtle
Coriander	Rosemary
Costmary	Rue
Mints	Sweet Woodruff

Evergreen Garden

Evergreen herbs can be used in mass plantings or alone as a centerpiece in a theme garden. They add drama to the landscape and a sense of security planted around the home. Evergreens combine well with ground cover herbs and create a fragrant hedge near and around the home. Be sure to plant hardy rosemaries in freeze zones. They can be shaped and trimmed for an outdoor Christmas tree or harvested for wreaths inside the home. Evergreen gardens are dramatic under lights. Revolving colored lights or spotlights will accent the beauty and simplicity of the family of evergreen herbs.

Bouncing Bet (Soapwort)	Rosemary (ARP, Hills
French Sorrel	Hardy varieties)
Germander	Roses
Lemon Thyme	Sage
Oregano (as ground cover)	Southernwood
Parsley, Cilantro	Thyme
Roman Chamomile	Yarrow (as a border)
(as ground cover)	

Ground Cover

For herbalists who enjoy using herbs for ground cover and in open spaces, the following herbs offer their fragrances. Use Roman chamomile, woolly thyme, Corsican mint, and pennyroyal as carpeting herbs. Plant them instead of grass for a fragrant footpath. The remaining herbs listed can be used in borders and as fillers in every garden where space is available. The ground cover herbs are excellent erosion barriers for areas where loose soil washes away easily.

Betony	Pennyroyal
Catnip (shade)	Prostrate Rosemary
Corsican Mint	Roman Chamomile
Germander	Sweet Woodruff (shade)
Lamb's Ears	Woolly Thyme
Munstead Lavender	

Lover's Garden

As we began in a romantic garden, we will end our visual journey in a lover's garden, where dreams create a new reality. Echoes of Shakespearean sonnets and footprints of fairies take us onto a stone pathway and under an arching trellis of a fairy rose with hanging clusters of tiny, pink flowers. Splashes of colors meet us as we walk toward a bubbling fountain with sparrows splashing around in circles. Soon our eyes follow a butterfly who visits every flower . . . pink dianthus surrounded by blooming silver thyme, curious columbines peeking over the pinks and blues of bachelor's buttons, the stately foxglove with freckles of fairy paths nestled near the night blooming evening primrose and highlighted by the silvery leaves of lavender that glow in the moonlight. White coneflowers bloom near a large rosemary believed to be visited by angels. Balm and lemon thyme are waiting to be touched . . . but where are the lovers? Invite one and be ready to celebrate with Mother Nature.

Bachelor's Buttons	Foxglove
Columbine	Lavender
Dianthus	Lemon Balm
White Coneflower	Lemon Thyme
Evening Primrose	Rosemary
Fairy Rose	Silver Thyme

Landscaping with Old Roses

Gardeners enjoy growing old roses with herbs to lend beauty, fragrance, and tradition; they are the perfect companions for organic herbs. There is a story behind each antique rose. They have been grown since ancient times. Hybridization of tea roses was initiated in 1867, turning a new page in the history of roses. Old roses connect us to the historical pleasures of almost every known culture. If there is one item in creation that all humankind has in common, it is a sense of awe for the exquisite beauty and fragrance of a rose. Their value in the landscape is paralleled by their low maintenance. They will delight you in their resilience and spectacular displays of blooms. Most were found in cemeteries and abandoned farms, blooming without human intervention.

Old roses are native to the entire northern hemisphere, from the equator to just outside the Arctic. They naturalize easily with minimal attention the first year. Many species are found in the wild and are naturalized by rosarians from a cutting of the original plant. Garden cultivation started in China about five thousand years ago, although roses have been around since prehistoric times. Original roses had five petals. They bloomed once and reproduced from seed. Old roses are both food for the soul and nourishment for the body.

In landscaping, old roses can be used in two ways. They can be separated in the landscape for a spectacular, singular display, or used as a supporting or background plant, a "mixer."

Plant old roses in full sun. They require six hours of sunlight to produce showy blooms. Good circulation, drainage, and slightly acidic soil will enhance the health of the roses. Old roses are heavy feeders. Include organic fertilizers, well-composted cow or horse manure, seaweed, fish emulsion, and alfalfa humus. Roses assimilate fertilizers every four to six weeks from February to October. Foliar feeding as well as root feeding is successful. Foliar feeding should be done in the early morning to allow the leaves to dry.

Place roses in well-drained soil with ample room for the roots to spread. Soak the roots one hour before planting. Wait until after the first bloom to begin fertilizing. Cut off dead wood and old blooms, cutting blooms to the fifth or seventh leaf stem to produce new blooms. Continue to apply organic amendments and soil conditioners two or three times a year, adding several inches of organic mulch to protect the roots. Deep-water during the hot summer or before the first freeze. Roses thrive on weekly deep waterings and remain disease-resistant when their leaves remain dry.

The rose looks fair, but fairer it we deem for that sweet odour which doth in it live.

—Shakespeare's Fourteenth Sonnet

Blackspot and powdery mildew can infect old roses. Foliar feeding with a dilution of baking soda or chamomile tea every few days is preventive. Dilute one tablespoon of baking soda to every gallon of water. Chamomile tea can be diluted by half for foliar feeding.

Many old roses are container size. They may require more frequent watering in the summer. Soil amendments, pruning, and maintenance are the same as ground varieties. Old roses in containers lend an attractive patio and balcony display of fragrant blooms.

Companion plant old roses with herbs and silvery foliage. Silvery foliage, such as lavenders, need less water and fertilization than roses. They companion plant best in well-drained soil. Munstead lavender makes an excellent border for an old rose garden. All varieties of dianthus, petunia, and geranium accent the gracefulness of shrub old roses. Hibiscus, hollyhock, foxglove, *hypericum* St. Johnswort, and gardenia create a striking display of color, scent, and variety. Background plants may include crepe myrtle and Rose of Sharon *(Althea officinalis)*.

Here is the story behind a few of my favorite old roses.

AUTUMN DAMASK *(Damascana bifera)* (1819) is the fragrant parent of the bourbon and hybrid perpetuals, the only repeat bloomer of the ancient Middle Eastern roses. Flowers are crumpled, double, pink, and contain the finest scent for perfume. Height may reach five feet.

CHEROKEE ROSE *(R. laevigata)* (1759) originated in southern China and has since become the state flower of Georgia. It easily grows to a height of fifteen feet with a spectacular display of early spring blooms. The flowers are pure white with golden stamens set into five petals. The thorns are huge, so consider growing Cherokee Rose as a background plant against a fence.

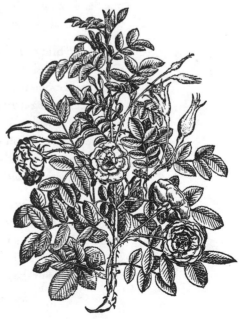

ROSES

LADY EUBANKSIA *(R. banksiae normalis)* (1796) is a vining old rose from China with slender canes and lightly scented, tiny, single white spring blooms. A double white variety became available in 1807 and a double yellow variety was introduced in 1824. All three Lady Eubanksia reach twelve to twenty feet in height, are thornless, and make a spectacular arbor or background plant. They flower better in a sheltered, sunny location, protected from strong wind and harsh weather.

FORTUNE'S DOUBLE YELLOW *(R. x Odorata pseudindica)* (1845) was discovered by Robert Fortune. She was brought to the west from a Chinese garden. She blooms once in the spring by covering her thorny ten-foot vine stalks with a profusion of salmon yellow flowers. Fortune's Double Yellow is best grown alone with support or as a background rose.

FORTUNIANA *(R. Fortuniana)* (1850) is the natural offspring of Cherokee Rose and Lady Eubanksia. She was found in a Shanghai garden by Robert Fortune. The blooms have a faint violet fragrance on large, thornless canes. An early spring one-time bloomer, Fortuniana produces white double flowers with a knotted center. Fortuniana is disease-resistant and thrives in poor soil, a blessing to any garden as a climber or a mounding shrub. She will spread eight to ten feet if left to her natural habits.

OLD BLUSH, hybrid of *R. chinensis* (1752), is better known as Parson's Pink China. Old Blush grows as a six-foot shrub or is available as a twenty-foot climber. She blooms in mass in the early spring with repeat performances until a hard freeze. She offers loose clusters of semi-double pink flowers with a soft tea rose scent. Orange rose hips form soon afterwards. Old Blush is of special interest to Americans because she is the rose that stood behind General Lee at Appomattox. Old Blush is spectacular as a border plant and equally beautiful standing alone.

LOUIS PHILLIPE (1834) was introduced by the French, but his parentage is unknown. It is a compact two-foot rose with loose semi-double blooms. The flowers bloom deep crimson to purple with white margins. It grows well in a container or garden spot in rich soil, with repeat blooms in the spring and fall.

ARCHDUKE CHARLES (before 1837) is another rose with unknown heritage. The flowers bloom crimson with pink centers, then turn crimson from the warmth of the sun. It blooms constantly and enjoys a garden spot or container home large enough to accommodate a three- to five-foot rose.

CHAMPNEY'S PINK CLUSTER (1811) was developed by John Champney of South Carolina by crossing the fragrant *R. moschata* with Old Blush. Champney's Pink Cluster became the first of the noisette roses producing quantities of pastel pink, highly scented flowers. Most are grown as climbers, displayed on a trellis or fence. Noisettes are well adapted to a southern climate.

JEANNE D'ARC (1848) is a vigorous six- to eight-foot rose with semi-double clusters of fragrant white flowers. She bears her strong musk fragrance in a spectacular fall bloom with red hips appearing at the same time. Be sure to save these and other old rose hips for a jelly or a tea.

QUEEN OF THE BOURBONS (1834) ushered in the popular fragrant Bourbon roses from the east coast of Africa. Although the parentage of the Bourbon roses is unknown, rosarians believe them to be a cross between Autumn Damask and Old Blush. They make an excellent hedge or climber roses. Queen of the Bourbons has flowers with mauve veins. She blooms in the south in the spring and fall, followed by rose hips before winter. Most of the Bourbon roses were developed after 1867 and enjoyed an immense popularity in nineteenth century gardens.

ENFANT DE FRANCE (1860) is a hybrid perpetual, an extremely fragrant rose. She is only three feet tall with silvery, double pink blooms. All hybrid perpetual roses have a multi-rose racial parentage.

VIRIDIFLORA (before 1845) is an everblooming green rose that turns bronze. It is a compact rose with a spicy fragrance. Viridiflora grows three to four feet tall and gives rosarians no hint of its heritage.

Healing from the Heart

ℰach flower has its own signature, inherent in the color, texture, and aroma of every bloom. Flowers bloom from internal stress. We are like flowers, blooming under grace, as we transcend and overcome each challenge life offers. All our treasures are in our hearts.

The heart is a symbol of the unifying life principle, the flowering of love. Herbs transcend the wisdom of reason, ruled by the head, to touch the wisdom of feeling, centered in the heart. Here is how the symbolism of the heart unfolds over the centuries and throughout various cultures and religions:

Culture/Religion	Heart Symbolism
Aztec	The heart is the center of man, his religion, his love. The heart sacrifice represented the liberation of life-giving blood to flow into eternity, a promise of constancy.
Buddhist	The heart represents purity and indestructibility, which cannot be disturbed.
Chinese Buddhist	The heart is one of eight precious organs of Buddha.
Celtic	The heart is kindness, generosity, and compassion.
Christian	The heart represents love, joy, courage, and sorrows. The flaming heart is religious zeal and devotion. A heart in hand portrays understanding and piety. The sacred heart of Jesus represents the unifying love of God, covering us with Grace.
Hebrew	The heart is the Temple of God.
Hindu	The heart is the divine center, symbolized by the lotus. The third eye is the eye of the heart, indicating transcendent wisdom.
Islam	The heart is the spiritual center, the absolute intellect, which is illumination.
Taoism	The heart is the seat of understanding. A sage has all seven orifices in his heart open, which leads to compassion and understanding.

The following flowering herbs have an affirmation of encouragement to fill the gardens of our hearts (from *Returning to the Source* [Herbal Essence, Inc., 1989] and *Romancing the Rose* [Herbal Essence, Inc., 1995]).

FLOWERING HERB	AFFIRMATION
African Violet	I am lifted up on the petals of love.
Amaryllis	I step out in faith to achieve my greatest good.
Anemone	The fullest melody of joy lies within me.
Baby's Breath	I am the beauty of innocence.
Bachelor's Buttons	I release past painful experiences.
Basil	As I accept myself, others fall into line.
Begonia	I trust my inner voice for guidance.
Borage	I learn to stand on my own.
Bougainvillaea	Unconditional love shatters the illusion of guilt.
Chamomile	I acknowledge my feelings to bloom in faith.
Daffodil	I overcome shyness with a smile.
Dandelion	My dreams set free the best in me.
Dianthus	Joy is all I know.
Dill	I am never alone.
Garden Mum	I let go of critical thoughts and accept love.
Gardenia	My relationships fulfill my deepest desire.
Geranium	The decision is mine; I am created perfect.
Iris	I bloom; therefore, I am.
Jasmine	Where order reigns, I am.
Lemon Grass	I choose loving partners.
Ligustrum	I burst forth into full bloom.
Lilac	I am the compassion of forgiveness.

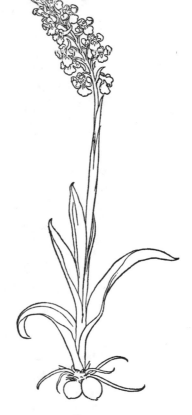

ORCHID

FLOWERING HERB	AFFIRMATION
Lily	I am the channel of love.
Magnolia	I appreciate myself.
Marigold	I love others as myself.
Morning Glory	I welcome change.
Narcissus	I bloom to share.
Onion	I am the flavor of friendship.
Orchid	I make peace with my past.
Pansy	I bloom to remind you that death is an illusion.
Penta	It is safe to love.
Peppermint	I am untouched by the fear of loss.
Periwinkle	I am the memory of creation.
Pine	I bury the past and look forward to the future.
Poppy	I look within to find happiness.
Primrose	I am the vessel of every kind and loving thought.
Ranunculus	Kindness is my fame.
Red Carnation	I am worthy of your affection.
Rosemary	I am the memory of peace.
Rose of Sharon	I am the benediction of peace.
Scarlet Sage	I am the seed of inspiration.
Soapwort	I am the rainbow of promise.
Stock	I step forward to declare the independence of unlimited mind.
Sunflower	I am the calling of peace, dissolving separation.
Sweet Annie	I am the simplicity of grace.
Tansy	I am the protector of gentle souls.
Thyme	I attract the magical qualities of Nature.
Verbena	I am the key to inner grinning.
Wisteria	Only beauty remains . . . .

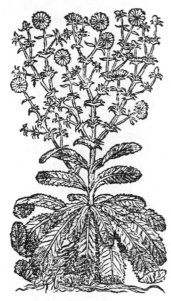

12

The Harvest
Mother Nature's Bounty

Mother Nature's secrets are revealed at harvest time.

Harvest time is the season to enjoy the fruits of the year's labor after a busy time of picking, hanging, drying, freezing, and storing herbs in a variety of ways. By the end of the harvest, you will be wondering how Mother Nature can be so prolific. The secrets to a successful harvest are in capturing the full flavor and quality of each herb harvested.

The following tips will help you harvest Mother Nature's bounty.

- Select leaves for drying before herbs flower to ensure full flavor. Harvest after 10 A.M., when dew dries and before the sunlight is most intense. Gather in a basket. Tie stems in small bunches and hang them upside down to dry in a well-ventilated, cool room until they crumble easily. Crumble the dried herbs in an airtight jar. Keep for six months to one year.

- Roots can be harvested with a sharp knife. Leave uninjured root-stock to continue growth. Soak and clean roots under running water and rub dry. Hang in a cool, well-ventilated room. You may have to cut large roots into pieces before drying, such as dock, comfrey, and echinacea.

The secrets to a successful harvest are in capturing the full flavor and quality of each herb harvested.

~

*Keep dried
herbs away
from heat
and light
to retain
their best
flavor.*

~

- To freeze fresh herbs, first dry them lying flat on a cookie sheet, then put them in freezer bags or containers for freezing. Leafy herbs freeze well in a Ziplock plastic bag. Basil may be blanched before freezing. The herbs will freeze well up to six months. Freeze delicate herbs, like dill and thyme, in sprigs. Freeze other fresh herbs, such as basil, dill, and parsley, by blending them with a tablespoon of water and then freezing them in ice cube trays, or making a paste in oil and water and refrigerating or freezing for later use.

- Preserve seeds and spices by cutting the blossoms and seeds right before they ripen and scatter. Tie them together in loose bunches and hang them upside down to dry. Spread a cotton towel underneath to catch the seeds as they ripen and fall, or as you shake them loose. You can also tie a paper bag around the stem and allow the seeds to fall into the bag. Use a sieve or colander to sift out the chaff. Store in an airtight container. Some examples are coriander, dill, fennel, and parsley seeds.

- Oven-dry herbs only when humidity is too high to air-dry. Keep the oven door slightly open and use only the heat from the pilot light to dry the herbs. When using an electric stove, use the lowest heat (140 degrees). Check frequently to avoid drying them to a crisp. Dry all herbs on racks. **Note:** Basil will discolor and lose some of its flavor if washed and then dried. Use a damp paper towel and wipe the leaves before drying.

- Dry unwashed parsley, coriander leaves, and rosemary in the refrigerator by closing them in a paper bag for a month.

- Keep dried herbs away from heat and light to retain their best flavor.

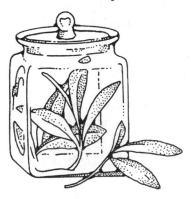

Herbs for Your Kitchen

*N*ow the herbs are ready to create a new taste sensation in your meals. Here are a few ideas to get you interested. Enjoy using your creative ideas to bring out the herbal gourmet in you.

Hints for Using Herbs

- Serving Rule: Two teaspoons of minced, fresh herbs will flavor four servings. One teaspoon dried herbs or seeds serves four. Delicately flavored herbs, like marjoram, can be used more liberally.

- For soups and stews, add fresh herbs during the last 20 minutes.

- To develop the flavor of freshly dried herbs, soak them for 10 minutes in lemon juice, stock, or oil before cooking.

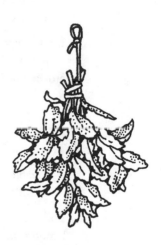

- Before cooking, rub fresh herbs between clean hands to release their unique flavor in the volatile oils. This will accelerate flavoring as your entrée cooks.

- Firmly press herbs into the flesh of meats, fish, or poultry before cooking to enhance aroma and taste. No sauce or further preparation will be necessary.

- Flavor salad dressing by soaking herbs in it for 30 minutes to an hour before serving. Use one teaspoon of herbs to one cup of dressing.

- Microwave: Whenever possible, sauté herbal blends in a small amount of liquid, stock, butter, or oil before adding to a microwave dish to assure flavor.

- Sugar can be flavored by layering 12–15 rose geranium or lemon rose geranium leaves on top of 1 pound sugar. Any flavor of geranium leaves will do. Keep covered until ready to use. Flavored sugars add a delicate flavor to biscuits, cookies, and muffins.

- A substitute for lemon peel in baked goods is finely chopped lemon balm, lemon thyme, or lemon verbena.

Tea Time

Here are a few of my favorite teas. They recall memories of cozy times with my children on cold winter days. The morning blend was created by my youngest son, Jason.

❧ *Mother Nature's Morning Blend* ❧

This is a refreshing tea to sip while watching the morning news or reading the paper.

- 2 tablespoons jasmine tea
- 4 tablespoons fresh applemint or peppermint

Brew 8 cups of water in a coffee pot using jasmine tea with fresh applemint or peppermint. (I'm always trying to use up some of my applemint. It's growing *inside* my back door!)

❧ *Mother Nature's Zesty Morning Blend* ❧

This tea will get you to work on time.

- 2 tablespoons green tea
- 1 tablespoon fresh or dried lemon grass

Boil 6 cups of water in a glass or porcelain tea pot. Steep green tea and lemon grass. Strain and enjoy.

❧ *Mother Nature's Nightcap Tea* ❧

Guaranteed to make you snooze.

- 1 tablespoon chamomile flowers
- 1 large passion flower
- 1 teaspoon fresh lemon balm or fresh or dried lemon grass
- 1 tablespoon dried catmint or catnip
- 1 drop pure vanilla extract

Steep in 1½ cups of boiled water, covered, for 10 minutes. Strain and add vanilla.

Herb Butters

Herb butters add a delightful flavor to vegetables, crackers, breads, and meats. They are quick and easy to prepare and turn an ordinary dinner into a meal to remember.

Hints:

- Use unsalted butter.

- Use lemon zest to enhance flavor.

- Mix into softened butter or simmer.

- Herb butters get stronger with time. Refrigerate 2–3 weeks. Freeze 2–3 months.

- Add nuts just prior to serving.

- Chop fresh herbs, cut with scissors, or food-process fully dry.

- Simmer herbs about 10 minutes. Do not bubble.

∾ *Mint Butter* ∾

Use on breads, muffins, carrots, and parsnips.

 3 tablespoons finely chopped fresh mint leaves
 1 stick unsalted butter
  lemon zest to taste
 2 tablespoons marmalade, preserves, or honey of choice

Simmer 10 minutes or less for a lighter flavor.

∾ *Lemon Butter* ∾

Add to vegetable dishes.

 ½ cup chopped lemon grass bulb or lemon balm, lemon thyme, or lemon basil
  lemon zest and juice of ¼ fresh lemon
 2 sticks unsalted butter

Melt herbs and butter together. Simmer lightly 5–10 minutes. Strain and refrigerate.

❧ *Rose Geranium Butter* ❧

Spread on toast, biscuits, or cakes. This butter can also be used to make biscuits and cakes.

1 pound unsalted butter
several fresh geranium leaves, finely chopped

Blend butter with geranium leaves and refrigerate.

Herb Vinegars and Oils

Combine your favorite herbs and spices in a delicious herb vinegar or oil to flavor salads, vegetables, pastas, and marinades. Add six 2-inch sprigs or 1 tablespoon of fresh leaves to every cup of heated vinegar or oil. Cool, cover and store in a glass bottle in a cool, dark place up to one year. I reuse vinegar bottles to store herb vinegars. When adding garlic, chilies or chives, use one for every cup of vinegar.

❧ *Salad Vinegar* ❧

The cucumber taste of burnet will heighten the taste of a simple green salad.

3 sprigs each sage, salad burnet, and shallots
1 cup heated red wine vinegar

Steep sage, salad burnet, and shallots in heated red wine vinegar for 30 minutes. Strain and serve or store in a glass bottle.

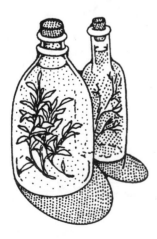

∾ *Vinegar Marinade* ∾

Use this vinegar as a marinade for fajita meats.

- 1 chili
- 1 garlic clove
- 3 sprigs oregano
- 1 cup apple cider vinegar

Steep chili, garlic, and oregano in apple cider vinegar overnight.

∾ *Fruit Salad Vinegar* ∾

Add this vinegar to a salad of oranges, apples, pears, peaches, and dates.

- 6 rose petals
- 6 violets
- 3 sprigs lavender, optional
- 1 cup heated rice vinegar

Steep rose petals, violets, and lavender in heated rice vinegar.

∾ *Pasta and Vegetable Oil* ∾

Season pasta salads and steamed zucchini for a hint of minty flavor.

- 2 (6-inch) sprigs each oregano, thyme, and spearmint
- 1 cup heated olive oil

Steep oregano, thyme, and spearmint in heated olive oil.

∾ *Herbal Oil for Salads and Sautés* ∾

Enjoy this spicy oil for Mexican salad and rice dishes, or add it to a fresh garden salad.

- 1 cup oil
- 3 (2-inch) sprigs each of oregano and basil or rosemary and thyme
- 1 tablespoon each fresh oregano and basil or rosemary and thyme
- 1 (¼-inch) piece ginger
- 1 chili
- ½ teaspoon seeds, crushed with mortar and pestle

Gently heat oil 3–5 minutes. Pour into a glass jar with six 2-inch sprigs of herbs for each cup of oil, or one of the following: fresh herbs, ginger, chili, or seeds. Cool, cover, and refrigerate up to six months. **Note:** Only add garlic to oils to be used within three days. Garlic forms a botulism in oil that can cause severe diarrhea.

～ *Marinade Oil* ～

Flavor rice, vegetables, and meat marinades.

   1 (¼-inch) slice ginger
   ½ teaspoon each crushed cardamom and coriander seeds
   1 cup safflower oil

Simmer ginger, cardamom, and coriander seeds in safflower oil for 3 minutes. Strain.

～ *Flavorful Oil* ～

Use this oil to flavor vegetables and baked potatoes, and brush on garlic bread before serving.

   1 tablespoon combined fresh lemon grass,
     lemon verbena, and lemon thyme
   1 cup heated almond oil

Steep and strain.

No-Salt Herbal Blends

Herbal blends add a flavor your salt shaker can never do. The following blends are beneficial in lowering dietary sodium while creating a whole new flavor with various herbal blends. The flavor of herbs is created from volatile oils that are natural preservatives for food. Try a teaspoon for each 4–6 servings and store any remaining dried herbal blends in airtight tins for up to 6 months. Prepare these blends in a mortar and pestle, blender, or coffee grinder for a new flavor sensation.

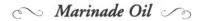

❧ *Egg Blends* ❧

Sprinkle on omelettes and scrambled eggs or egg whites.

1. Mince 1 teaspoon each dill, chives, parsley; ¼ teaspoon paprika.
2. Mix ¼ teaspoon freshly grated dry mustard or cayenne.
3. Mince 1 teaspoon each fresh marjoram, garlic, thyme.

❧ *Green Vegetable Blends* ❧

Sprinkle on green beans, zucchini, and asparagus before serving.

1. Mix 1 teaspoon each savory, parsley, oregano; 1 onion.
2. Mix 2 teaspoons each lemon basil, lemon thyme;
   1 teaspoon marjoram; ½ teaspoon allspice.

❧ *Yellow or Orange Vegetable Blends* ❧

Carrots, squash, and sweet potatoes will benefit from a teaspoon of one
of these blends.

1. 1 teaspoon each: thyme, cinnamon, orange zest, 1 dash nutmeg
   or allspice. Add the last few minutes of cooking.
2. 1 teaspoon ginger, allspice, maple sugar. Flavor before cooking.
3. 2 teaspoons fresh bee balm, thyme, 1 teaspoon fresh applemint.
   Sprinkle before serving. The aroma will precede you to the table.
4. 2 teaspoons fresh perilla or mint leaves, crushed; 1 teaspoon
   tarragon; 1 teaspoon combined ground cumin, coriander, and
   cinnamon. Blend into the vegetables before serving.

❧ *Beef, Lamb, or Pork Blends* ❧

Change the flavor of your meat and create a new twist to your main
entrée. Serve vegetable blends that are seasonally compatible.

1. Mix 1 teaspoon each lemon thyme, rosemary, ground ginger,
   and lemon zest for each pound of meat.
2. Mix 1 teaspoon each marjoram, thyme, orange peel;
   ½ teaspoon ground cloves; and ½ teaspoon minced
   garlic for each pound of meat.
3. Mix 1 teaspoon each ground chili powder, minced onion,
   spicy Mexican oregano and ½ teaspoon yellow mustard
   seed for each pound of meat.
4. 1 tablespoon mint, such as applemint, spearmint, or
   cinnamon basil. This is especially tasty on lamb.

❧ *Chicken Blends* ❧

Dredge chicken pieces in an herbal blend and bake, broil, or grill.

1. Mix 2 teaspoons each ground sage, parsley, minced ginger or ground ginger, and 1 teaspoon each orange thyme and orange zest for each pound of chicken.
2. Mix 1 teaspoon curry powder, ½ teaspoon cumin, and ½ teaspoon each minced garlic, minced onion, crushed mustard seed.
3. Mix 2 teaspoons each rosemary, chopped lemon grass; 1 teaspoon each marjoram and zest of lime.
4. Mix 2 teaspoons fresh tarragon or marigold mint, 1 teaspoon each minced spearmint and lemon zest.
5. Mix 2 teaspoons each basil, rosemary, lemon balm; add 1 teaspoon zest of lemon.

❧ *Fish and Shellfish Blends* ❧

Combine an herbal blend in a tablespoon of butter, ghee, or oil and baste onto the fish or shellfish as it cooks.

1. Mix 2 teaspoons each crushed dill seed and chopped parsley or coriander; 1 teaspoon each crushed mustard seed and lemon zest.
2. Mix 2 teaspoons each lovage or chervil and crushed celery seed; 1 teaspoon each cayenne or black pepper and zest of lemon.
3. Mix 2 teaspoons each crushed fennel seed, lemon grass, lemon thyme; 1 teaspoon ground paprika.

Herbal Scents for Honey

Add herbs to honey or grow them near hives to produce flavored honey. Do not heat honey. To produce the flavor of your choice, steep herbs in honey for three weeks and strain. Add one tablespoon of herbs for each cup of honey. Here are some herbs for honey to tempt your sweet tooth.

- thyme, lemon thyme, or orange thyme, equally blended or separate

- lemon balm, chopped lemon grass bulb, and lemon verbena blended in equal parts or alone

- 1 tablespoon curry leaves, 1 tablespoon candied ginger

- 1 tablespoon rosemary flowers

- 1 tablespoon lavender leaves and flowers

- 1 cinnamon stick, 1 tablespoon chocolate mint, and a few drops of vanilla extract

- scented geranium leaves, such as lime, peppermint, or strawberry

- 1 tablespoon marjoram, 1 teaspoon lemon geranium leaves

- 1 tablespoon licorice mint, 1 teaspoon hyssop

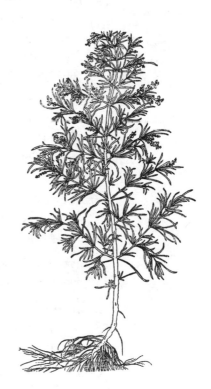

ROSEMARY

Herbs for Your Medicine Cabinet

Many of these herbs may be growing in your garden.

∾

Working with herbs increases all levels of consciousness, which is necessary to overcome chronic problems within our bodies. It takes one to three years to change chronically diseased systems. Listed below are some simple herbal aids used by our ancestors as folk remedies. The herbs used here were brought to America by colonists and grown locally—many of them may be growing in your garden. Herbs are most beneficial as nutrients. Consult your physician for diagnosis and treatment of disease states.

ACNE: Locally apply a compress of washed and bruised fresh comfrey leaves to any skin lesion. Simmer several leaves in a pint of water about 10 minutes. The water turns a brown color. Strain and apply locally, warm or cool. Refrigerate the remaining liquid from 1 to 3 days and reapply 1–2 times daily.

ATHLETE'S FOOT: For Liniment of Peppermint, combine 1 teaspoon of menthol crystals, 1 teaspoon camphor flowers, and 1 pint of oil. The above items are available through your druggist. Heat until dissolved (do not boil) and add 1 teaspoon peppermint oil. Strain into a glass jar and refrigerate. Apply locally to the affected area 2–3 times daily.

BLEEDING: Apply ice and pressure directly for 10 minutes, then apply cayenne pepper to the affected area. Dampened and bruised yarrow leaves applied locally will also stop bleeding.

BRUISES: Locally apply washed and bruised fresh comfrey, costmary, or violet leaves for 15 minutes. This can be reapplied several times daily.

BURNS AND SUNBURNS: Apply a cold water compress with undiluted aloe vera gel and 2 drops of lavender essential oil for 15–20 minutes. Reapply as necessary.

COLDS: Drink several cups of lemon balm and peppermint tea as an infusion daily. Add a dash of ginger to alleviate chills or induce sweating. This is safe for children and may be sweetened as desired.

COUGHS: Combine 1 tablespoon marshmallow root *(Althea officinalis)* in 6 cups of cold water and allow to stand at room temperature for 1 hour. Bring to a boil and simmer to reduce the liquid by half. Sweeten to taste, strain, and bottle. Drink 1 cupful 3 times daily to alleviate coughs and scratchy throats.

DIARRHEA: Make a very strong tea of ½ cup of blackberry leaves in 1½ cups of water. Steep 10 minutes and strain. Add 1 tablespoon or less of carob powder and drink it 3 times daily to promote homeostasis.

FACIAL: For all skin types. Mix equal parts of rose petals, comfrey leaves, peppermint, and lemon balm leaves, about a handful each. Chamomile flowers can be added to soothe rough and chapped skin. Simmer in a pint of water, covered, for 5 minutes. Remove from heat and bend over the pot with a towel covering your head and shoulders. Steam your face for 5 minutes and rinse with cold water. The solution can then be strained and added to bath water.

HEADACHES: Make a tea with rosemary leaves. Apply it as a compress.

INSECT REPELLENT: Make a strong tea of pennyroyal leaves or dilute pennyroyal oil in a pint of water. Spray the infusion around the area. This is harmless to animals and plants. Make a strong tea of citrus rinds, especially lemon and orange rinds. Spray directly on areas inhabited by ants as a repellent. Use a half cup of chopped rinds for each cup of water. Simmer 20 minutes. Cool and strain.

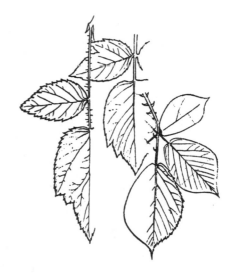

LINIMENT: For aches, pains, stiffness, sore muscles, or swollen glands, combine 2 tablespoons marjoram or oregano leaves, 1 tablespoon thyme, and 1 pint safflower or sesame oil. Simmer the herbs in the oil 5–7 minutes. Strain and apply locally to the affected area for 15–30 minutes. A ginger compress can also be used.

BLACKBERRY LEAVES

SINUS CONGESTION: Drink or apply a compress of an infusion of sage leaves. Pour 2 cups of boiling water over 1 tablespoon fresh sage leaves. Cover and steep 20 minutes. Strain and add 8 tablespoons or less of honey and refrigerate. Take 1–3 tablespoons daily. A ginger compress will also disperse congestion. Do not drink sage tea if nursing; a strong infusion can dry up mammary secretions.

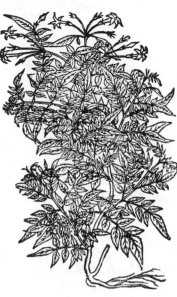

JASMINE

13

How to Use Essential Oils and Flower Essences

Bloom with the roses and promote world harmony.

The body is a rainbow of color, scent, and sound. One's body reads taste, smell, color, shape, and touch as the same language. Flower essences, essential oils, and natural fragrances are messengers that touch our soul. A flower essence or essential oil is a glimpse of the soul of a flower. Even a fragrance-free flower essence imparts a message to the soul. Every flower can affect the chemical messengers we refer to as emotions. On a deeper level, flowers can affect the attitudes causing emotions and promote the growth necessary for self-mastery. Self-mastery is being responsible for our choices, attitudes, and how we treat others. On a physical level, self-mastery is learning how to best nurture the body with lifestyle habits that support radiant health down to paying the bills in a timely fashion. To live a life manifesting high ideals, it is necessary to be grounded. This is where our chakras come into play. (Chakra information is from *Healing from the Heart* [Herbal Essence, Inc., 1985].)

Flower essences, essential oils, and natural fragrances are messengers that touch our soul.

~

The Centers of Consciousness: Chakras

Flower essences were discovered by ancient, prehistorical cultures and used by the rishis of India to balance the chakras. Chakras are large nerve centers aligned to the spinal column that code messages to the brain.

They create an image of an open flower whirling in a clockwise motion. Emotional imbalance and stress immobilize their free flowering, creating an illusion of separation and fear in the personality's perception of life. Each chakra responds to an essence like a flower blossoming in a song of self-harmony. The aroma also attracts other people of like mind. Essences are applied to the central point of the chakra, on the wrist, temples, throat, or inner right ear, to promote inner peace and union with the soul. A blend of high, middle, and base note essences can be worn, as well as individual essences and colors to enhance creative potential.

Chakra balancing is especially helpful when an individual feels stuck —dense clouds, no rain. When the chakras are harmonious, the individual becomes constructive, creative, and focused.

The following chakras—the crown, visual, throat, heart, vital energy, sacral, base of the spine, and unnamed—have specific needs for being grounded. They are considered primary to promoting health and feelings of well-being.

The Source

The secret of immortality is found in the purification of the Heart . . . for immortality is Union with God.

—The Upanishad, "Katha"

~

The physical body is a garden blooming with the flowers of our senses: sight, taste, touch, and smell, all permeating matter with eternal light. Matter is a partial expression of spirit, the Unlimited as limited. The difference proceeds from the rate of vibration, or frequency. Each individual has a vibratory signature of his or her own state of consciousness, conveying thoughts, feelings, and desires.

The soul is a channel through which love flows uninterruptedly to express perfect faith, peace, and wisdom. As the power of the soul awakens, the awareness of cosmic consciousness of Oneness emerges. The soul's purpose is to bring the consciousness from a state of ignorance to the realization of truth, as the only remedy for ignorance is truth.

The spirit is the creative power of life-giving energy charging all feeling, will, and thought; an unchangeable state of awareness free from restrictions and duality. Spirit is the realization of truth, the "I Am" consciousness in chakra terminology.

Disease manifests from inactivation of the vital life force within. Healing begins as the will directs the vital life force to every body part. As above, so below. Decorate and arrange your thoughts to concentrate and enhance the dynamic force of Aum, the creative life force.

The human body is a column of light, vibrating to the sound of color. The chakras emit a sound and color that precede emotions and produce an energy field that affects chemical changes in our nerve endings. Stress and tension block the smooth flow of energy throughout the human body, depleting our energy and altering our chemical and hormonal response to life.

Plants are extremely sensitive instruments for measuring our emotions. The energy fields they radiate benefit us in many ways to alleviate toxic, nutritionally deficient, and stress-dominated systems.

Each chakra is a "wheel" or vortex of energy related to major nerve plexus and endocrine glands. Balancing the chakras intensifies, fine-tunes, and focuses energy to the related areas and organs. Flower remedies harmonize the energy flowing in, out, and between the chakras to enhance the higher states of spiritual realization.

Each chakra harmonically resonates and vibrates to frequencies of sound and light (color) to induce certain emotions and consciousness. The soul searches the harmonious unity within the spheres of cosmic consciousness as all chakras become purified receivers and transmitters of this energy. Love is the universal power that will transfigure every aspect of our lives. We incarnated to create happiness, rather than seek it outside of ourselves.

All of the eight chakras are described on the following pages. A chart in each section lists location, color, musical note, music, jewel to be worn, dietary guidelines, enfleurages/oils, and flower essences that support the flowering of this center.

The Crown Chakra

The crown chakra is above the head, flowing energy into the body from a fountain of light. This chakra is where the union of spiritual ideals and physical realities occurs. As this thousand-petalled flower opens, a receptivity to higher intuition and guidance begins. The personality joins the spiritual self. Actions and decisions will benefit everyone. In the body, this center releases endorphins to keep the individual tuned within. The inner reality is now more important and real than the outer world. Rhythm and order release an energy flow in a figure-eight pattern from the base chakra to the crown. The color is white, resonating to illumination.

Location	Directly above the top of head
Color	White
Musical Note	Key of B
Music	Sacred music
Jewel to be Worn	Sapphire or diamond
Dietary Guidelines	Lipoic acid available in flowering plants

| ENFLEURAGES/OILS | Lavender, white ginger, African blue basil |
| FLOWER ESSENCES | Orchid, ranunculus, sunflower, verbena, Silver Moon antique rose, Yellow Peace rose, dill, echinacea pupura, Cherokee rose |

The Visual Chakra

The visual chakra is located in the center of the forehead. It is referred to as the brow chakra. This center relates to the ability to visualize and create from the imagination. Before beginning a new plan of action, this center can best be utilized by visualizing what is desired. See it, feel it, and allow that seed to be planted in the mind; for example, the principal of "think thin" is a visualization from the imagination. Our inner vision is as real as our external world, for our external world is the result of our thoughts and attitudes as well as our actions. However, this center is activated by feeling the desired result at the same time it is visualized.

This chakra is also useful for introspection, an inner vision that encourages a closer look at our motives and actions. The visual center projects from the pineal, pituitary, and hypothalamus glands. This trinity masterminds much of the body's chemical and hormonal responses from the brain center. It is the decision maker that qualifies emotions and attitudes. The color is indigo violet, the color of fulfillment and knowledge. When the third eye opens, the imagination is activated from the love that created us and prophetic dreams occur.

LOCATION	Center of forehead
COLOR	Indigo violet
MUSICAL NOTE	Key of A
MUSIC	Melodies
JEWEL TO BE WORN	Pearl
DIETARY GUIDELINES	Vitamin K, manganese, full spectrum light (See nutrient charts, page 327)
ENFLEURAGES/OILS	Old Blush antique rose, Rose Gardenia antique rose
FLOWER ESSENCES	Iris, red carnation, Madame Alfred Carrier antique rose, Maggie antique rose, kolanchoe

The Throat Chakra

The throat chakra is the power center of the spoken word. The color is royal blue, the color of creativity. Its purpose is to stimulate artistic and creative faculties, balancing the communication between the heart and cortical brain. Latent talents may be discovered and explored as the spoken word manifests into co-creation. The individual will often become an authority in his or her career as this sixteen-petalled flower opens. "I speak only what I want to see manifest."

LOCATION	Anterior part of the neck
COLOR	Royal blue
MUSICAL NOTE	Key of G
MUSIC	Romantic
JEWEL TO BE WORN	Amethyst
DIETARY GUIDELINES	Increase metabolism with foods containing iodine and vitamin A, vitamin B_1, thiamine, vitamin B_2, riboflavin, chromium (See nutrient charts, page 327)
ENFLEURAGES/OILS	Alfredo de Damas, damask rose, Lady Eubanksia antique rose, Fortune's Double Yellow antique rose
FLOWER ESSENCES	Red crepe myrtle, azalea, pansy, white petunia, white hyacinth, red rose, marigold, meadow sage, chamomile

The Heart Chakra

The heart chakra is centered in the chest. It relates to compassion, forgiveness, and faith. As the twelve-petalled flower opens, the joy of the heart's desire begins. The color resonance is green, the color of balance and of allowing intimacy to be fulfilled through touch. Surrender is necessary for the heart chakra to open and faith to flow through compassion. As the heart opens, the diaphragm releases and the breath becomes easier. Self-trust is secure as the heart's desire moves the individual into action.

LOCATION	The center of the chest
COLOR	Green
MUSICAL NOTE	Key of F
MUSIC	Elevator music

Jewel to be Worn	Emerald or jade
Dietary Guidelines	Increase greens, chlorophyll, inositol, vitamin D, vitamin F, calcium, copper, potassium (See nutrient charts, page 327)
Enfleurages/Oils	Marigold mint, Sweet Annie, wisteria, lilac, gardenia, geranium, eucalyptus, anise, hyssop
Flower Essences	Wisteria, lilac, daffodil, penta, narcissus, periwinkle, tiger's jaw cactus, white rose, Lady Eubanksia antique rose, Marquise Bocella antique rose, Autumn Damask antique rose, Louis Phillipe antique rose, Archduke Charles antique rose

The Vital Energy Chakra

The third chakra resonates with the digestive organs surrounding the navel. Digestion and assimilation of proteins and nutrients vitalize the body and increase metabolic processes for heat and energy. Once the umbilical cord is cut, our diet provides the nutrients for longevity. The vital chakra is responsible for transporting the essence of each nutrient through circulating blood and bodily fluids. Muscle strength as well as the energy level of the entire body is supported by this center. The chakra resonates to a vibrant yellow, the color of vitality. On a personality level, a success consciousness and sense of self-appreciation is enhanced: "I can do it!" As the ten-petalled flower opens, the individual begins to desire much more than enjoying a good meal. A sense of community spirit encourages the person to learn and teach ways to better our environment and community. A healthy body creates a healthy mind that desires to live in a healthy environment. There is a sense of oneness with all that is created.

Location	Navel or midpoint of the body
Color	Yellow
Musical Note	Key of E
Music	Stimulating
Jewel to be Worn	Topaz

DIETARY GUIDELINES	Vitamin C, vitamin K, vitamin P, pantothenic acid, B_5, pangamic acid, B_{17}, paba, para amino benzoic acid, choline, biotin (See nutrient charts, page 327)
ENFLEURAGES/OILS	Magnolia, peppermint, thyme, sage, rosemary, lemon grass, fennel, chamomile, lemon balm
FLOWER ESSENCES	Crossandra, catnip, ligustrum, onion, morning glory, peppermint, pink geranium, primrose, white carnation, Gröss Aachen antique rose, fennel, Madam Louis Levique antique rose, Fortune's Double Yellow antique rose

The Sacral Chakra

The sacral chakra is centered in the pelvis, below the navel, cradled by the sacrum. By measurement, it is four inches above the base of the spine. It works with the part of the body's intelligence that provides self-protection and inner guidance. The urinary, genital, and adrenals are the related organs. In Oriental medicine, the ancestral chi, or genetic inheritance and vitality, is stored in the memory bank of the adrenals. The adrenals kick off the immune system in the fight-or-flight syndrome. Orange, the color of regeneration and sexuality, resonates to this chakra. When this six-petalled flower opens, the body responds with a renewal of joy, enhancing the endocrine system. The health of the endocrine organs relates to our emotional well-being. The inner guidance is translated into a sense of knowing: "I know what to do; I have direction; I know how to take care of myself." The roller coaster of emotional responses harmonizes to an inner feeling of peace: inner grinning! This sense of well-being and security enhances immunity by lowering the stress response. Sexual function and reproduction are nurtured by this chakra.

LOCATION	Four inches above the base of the spine, cradled in the sacrum
COLOR	Orange
MUSICAL NOTE	Key of D
MUSIC	Songs that evoke deep feelings
JEWEL TO BE WORN	Gold

DIETARY GUIDELINES	B_3, niacin, magnesium and B_6, pyridoxal phosphate (See nutrient charts, page 327)
ENFLEURAGES/OILS	Jasmine, cinnamon, cinnamon basil, iris, Mexican oregano
FLOWER ESSENCES	Bachelor's buttons, basil, bellaparone (the shrimp plant), Old Blush antique rose, lily, Cecile Bruner antique rose, Country Marilou antique rose, amaryllis, bamboo, begonia, white petunia, snapdragon, the fairy rose, Indian paintbrush

The Base of the Spine Chakra

At the base of the spine, the body's consciousness relates to self-identity and trust issues. It works with the sexual identity that relates to self-acceptance and personal power. Survival memories are also stored in the coccyx. The base chakra resonates to red, the color of energy and enthusiasm. The East Indians describe this chakra, the seat of kundalini, as a four-petalled lotus flower. When this flower or vortex of whirling energy opens, the regenerative powers of the body begin. The personality is endowed with a sense of destiny and self-esteem replaces timidity. As circulation increases, the quality of blood is enhanced and metabolic wastes are filtered to the kidneys. On a personal level, the individual feels a sense of well-being through increased vitality. The will to live is increased.

LOCATION	Coccyx
COLOR	Red
MUSICAL NOTE	Key of C
MUSIC	Marching
JEWEL TO BE WORN	Ruby
DIETARY GUIDELINES	Increase oxygenating foods high in iron, B_{12}, folic acid, vitamin E, phosphorus, zinc (See nutrient charts, page 327)
ENFLEURAGES/OILS	Vanilla, sandalwood, oak moss

Flower Essences
Viridiflora, stock, Wandering Jew, dianthus, baby's breath, fimbriata, salvia, bluebonnet, Champney's Cluster antique rose

The Unnamed Chakra

The unnamed chakra is union with the soul. It is a blend of color creating a golden hue. This silent center is where enlightenment occurs, harmony with all that is divine. This is a very unique, personal experience where unconditional love is the only reality. Pursue happiness from within.

The Nature of Flower Essences and Essential Oils

A flower essence is an extraction of the chemical hormones that make a flower bloom. In the physical body, it relates to lipoic acid, a natural liver cleanser and purifier. Since flowers bloom under stress, flower essences can be worn as an affirmation to help us bloom to our fullest creative expression.

Flower essences are derived from the water condensed from an essential oil. When an essential oil is made, the flowers of herbs are ground and cooked in water. The heat causes condensation of the flower water and any essential oil will follow.

An essential oil is the volatile oil in herbs and flowers that give the plant a characteristic odor. It takes a large volume of flowers and herbs to produce a small quantity of essential oil. For example, several hundred roses may produce one dram, or one teaspoon, of essential oil through a condensation process. A still is required, with a condensing flask and tube, to produce essential oils. The essential oil floats on top of the flower essence water and is separated without hexane or unnatural processes. If the flowers or herbs have been grown conventionally with chemicals, the essential oil or flower essence will also have that characteristic or signature.

There is another difference between essential oils and flower essences. Flower essences affect the awareness through the electrical and magnetic charges of the body that are often referred to as the aura. They also affect the electrical charges firing the central nervous system, rather like a battery charger. Every organ, muscle, bone, and tissue has an electromagnetic quality. Flower essences can enhance the system and catalyze the personality into constructive action. The body reads the application of a

An essential oil is the volatile oil in herbs and flowers that give the plant a characteristic odor.

∿

properly made flower essence as a message of empowerment to the part of us immobilized or adversely affected by fear, anger, or disappointment. They gently encourage self-nurturing from the soul, the part of us connected with the harmony pervading creation. It is a very different way that Mother Nature feeds us. She always sees us as a complete self-healing system of checks and balances. Flower essences are very cooling to the emotions, breaking down "crystallized" attitudes that no longer serve our growth.

Essential oils are heavier, denser, and warmer than flower essences. Their aroma rises immediately to the highest centers of the brain to produce a chemical response from hormones flowing through the bloodstream. Essential oils are highly concentrated natural fragrances, unlike chemical reproductions. They are used for topical healing and utilizing the skin to trigger the immune system.

Note: The definition of a flower essence is a traditional one, handed down throughout many cultures. Commercially made flower essences are made in the Bach tradition, a very different method than the handmade process.

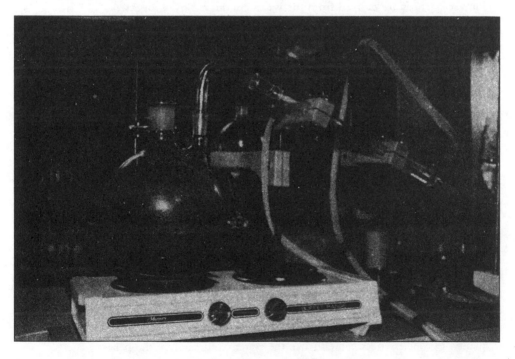

DISTILLATION UNIT FOR MAKING ESSENTIAL OILS.

How to Distill Essential Oils and Flower Essences

Many essential oils and flower essences are best extracted by steam distillation. The practice of steam distillation was used as early as five thousand years ago by Mesopotamians and other major cultures for medicinal, cosmetic, and ceremonial purposes. For example, the Egyptians distilled oils for mummification and the Arabs treated patients by applying essential oils to the chakras. From 1500 to 1700, Europeans distilled over one hundred essential oils for medicinal and cosmetic purposes.

To make an essential oil, plant leaves and flowers are gathered at peak times of oil production, usually when they bloom. Plant material is stripped from any woody portion of the plant and blended with distilled water to form a pulp. The pulp is poured into a glass flask, which sets on a burner. As the material is heated, steam is produced. The droplets of essential oil are carried by the steam into a glass condensing tube, which is kept cool by cold running water. Pressure and temperature are adjusted for each plant's requirements. The oil is usually the first to condense and a pure distilled water follows.

Essential oils must then be separated from the water in a glass separator. This is a lengthy process and many producers use highly toxic petroleum-based hexane to facilitate separation.

The water that is separated can be used as floral water and, when only flowers are used, becomes a true flower essence. A flower essence is the water that condenses from steam distillation.

The plant material used must be picked during the herb's highest amount of oil production. Learning when to produce the essential oil of each herb is an art learned by experience. For thyme, it is when it blooms. Midsummer is the best time to gather rosemary for essential oil production. Roses can be gathered in the spring or fall, but produce very little oil. It may take five hundred pounds of roses to produce one pound or less of steam-distilled rose oil.

Therefore, the enfleurage method has been used since the earliest times to produce fragrances and oils from flowers, such as rose and jasmine, which yield poor results from steam distillation. To make an enfleurage, freshly picked flowers were saturated in animal fat or oil repeatedly until the fragrance was absorbed by the fat. The flowers were pressed into pork fat between two sheets of glass for two to three days and then replaced with new blooms. Homemade enfleurages were created by repeatedly saturating animal fat with fresh, fragrant blooms. The fragrant animal fat was applied to the body like a fragrant perfume.

Essential Oils

The following list details a few of the most important essential oils. Local, organically grown and nonchemically processed essential oils are well suited for therapeutic purposes.

BASIL OIL *(Ocimum basilicum).* Reduces headaches, calms the mind, and repels flies! It opens the highest creative center in the brain. Basil has stimulating effects on lusterless hair.

EUCALYPTUS *(Citriodora).* A disinfectant, enhances breathing and mental concentration, opens the sinus passages, reduces coughs, muscle spasms, fevers, and scares away even Texas-sized mosquitoes. Dilutions reduce large pores, blemishes, and dandruff.

GERANIUM *(Pelargonium odorantissimum).* First used to repel insects, soon it was obvious that the aroma reduced depression and anxiety. Menopausal women especially notice its balancing effect. In a lotion, geranium oil has been used to reduce facial neuralgia and "traveling" rheumatic pain.

LAVENDER *(officinalis* and *latifolia).* Reduces stress, mood swings, nervousness, and irritability. Relieves headaches, bee and wasp stings, burns, hair loss, earaches, and bronchial conditions. A natural deodorizer, apply lavender to linen and pumices to repel moths.

LEMON GRASS *(Cynbopogon citratus).* A cooling, stimulating tonic and a cleansing antiseptic for oily skin, this refreshing fragrance also awakens concentration. In massages, it increases lymphatic drainage, decreases fluid retention, and reduces varicose veins.

MEXICAN MARIGOLD MINT *(Tagetes foeniculum).* A sweet fennel aroma, this fragrance is calming for children and colicky babies. In massage and skincare products, it soothes inflamed skin and reduces cellulite and small wrinkles.

PENNYROYAL *(Mentha pulegium).* A smooth muscle relaxer, its strong scent can repel insects and relieve itchy, watery eyes. Keep out of reach of small children.

PEPPERMINT *(Mentha piperita).* Stimulates pleasant memories while reducing joint and muscle stiffness, weather sensitivity, and headaches. Deep massage increases digestion and natural detoxifying processes.

Rose *(damascena)*. Evokes feelings of faith and love. Roses picked at daybreak yield a fragrance that is comforting in times of sorrow. Rose oil has been used for heart arrhythmias and female hormone balancing. Dilute in honey to reduce gingivitis or teething pain for infants. As a moisturizing beauty aid, rose oil is most protective.

Rosemary *(Rosemarinus officinalis)*. An uplifting nerve tonic that can increase mental awareness and memory. The oil has antioxidant and antiseptic properties that balance oily or problem skin and hair. Rosemary is beneficial to asthmatics and those who suffer during the flu and cold season. In massages, it can increase circulation to reduce PMS and tension headaches. Ancient Egyptians used rosemary for ritual cleansing, and early European cultures sprayed rosemary oil in their homes to attract beneficial spirits and lift depression.

Sage *(Salvia officinalis)*. Sage works well in a bath, compress, or massage. In a bath, it relaxes muscles; as a compress, it relieves sinus congestion, heat flashes, fluid retention, and sore throats. The earthy aroma is very masculine.

Thyme (white *Thymus vulgaris*). Enhances stamina in troubled times, reduces chronic fatigue, and protects against infectious diseases. The antibacterial properties increase white blood cells and destroy staphylococcus bacteria. Antiviral properties reduce flu, bronchitis, sinusitis, sore throats, coughs, and athlete's foot. Thyme diffuses easily in an aroma lamp or mister.

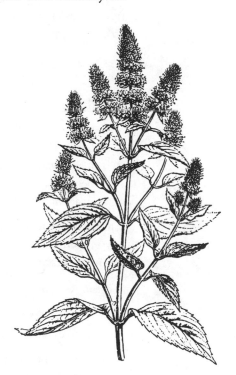

PEPPERMINT

Aromatherapy from Head to Toe: Herbal Skincare

For those who love to indulge in herbal luxury, begin by cleaning your face and removing all makeup.

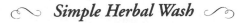

Simple Herbal Wash

Use this simple herbal wash to clean your face.

- ½ cup chamomile or lavender flowers
- ½ cup crushed fennel seeds
- 2 cups boiled water

Infuse chamomile or lavender flowers and fennel seeds in boiled water. Steep 20 minutes, strain, and splash on your face.

Herbal Facial Steam

After the herbal wash, prepare an herbal facial steam and get ready to relax.

- 8 tablespoons of a combination of any of the following herbs: mint leaves, chamomile flowers, rose petals, scented geranium leaves, lemon verbena, lemon balm, lemon grass, thyme, sage, eucalyptus, bergamot, jasmine, gardenia or honeysuckle flowers
- 1 quart boiling water

Simmer herbs in a covered glass quart of water. After 10 minutes, uncover your herbal facial and cover your head with a towel to catch the steam. Steam your face about 5 minutes to remove any impurities.

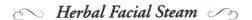

Cool Mint Pack

Next, prepare and apply a cool mint pack for a refreshing interlude.

- 1 cup fresh mint leaves
- 1 cup cold water

In a blender, blend mint leaves in cold water for 1 minute. Refrigerate for 10 minutes. Pour onto a clean hand towel. Lie down and relax while applying the pack to your face for up to 10 minutes.

❧ *Herbal Mask* ❧

Now apply the following herbal mask and allow it to set for 10 minutes.

- 1 tablespoon comfrey leaves, chopped
- 1 tablespoon chamomile, chopped
- ½ cup boiled water
- 3 tablespoons yogurt or powdered oatmeal (grind in a blender or coffee grinder)

Infuse comfrey leaves and chamomile in boiled water. Cover and steep 10 minutes before straining. Add to yogurt or oatmeal and apply liberally on your face and neck. Lie down and cover your eyes with a cotton ball dipped in the leftover infusion (put on a relaxation tape with soft music as you wait for it so set). Rinse and apply an herbal toner.

❧ *Herbal Facial Infusion* ❧

Use this infusion in toners and moisturizers.

- 2 tablespoons fresh herbs (rosemary, lavender, fennel) or roses
- ½ cup boiled water

Steep herbs or roses in boiled water for 10 minutes, strain, and apply with cotton balls.

❧ *Herbal Moisturizer* ❧

I don't like to use lanolin, so here's an easy moisturizer you can make at home.

- 2 tablespoons herbal infusion (rose, lavender, marigold mint)
- 1 teaspoon honey
- 1 tablespoon vegetable glycerine or 2 tablespoons cocoa butter a few drops essential oil (any kind), optional

To an herbal infusion, add honey and vegetable glycerin or cocoa butter. You can add a few drops of essential oil of your choice. Choose an herb to infuse from the list of simple herbal skin fresheners (page 310).

∽ *Herbal Toner* ∽

Here's a recipe for a simple toner to be used within 3 days.

For sensitive and mature skin:
½ cup rose, lavender, or calendula water infusion*
1 teaspoon vegetable glycerine
½ cup witch hazel

For oily skin:
½ cup sage leaves, or
½ cup lemon balm, lemon grass, and lemon verbena, or
½ cup rosemary
1 teaspoon vegetable glycerine
½ cup witch hazel

*For an infusion, steep 2 tablespoons fresh herb (or a combination of herbs to equal 2 tablespoons) in half a cup of boiled water in a covered glass or porcelain container for 10 minutes. Strain before using.

For sensitive and mature skin, combine rose water, lavender water, or calendula water as an infusion with vegetable glycerin and witch hazel. Apply with a cotton ball. For oily skin, infuse any of the herbs in half a cup of boiled water for 10 minutes and strain. Add glycerine and witch hazel. Refrigerate after using. After the toner dries and sets, apply a moisturizing cream or lotion.

∽ *Light Herbal Moisturizer* ∽

This will tighten, nurture, and moisturize sensitive or oily skin.

1 cup milk
3 tablespoons lavender or violet flowers

Heat, but do not boil, the milk and lavender or violet flowers. Cover, remove from heat, and steep 30 minutes before straining. Apply lightly to sensitive skin.

✎ *Rose Oil Skin Softener* ✎

This lovely handmade lotion can be applied to pumiced elbows, knees, and feet.

- 4 tablespoons vegetable glycerine
- 1 cup rose water
- 4 tablespoons cornstarch
- 5 drops rose oil, optional
- 2 drops lavender, optional

Combine vegetable glycerin, rose water, and cornstarch, and heat over a double boiler to thicken. Cool, add rose oil and lavender (optional). Stir and apply to chapped or dry skin. Bottle any leftovers.

✎ *Herbal Nail Strengthener* ✎

Remember to nurture your nails with an herbal infusion.

- 2 tablespoons chopped horsetail or crushed dill seed
- 1 cup boiled water
- 1 tablespoon almond oil

Infuse chopped horsetail or crushed dill seed in boiled water. Cover and steep 20 minutes. Strain and pour into 2 small bowls. Soak your nails for 10 minutes or longer. Massage 1 tablespoon of almond oil into the nails and cuticles. Use the infusion to soak the toenails and massage any leftover oil into the toenails.

As evening beckons, it's time to step into an herbal bath and finish the beauty treatment with a good twenty-minute soak. Infuse 2 cups of herbs in 4 cups of boiled water for 30 minutes. Strain and add to a warm bath. Suggestions are chamomile, lemon balm, Mexican marigold mint, catnip, Sweet Annie, violets, roses, lavender, or lemon grass.

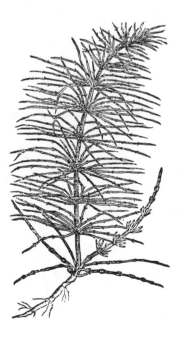

HORSETAIL

Simple Herbal Skin Fresheners

Make the tea with any of the following herbs by steeping 1 tablespoon of herb in 1 cup of boiled water for 15 minutes, covered. Strain and apply to the skin after it cools, using a cotton ball or clean cloth.

- Chamomile flowers soothe the skin and reduce puffiness around the eyes.

- Comfrey soothes inflamed skin and reduces blemishes.

- Eucalyptus reduces pores and sinus congestion.

- Fennel cleans and tones the skin.

- Hyssop, sage, and thyme are antiseptic.

- Lemon balm or lemon grass increases circulation and lightly astringes the skin.

- Mexican marigold mint deep-cleans and reduces large pores.

- Rose petals, violets, and salad burnet leaves reduce fine lines and soften the skin.

- Rosemary reduces oily skin.

Aromatherapy Applications

Allow the following combinations to free the mind and promote self-healing. The topical use of the ancient memories inherent in each fragrance will also tap into the innocent child residing in the heart.

Symptom	Application of Oil
Appetite stimulant	Apply a few drops of lemon grass to the throat.
Appetite suppressant	Apply a few drops of geranium or lavender to the temples.
Arthritic, rheumatic pain	Dilute 5 drops of sage or ginger in 1 ounce of carrier oil and apply locally. A combination of 3 drops each of peppermint and sage with 1 drop of ginger can be diluted in 1 ounce of carrier oil also.
Rheumatic pain that moves	Combine 2 drops each of pennyroyal and rosemary to 1 ounce of carrier oil and apply locally or use undiluted in a compress.

Arthritis, rheumatoid	Apply a few drops each of lavender and geranium in 1 ounce of carrier oil and rub into the joints twice daily. The essential oils may also be added to a lotion instead of a carrier oil in the same proportions.
Angina pain	Combine 3 drops each of eucalyptus and wisteria in 1 ounce of carrier oil and apply to the chest and down the arms every 30 minutes until you see your doctor. Three drops of sandalwood alone may also be used.
Anxiety	Combine 3 drops each of basil and white ginger in 1 ounce of carrier oil and apply to the throat. Two drops of vanilla or sandalwood alone may also be used.
Asthma	Rub the front and back of the chest with 5 drops each of lemon grass, eucalyptus, and lemon balm diluted in 1 cup of warm water or carrier oil.
Colic	Dilute 5 drops each of marigold mint and peppermint or 5 drops of dill alone in 1 cup of warm water. Apply to a clean cloth or washcloth and apply warm to the tummy. Cover with a plastic bag wrapped around a heating pad when applicable.
Dandruff	Rinse your hair with 3 drops each of rosemary and peppermint diluted in 1 cup of warm water. Protect your eyes.
Depression	Combine 2 drops each of rose and lavender essential oil. Dilute in ¼ cup of water to spray on face and hair. Combine 3 drops of lemon grass essential oil and lemon balm enfleurage to apply to temples and nape of the neck undiluted. Inhaling peppermint essential oil a few times may lift your spirits too: apply 3 drops to a clean hankie and hold near your nose to catch the aroma.
Burns, sunburn	Apply undiluted lavender oil.
Digestion	Dilute 5 drops of peppermint oil and 3 drops of marigold mint essential oil in 1 cup of warm water. Saturate a clean cloth with the fluid and apply to the tummy as a compress for 15 minutes before or after eating. This will increase circulation and digestion and reduce flatulence.

Symptom	Application of Oil
Eczema	Mix 3 drops each of geranium and rose essential oil in 2 tablespoons of melted cocoa butter or coconut oil and apply locally to the affected area. Keep the skin coated to prevent breakout.
Flus, colds, coughs	Thyme and sage essential oils can kill most viral germs and have antiseptic properties. Sage is also a decongestant useful for coughs and sinus congestion. Dilute 2 drops of each in 1 ounce of jojoba oil and apply to the forehead and temples. Make a tea from fresh leaves to drink.
Headaches	Apply a drop of peppermint, lavender, or rosemary oil to the temples.
Herpes Simplex I	Dilute 2 drops of lavender oil and 1 drop of lemon balm enfleurage in 1 tablespoon of jojoba oil. Or, combine 2 drops of myrrh essential oil and 2 drops of thyme oil in ¼ cup of jojoba oil. Apply to sores with a cotton swab.
Hiccups	Apply 2 drops of undiluted lavender oil to the diaphragm area in the center of the chest or the throat, or use the same amount of diluted marigold mint essential oil in a few drops of water.
Insect bites	Apply undiluted lavender oil.
Insomnia	Combine 2 drops each of Lady Eubanksia and white ginger enfleurage and apply to the temples before bedtime. Combine 2 drops each of lavender and rose essential oil in an aroma lamp or dilute in a teaspoon of jojoba oil and apply to the temples and nape of the throat.
Energy	Apply Old Blush enfleurage to the temples and neck or dilute a few drops of peppermint oil or lemon grass oil in a teaspoon of jojoba oil and apply to the same places. Even inhaling peppermint or lemon grass oil or spraying them in a room can liven the party!

Immunity | Wearing or inhaling lavender, rosemary, or thyme may reduce the tendency to catch colds or viruses. Spraying a room or using an aroma lamp may cleanse a large area. Dilute 2 drops of an essential oil of your choice in 1 teaspoon of carrier oil to wear on the nape of the neck or dilute 2 drops in an ounce of water and spray in a room. Apply 2 drops of essential oil to a warm aroma lamp.

Menopause | The transition may be easier by using 5 drops each of rose and geranium essential oils in baths, 2 drops of each in an ounce of vodka for a cologne, or 5 drops of each in 2 ounces of lotion.

Neuralgic aches | Combine a few drops each of rosemary and peppermint oils, 1 drop of lavender, and dilute in ½ cup of jojoba oil or a lotion.

Sinusitis, congestion | Eucalyptus oil will help open the lungs and facilitate the drainage of congestion. Dilute 2–5 drops in 1 ounce of jojoba oil and apply to the chest and back. Dab a little on the temples, forehead, and nape of the throat for easy breathing. Apply a few drops to a cotton ball and place it on the outside of a cool mist vaporizer.

Aromatherapy for Pets

The following essential oils can be used singly or in combination. For every 5 drops of essential oils, dilute in 1 cup of water. Spray or rub the combination on your pet as needed to repel insects and reduce pet odor. Do not apply to abrasions or broken skin.

Eucalyptus

Lavender

Lemon grass

Mexican marigold mint

Pennyroyal

Rosemary

Sage

Thyme (white thyme essential oil is safest)

Pet Tips

- To reduce fleas and ticks and promote a shiny coat, spray a dilution of either lemon grass, thyme, eucalyptus, sage, pennyroyal, or lavender on the pet's coat. Either use 3 drops in a cup of water or combine 3–5 drops of two to three oils in 1 cup of water and spray.

- Any citrus essential oil or infusion can be used to repel fleas as well as other insects. Dilute 3 drops of oil in a cup of water or simmer several orange or lemon peelings in 2 cups of water for 15 minutes before straining and spraying. **Caution:** Do not apply undiluted essential oils on a pet. This could cause burning or skin irritation.

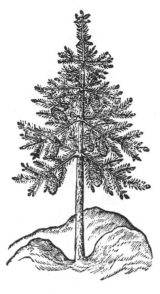

FIR

Epilogue

The Arms of Mother Nature

Step into the enchanted world of Mother Nature,
where flowers talk and Nature sings.

To the ancients, trees were the center of the world. They join spirit and matter, allowing communication between heaven and earth. Trees represent the feminine principle, rooted deep into the earth, nourishing and protecting, enlivened by solar power. Branches reach up to the heavens to behold eternity. Each year another ring is added, encircled by the World of Time.

Trees were sacred in ancient lands. Each tree represented heavenly protection. As a symbol of unity, the evergreen tree represented the immortality of an undying spirit. An affirmation of diversity, the deciduous tree represented the constant renewal of life, the resurrection. Trees bearing fruit were always sacred, a reminder of the compassion of creation.

As a mouthpiece of divinity, trees were also sought as oracles. Groves were customarily planted around temples and altars and decorated by sweet-smelling herbs such as marjoram, roses, crocus, and chrysanthemums. Myrrh trees were imported and planted around the Egyptian temple of Amon for religious ceremonies. The fragrance of their burning branches was believed to ascend to the heavens and please the gods.

To the original civilizations, there was only good, represented by the World Tree. The Australian aborigines have a World Tree that supports

Trees join spirit and matter, allowing communication between heaven and earth.

~

heaven. The stars stud the branches, drawing spiritual sustenance from Nature and Earth. Spiritual sustenance gave them real strength and power for such long endurance. The natives celebrated the land and their closeness to it, even oneness with it, through various ceremonies that bound them together on the deepest religious level. Their strength was bringing the people of the present into contact with their past and their dreamtime. All of these religious practices had their roots in the land and the trees. The people were part of the land and the land was part of them.

Many cultures had a Tree of Life and a Tree of Knowledge. The Tree of Life represented regeneration and a return to perfection through immortality. The Tree of Knowledge represented duality and the resulting good or evil resulting from the fruits of the intellect.

Every culture found a Tree of Life growing in their land. To the Egyptians, the sycamore was the Tree of Life. Hathor is portrayed as the tree distributing nourishment from her branches. The Mexicans discovered the agave milk-giving cactus to be their provider. In Japan, the bonsai represent Nature in all its wisdom. For the Mithraic, the honors belonged to the ancient pine. Scandinavians called the ash Yggdrasil and rooted their Tree of Life in the fate of the universe. The ancient civilizations of Chaldea, Phoenicia, and Babylonia held the palm in high esteem. Teutons revered the fir of Woden, later to become the Christmas tree. Through the Christian tradition of Christmas, the tree remains the image of humankind and has the ability to produce both good and evil.

To the Celt, every tree was sacred. When threatened by the forces of darkness, these forest giants came to rescue humanity. In veneration, Celtic priests took the name "Druids," the Celtic word for oak, as their own and based their alphabet on the names of other known trees.

The Eihwag, or yew tree, has red berries that will sustain you. As you meet obstacles on your way, call each one teacher and friend.

Oak and mistletoe represent male and female power. Magical power was realized in rowan, willow, alder, holly, and yew. Rebirth and fertility reign in birch.

Everywhere ancients looked, they found evidence of divinity in Nature. In art and later in literature, plants came to represent the gods ruling the heavens, earth, seas, and the underworld.

Today we seek not only our roots in the tradition of plant life, but also knowledge of the unknown. Trees, herbs, and flora remain the mediators between heaven and earth and the promise of rebirth, for what is divine cannot be separated from its source.

What is divine cannot be separated from its source.

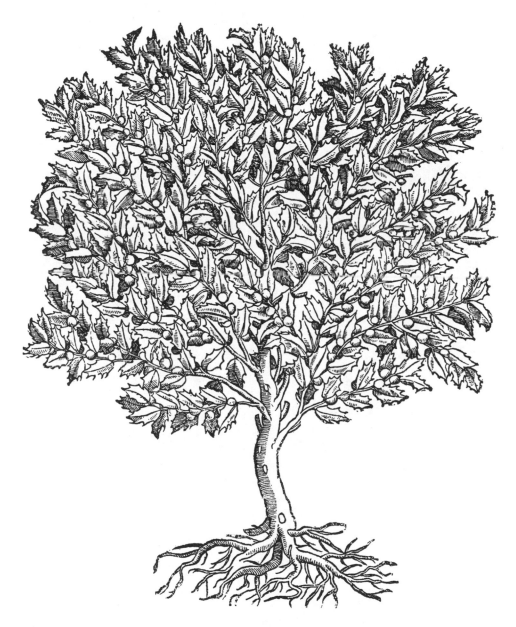

KERMES OAK

SECTION III

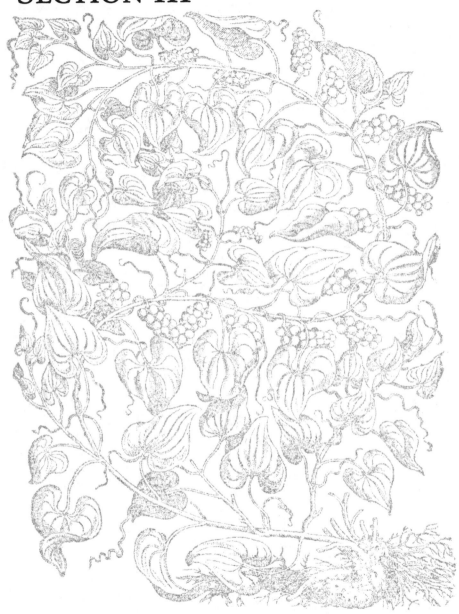

Appendices

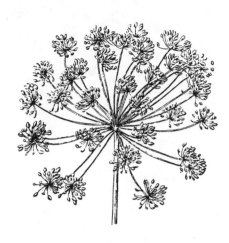

Dill

I

Growing Chart

Prepared by Theo De Maere

Herb	Type	Location	Uses
Aloe	tender perennial	sun, winter protection	medicinal
Basil blue bush, cinnamon, spicy globe, sweet	annual	sun	culinary
Bay laurel	tender perennial	shade, humidity	culinary
Bee balm	perennial	part shade, moist soil	ornamental, culinary, oswego tea
Borage	annual	full or part sun	ornamental, culinary
Caraway	biennial	sun	culinary
Catmint	perennial	part shade	medicinal
Catmint Six Hills Giant, nepeta	perennial	part shade	ornamental, tea
Catnip	perennial	part shade	medicinal, culinary

Herb	Type	Location	Uses
Celeriac	annual	sun	culinary
Chamomile German	annual	part shade	culinary, medicinal
Chamomile Roman	perennial	sun, part shade	ground cover
Chervil	annual	part shade	culinary
Chives garlic, onion	perennial	sun	culinary
Cilantro	annual	part shade	culinary
Comfrey	perennial	part shade	culinary, medicinal
Coneflower pink, purple (echinacea)	perennial	full sun	medicinal, ornamental
Curry	tender perennial	part shade, winter protection	culinary
Dandelion	perennial	full sun or part shade	culinary, medicinal
Dill	annual	sun	culinary, medicinal
Dittany of Crete	tender perennial	part shade, winter protection	culinary
Epazote	annual	sun	culinary
Eucalyptus (all)	tender perennial	sun, moist soil, winter protection	medicinal
Fennel	annual	sun	culinary
Geranium scented (all)	tender perennial	part shade	cosmetic, aromatic, culinary
Gotu Kola	tender perennial	part shade	medicinal
Horehound	perennial	sun	medicinal
Hyssop	perennial	full sun	culinary, antiseptic
Lamb's Ears	perennial	full sun, part shade	medicinal, ornamental
Lavender French	tender perennial	sun, part shade	aromatic, medicinal
Lavender *Lavandula*	perennial	sun, part shade	aromatic, medicinal
Lavender *Munstead*	perennial	sun, part shade	aromatic, medicinal

Herb	Type	Location	Uses
Leek	annual	sun, part shade	culinary
Lemon balm	perennial	part shade	culinary
Lemon grass	tender perennial	sun	culinary
Lemon verbena	tender perennial	part shade	aromatic, culinary
Lippia Dulcia	perennial	part shade	culinary
Lovage	annual	part shade	medicinal, culinary
Marjoram, sweet	tender perennial	sun, part shade	culinary, aromatic
Mint orange, wintergreen, peppermint, pineapple, Mexican marigold	perennial	sun, part shade	culinary, medicinal, aromatic
Mullein	bi-annual	sun	medicinal
Oregano Cuban	container perennial	sun, winter protection	culinary
Oregano Greek, Italian	perennial	full sun	culinary
Oregano Mexican	perennial	sun	culinary
Parsley curled, flat leaf	biennial	part shade	culinary, medicinal
Pennyroyal	perennial	part shade	aromatic, medicinal
Peppermint	perennial	sun, part shade	culinary, medicinal
Peppermint black stemmed	perennial	sun, part shade	culinary, medicinal
Peppermint chocolate	perennial	sun, part shade	culinary
Perilla	annual	sun, part shade	culinary, medicinal
Powis Castle *Artemisia* *Absinthium*	perennial	sun	antiseptic, ornamental
Rosemary officinalis, hardy ARP	tender perennial	sun, part shade	cosmetic, culinary, medicinal
Rue	perennial or annual	sun, part shade	ornamental

Herb	Type	Location	Uses
Sage Bergarten, garden, golden or variegated, purple	perennial	full sun	culinary, medicinal
Sage, Pineapple	tender perennial	winter protection	culinary
Salad Burnet	perennial	sun	culinary
Santolina Green, grey	perennial	sun	ornamental
Sorrel French	perennial	sun, part shade	culinary
Spearmint	perennial	part shade	culinary
Summer Savory	annual	sun	culinary
Sweet Woodruff	tender perennial	shade, winter protection	aromatic
Tansy	perennial	sun	insecticide, ornamental
Tarragon French	tender perennial	sun	culinary
Tarragon Russian	perennial	sun	ornamental only
Thyme, all	perennial	full sun	aromatic, culinary, medicinal
Viola Odorata	perennial	shady, moist	cosmetic, medicinal
Winter Savory	perennial	sun	culinary
Wood betony	perennial	sun, part shade	medicinal, culinary
Yarrow	evergreen	sun	medicinal, cosmetic, ornamental

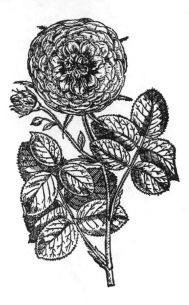

II

Origins of Old Roses

ROSE

EUROPEAN. *R. canina*, "Dog Rose" or "White Rose of York"

R. eglanteria
R. villosa
R. arvensis
R. pimpinellifolia, formerly R. spinosissima
R. gallica, best known as the apothecary rose
R. moshata, musk roses

AMERICAN. *R. virginiana*, golden fall foliage

R. nitida
R. palustris, Swamp Rose
R. setigera, Prairie Rose
R. carolina
R. blanda, 5-petalled single cherry-colored rose
R. foliolosa

ASIAN. *R. chinensis,* formerly *R. indica,* pink ever-blooming

> *R. laevigata* climber; "anemone" rose
> *R. bracteata* climber, single pure white bloom on a golden stamen
> *R. bansksiae* vining climber, white, yellow
> *R. multiflora* fencing rose with multiple blooms
> *R. wichuraiana* ground cover rose
> *R. rugosa,* native to Siberia, Alaska, Japan; very cold hardy roses
>   with hips. Rugosas sucker and spread
> *R. moyessi*
> *R. sweginzowii*

MIDDLE EASTERN. *R. pimpinellifoliae* yellow species

> *R. foetida*

UNKNOWN ORIGIN. *R. damascena* and hybrids (possibly Middle Eastern)

> *R. centifolia* and hybrids

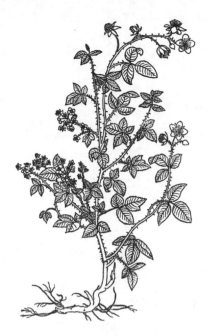

BLACKBERRY

III

A Guide to Nutrients

NUTRIENT	RELATED BODY FUNCTIONS
Vitamin A	repair of body tissue, production of visual purple (for night vision), antioxidant
B Complex	energy, metabolism, muscle tone, maintenance of gastrointestinal tract
Vitamin B_1	appetite, blood building, carbohydrate metabolism, circulation
Vitamin B_2	antibody and red cell formation, cell respiration, metabolism
Vitamin B_6	antibody formation, digestion, fat and protein utilization
Vitamin B_{12}	appetite, blood cell formation, cell longevity, prevents pernicious anemia
Biotin	cell growth, fatty acid production, vitamin B utilization
Choline	lecithin formation, gallbladder regulation, nerve transmission
Folic Acid	appetite, body growth and reproduction, red blood cell formation

Nutrient	Related Body Functions
Inositol	retards artery hardening, cholesterol
Niacin	circulation, sex hormone production, growth, metabolism
Pantothenic Acid	antibody formation, carbohydrate, fat, and protein conversion
Para Amino-Benzoic Acid	blood cell formation, graying hair
Panagamic Acid	cell oxidation and respiration, glandular system stimulation
Vitamin C	bone and teeth formation, collagen production, digestion, antioxidant
Vitamin D	calcium and phosphorus metabolism (bone formation), heart action
Vitamin E	aging retardation, anti-clotting factor, fertility, male potency, antioxidant
Vitamin F	arterial health, blood coagulation, glandular activity
Vitamin K	blood clotting (coagulation)
Vitamin P	blood vessel wall maintenance, minimizes bruising, antioxidant
Calcium	bone and tooth formation, blood clotting, heart rhythm
Chromium	blood sugar level, glucose metabolism, energy
Copper	bone and tooth formation, blood clotting, heart rhythm
Iodine	energy production, metabolism, physical and mental development
Iron	hemoglobin production, immunity
Magnesium	acid/alkaline balance, blood sugar metabolism, keeps calcium in the bones, smooth muscle relaxer
Manganese	enzyme activation, reproduction and growth, sex hormone production, blood sugar regulation

NUTRIENT	RELATED BODY FUNCTIONS
Phosphorus	bone/tooth formation, cell growth and repair, kidney function
Potassium	heartbeat, muscle contraction, nerve tranquilization
Sodium	electrolytes and normal cellular fluid level, proper muscle contraction
Zinc	cellular regeneration, carbohydrate metabolism, prostate gland function, secondary sexual characteristics, metabolism of vitamin B_I, phosphorus, and protein, immunity function

NUTRIENT	FOOD SOURCES OF NUTRIENT
Vitamin A	yellow and green fruits and vegetables, milk, fish liver oil
B Complex Vitamins	Brewer's yeast, liver, whole grains
Vitamin B_I	blackstrap molasses, Brewer's yeast, brown rice, fish, wheat germ
Vitamin B_2	blackstrap molasses, nuts, whole grains
Vitamin B_6	blackstrap molasses, Brewer's yeast, wheat germ
Biotin	legumes, whole grains
Choline	brewer's yeast, legumes, soybeans, wheat germ, lecithin
Folic Acid	green leafy vegetables, milk, whole grains, oysters
Inositol	blackstrap molasses, citrus fruits, Brewer's yeast, meat, vegetables
Niacin	Brewer's yeast, seafood, lean meats, milk, poultry, desiccated liver
Pantothenic Acid	Brewer's yeast, legumes, whole grains, salmon
Para Aminobenzoic Acid	blackstrap molasses, Brewer's yeast, liver, wheat germ
Panagamic Acid	Brewer's yeast, brown rice, meat, seeds, whole grains

NUTRIENT	FOOD SOURCES OF NUTRIENT
Vitamin C	citrus fruits, cantaloupe, green and red peppers, watermelon, white potatoes
Vitamin D	egg yolks, fortified milk, sunlight
Vitamin E	dark green vegetables, eggs, liver, desiccated liver
Vitamin F	vegetable oils (safflower, soy, corn, wheat germ, sunflower seeds)
Vitamin K	green leafy vegetables, safflower oil, blackstrap molasses, yogurt
Vitamin P	fruits (skin and pulp), apricots, cherries, grapes, grapefruit, berries
Calcium	milk, cheese, molasses, yogurt, almonds, cooked carrots, broccoli
Chromium	Brewer's yeast, clams, corn oil, whole grain cereals
Copper	legumes, nuts, seafood, raisins, molasses
Iodine	seafood, seaweeds, iodized salt
Iron	blackstrap molasses, eggs, fish, red meats, poultry, wheat germ, raisins
Magnesium	bran, corn, honey, green vegetables, nuts, seafood, spinach, seaweeds
Manganese	bananas, bran, celery, whole grains, egg yolks, green leafy vegetables, green tea
Phosphorus	eggs, fish, grains, poultry, yellow cheese
Potassium	dates, figs, peaches, tomato juice, blackstrap molasses, peanuts, apples, melons, white potatoes
Sodium	salt, milk, cheese, seafood, miso
Zinc	Brewer's yeast, liver, seafood, soybeans, spinach, mushrooms, sunflower and pumpkin seeds, red meat

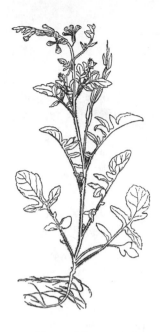

BLACK MUSTARD

IV

Purchasing Guide

Antique Roses

ANTIQUE ROSE EMPORIUM

9300 Lueckemeyer Road
Brenham, TX 77833

800 / 441-0002
Fax 409/836-0928

Send $5 for a 100-page, full color catalog with over 300 varieties of vegetative cuttings of original old roses. They ship December through mid-May.

Chinese Herbs

ALTERNATIVE MEDICINE, INC.

4612 Saldana
Fort Worth, TX 76133

817/292-2155
Fax 817/292-3335

This is where I buy my Chinese herbs. Chris Geng, their acupuncturist, gets the herbs directly from China.

Composting and Amendments

Rabbit Hill Farm   Route 3, Box 2936
Corsicana, TX 75110

Brown Nose earthworms for vermi-composting, earthworm castings, organic soil amendments, and organic herbs. Please send for catalog.

Dried Herbs

Simply Natural   P.O. Box 84
Aledo, TX 76008

817/441-6201

Carries dried herbs in bulk or small quantities, encapsulated herbs, and potpourri and supplies.

Flower Essences, Essential Oil Products, Natural Skincare

Herbal Health, Inc.   Box 330411
Ft. Worth, TX 76163

817/293-5410
Fax 817/293-3213
www.AromaHealthTexas.com

Organically grown and handprocessed. Petite Fleur Essences, Texas flower essences, essential oil blends, enfleurages, skincare, herbal tonics for longevity and radiant health, correspondance course on flower essences and tonic herbs by Judy Griffin.

Organic Seeds

Seeds of Change   P.O. Box 15700
Santa Fe, NM 87506
505 /438-8080

(to order catalog toll free) 800 /95-SEEDS
(to order toll free) 888 / 762-7333
Fax (toll free) 888 / 329-4762
Fax 505 /438-7052

One hundred percent of their seed is certified organic (certification from Oregon Tilth, one of the premier agencies in the country), open pollinated, and grown by a network of organic family farms and their own research farms. They also carry gardening merchandise, informational books on gardening, cookbooks, books for kids, and more.

Glossary

ABATE: To decrease or stop, i.e., symptoms of a disease.

ACTINOMYCETE MICROORGANISMS: Nitrogen-producing microorganisms available commercially to accelerate decomposition in compost.

ACUPUNCTURE: The activation of neural impulses by inserting needles into specific points along the body to move energy, promote circulation, inhibit pain, increase the immune response, reduce swelling, and promote healing in the body and mind through inner harmony.

ACUTE: The sudden onset and short duration of a disease, such as a cold or flu.

AERATE: To break up dense clay-like soil, allowing oxygen to be supplied to the loosened soil.

AERIAL (portion of plants): Above-ground portion of plants.

AFFIRMATION: A positive statement; a declaration of truth.

AGHIS OF RHODES: The first Greek chef recorded, renowned for using aromatic herbs.

AGUE: An old folk term for an intermittent fever.

ALCHEMY: A transformation process whereby the final result exceeds the initial product.

ALCOHOL: Organic compounds formed from hydrocarbons by substituting any number of hydroxyl (OH) groups for the same number of hydrogen atoms.

ALDEHYDE: The oxidation production of an alcohol, with a characteristic CHO. Example: acetaldehyde is CH_3CHO.

ALLANTOIN: A nitrogenous organic compound found in comfrey; used to heal and regenerate skin.

ALLOPATHIC: Western medical practices, employing chemically derived drugs therapeutically to alleviate symptoms.

ALTERATIVE: Blood purifier, such as echinacea root, that removes metabolic waste and toxins from the bloodstream.

AMEND (the soil): To enrich the composition and pH of the soil by adding organic matter, such as compost.

ANALGESIC: Pain reliever, i.e., a sedative or narcotic herb such as wild lettuce or valerian root.

ANASAZI: The "ancient ones," named by the Navajo Native Americans, who lived in Pueblos of the Arizona and Colorado desert.

ANNUAL: An herb that produces seeds and dies every year, usually at the first freeze, such as basil or epazote.

ANTISEPTIC LIQUOR: An alcoholic beverage made from herbs that destroys germs; a medicinal drink.

ANTISEPTIC: Disinfectant herbs, such as thyme, sage, and lavender.

AROMASIGNATURES: The color, shape, and fragrance that is unique to an aroma molecule inherent in every plant.

AROMATHERAPY: The use of essential oils to catalyze, balance, and strengthen the vital self-healing energies in the body, mind, and emotions.

ASHCAKES: Edible cakes made from mixing wood ashes with water to cook on an open fire during colonial and revolutionary times.

AURA: A distinctive, intangible quality surrounding a person, which creates an atmosphere mirroring the energy of an individual, often with color.

AYURVEDA: The ancient healing system of India.

AYURVEDIC: The ancient healing system of the East Indian sages, balancing the body, mind, and spirit.

BACILLUS THURINGIENSIS: A rod-shaped bacteria that is disease-producing, specifically to worms, moths, and butterfly larvae. It is harmless to beneficial insects (except butterfly larvae) and is generally sprayed onto plants to destroy worms.

BALM: A soothing ointment or lotion made from vegetable or animal fat infused with medicinal herbs.

BIENNIAL: An herb that blooms, produces seeds, and dies every two years, such as foxglove or parsley.

BILIARY: Pertaining to the liver and gallbladder, which produce and process bile into the intestines to digest fats and increase peristalsis for bowel movements.

BLOOD: The red blood cells and fluid processes of the body that are nutritive.

BOLT (as in plants bolting): A seed that suddenly sprouts, pushing itself up and out of the earth to greet the sun.

CALUMET: The stem of the peace pipe, carved from light wood and decorated with feathers, carvings, and beadwork. Calumet is of French origin, *chalumeau*. People of the Calumet are Algonkian tribes who migrated west from the northeast North American coast to the Great Lakes and south to Illinois and the Mississippi Valley.

CANCHA: Toasted corn eaten by Peruvians and Incan soldiers as a snack.

CANES (roses): A branch on a climbing rose.

CARDIOTONIC: An herb that enhances circulation, such as gotu kola or hawthorn berries.

CATALYZE: A substance that facilitates a chemical reaction or a change from one state into another, i.e., to encourage healing.

CELT: A member of an ancient Gaelic order of priests and sorcerers. They wore a serpent's egg badge for identification.

CHAKRAS: Vortices of subtle energy beside the spinal column that open and close like a fan. These were identified by ancient Rishi East Indian seers. Each of the seven chakras relates to particular organ functions and spiritual awakening in an individual.

CHANNA DAL: Yellow split peas.

CHRONIC: Frequent occurrence over a long period of time.

CLANS: The offspring and descendants from a common ancestry. Native American clans were matriarchal.

CLOISTER: A covered walkway with an open courtyard leading to another building in a monastery during medieval times.

COCINA COSTARRIQUEÑA: Costa Rican cuisine; literally Costa Rican kitchen.

COLD FRAME: A covered wooden box used to transition seedlings before they are planted in the garden. It shelters herbs from cold wind in the early spring and late fall.

COLIC: Sharp, sudden abdominal pain, usually involving cramping from gas.

COMMUNAL HOUSE: Multi-family lodging used by the Iroquois Native Americans.

COMPANION PLANTING: Arranging and interplanting herbs for their mutual benefit. There will be less competition for water, nutrients, and sunlight. The herbs will repel pests, improve their flavor, and attract predator insects.

COMPOSITAE FAMILY: Daisy family of herbs, echinacea, curry, and chamomile.

COMPOST: The product of accelerated decay of organic matter, such as decayed leaves, vegetable matter, and shredded bark, used to enrich soil composition.

COMPRESS: A clean cloth or pad soaked in a strong medicinal herbal tea and applied locally to an affected part of the body.

CONDIMENT: Herbs, spices, or seasoning added to flavor food.

CONSERVE: A preserve prepared from fruit.

COSMIC CONSCIOUSNESS: A release from the physical world of limitations, returning to the Source of Creation.

CREOLE CUISINE: A mixture of French, Spanish, and African-American seasoning, generally characterized as hot and spicy.

CRONES: Women beyond the child-bearing age, often referred to as wise women or herbalists.

CRUCIFERAE: Mustard family, including horseradish and black mustard.

DAMPEN OFF: A fungal virus that affects the roots of seedlings, causing them to suddenly wilt and die.

DECIDUOUS: A tree, shrub, or herb that loses its leaves during the winter.

DECOCTION: Drawing the medicinal qualities from herbs by cooking and steeping.

DEFICIENT: A chronic condition in the body, lacking nutrients, blood, or moisture, causing hypofunctioning of an organ or physiological system.

DEMULCENT: A soothing, healing herb, such as marshmallow root, which coats and sedates the skin and internal tissues.

DIAPHORETIC: A herb that has the ability to increase perspiration, i.e., boneset or sage.

DIATOMACEOUS EARTH: An agricultural grade of silica that repels or destroys many crawling insects, such as slugs, ants, and cutworms.

DIFFUSION: To reduce an herbal tea to a lower concentration.

DISTILLATION: The process of purifying a liquid through evaporation and condensation. Water is often used to produce steam to facilitate condensation. The distillation method is used to produce many essential oils.

DIURETIC HERBS: Herbs, such as parsley, corn silk, and dandelion leaves, which stimulate kidney sensory nerves to promote urination. They are generally high in potassium.

DOCTRINE OF SIGNATURES: A cross-cultural belief of indigenous natives that an herb's shape, size, and color identifies its medicinal property. A kidney bean is shaped like a kidney and facilitates urinary function.

DRIP IRRIGATION: Conserving water evaporation by slowly watering, drop by drop, into the soil.

DRUID: A member of an order of priests in ancient Briton and Gaul who appears in Irish legends as prophets and sorcerers.

ECLECTICS: Those who followed Galen's herbal practice during the Middle Ages.

ELIXIR: A panacea or cure-all.

EMETIC: A substance used to induce vomiting, such as ipecac. Emetics were used by Native Americans before fasting. Today, emetics are used to remove an ingested toxic substance, such as a poisonous mushroom, from the system.

EMOLLIENT: A product or herb that is soothing to the skin or mucous membrane, such as comfrey or cocoa butter.

ENDOCRINE: The organs in the body that produce hormones, i.e., pituitary, pancreas, adrenals and thyroid glands.

ENFLEURAGE: The saturation of animal or vegetable fat with fresh, fragrant flowers and herbs to produce an aromatic compound.

EROSION: To diminish by degrees; the gradual wearing away of soil.

ESSENCE: The most subtle, refined form of a flower plant.

ESSENTIAL OIL: A complex, highly volatile aromatic oil. The aroma is formed in the chloroplasts of the plant's leaves, containing alcohols, esters, terpenes, ketones, and aldehydes. Unlike fatty oils, such as jojoba and sesame oil, essential oils evaporate into the air or skin, releasing their aroma.

ESTER: A compound formed by an organic acid with an alcohol-eliminating water.

EURASIA: The continents of Europe and Asia.

EXCESS: Congestion of too much mucous, fluid, fat, or toxins in the body or the hyperfunctioning of an organ or physiological system.

EXTERNAL: Affecting the superficial tissues, such as hair, skin, muscles, vessels, and peripheral nerves and circulation.

FIREPOT DISHES: Cuisine cooked in a communal pot over an open fire in Manchuria and Mongolia.

FISH EMULSION: A blend of partially decomposed fish, high in nitrogen, used by organic gardeners to fertilize their gardens and plants. Dilution directions are on the label.

FIVE CHINESE ELEMENTS: Wood, fire, earth, metal, and water pertain to specific organ systems and characteristics in the body, derived from nature.

FLAT: Twelve to twenty-four plants of the same variety, i.e., a flat of thyme.

FLOWER WATER TONIC: A cold water infusion of a flower drunk to cool the mental, emotional, and physical nature of the recipient.

FLUSHING: The use of running water to flush salts out of topsoil. Salts are particularly prevalent in chemically fertilized soil.

FOLIAR FEEDING: Fertilizing plants by spraying the leaves with a water-based nutrient, such as seaweed or fish emulsion.

FOUR HUMOR THEORY: A medieval classification of food's energy: hot, hot and moist, cold and dry, and cold and moist.

FULFILLMENT: Realizing the heart's desire.

FUMIGANT: A vaporous substance used to treat an area by saturation. Odors can be treated with fumigants.

FUNGICIDE: A substance, such as chamomile tea, that stops the growth of fungi on plants. Fungal growth may cause seedlings to wilt and die prematurely.

GALLS: Knotty swellings on plant roots that inhibit nutrient uptake resulting in stunted growth, wilting, and death.

GERMICIDAL: Disinfects and destroys virus and germs. Example: eucalyptus, thyme.

GERMINATE: To sprout. As seeds germinate, they sluff an outer, protective coating and push up through the soil to grow toward sunlight.

GILL (in recipe for Rice "Woffles"): A measurement used by American colonists to equal half a cup.

GINSENG COOKER: A ceramic container designed with a fitted, flat lid and a dome lid that fits on top of it. The container may hold one to three cups of water to cook herbs placed in another pan of boiling water, like a double boiler.

HARDEN OFF: A transitional process for seedlings about to go into the garden after six to eight weeks of sprouting. They are moved from a protected environment into a cool, shady outside area for several days before planting them in the garden to prevent wilting and shock.

HARMONY: The balance of beauty and creativity in the nature of an individual, often described as a state of grace.

HATHOR: The Egyptian goddess of love, mirth, and joy.

HEMOSTATIC: A herb that arrests bleeding, such as yarrow (topically) or shepherd's purse (internally).

HEMOTONIC: Blood tonic, building and fortifying the red blood cells, such as yellow dock.

HEPATIC: Pertaining to liver function.

HERB: A seed plant that is not hardwood and may have medicinal, aromatic, or culinary properties.

HIGHER INTUITION: Divine guidance.

HOMEOSTASIS: A state of balance in the body.

HONEYDEW: The excretion of aphids and mealybugs that has a sticky residue. Ants guard these insects and eat the honeydew.

HUMUS: The organic part of topsoil formed from decaying matter. It holds moisture and nutrients in the soil.

HYBRID: The offspring of genetically different parents, as in old roses.

ILLUMINATION: Enlightened awareness.

IMMUNE STIMULANT: A herb that increases the white blood count in an individual, mobilizing the proper immune response. Example: echinacea root.

INFUSION: To steep an herbal tea without boiling.

INITIATE: A person who undergoes special instruction and ceremony to be indoctrinated into a certain group. The Ojibwa Grand Medicine Society initiated members and taught them the medicinal properties of herbs.

INNATE: Inborn, naturally occurring.

ION: An electrically charged particle.

JAGUAR CULT: Followers of the mythological jaguar god throughout Middle and South American religions.

JOHNNY CAKES: A light cornbread enjoyed by American colonists.

KETONE: The oxidation process of a secondary alcohol, such as $(CH_3)_2CO$, acetone, containing the carbonyl group (=CO). Ketones in the physical body are the end product of fat metabolism.

KIDNEY YANG: Adrenal cortical function, enhancing vitality and reducing inflammation.

KIDNEY YIN: Adrenal medulla function, enhancing nutritive and electrolyte balance in bodily fluids.

KITCHEN COMPOST: An inside compost contained in a margarine tub for small, nonanimal kitchen scraps.

KIVA: Secret, subterranean ceremonial room decorated with wall paintings of images and spirits for the use of Native American men.

KNOT GARDEN: A symmetrical, enclosed garden with wheels of interconnected herbs patterned in a knot. Knot gardens were popular during medieval and Elizabethan times.

LACERATE: To roughly tear.

LEGUMES: The bean family, highly nitrogenous plants eaten for their high protein content. They require a grain in a 1 to 2 proportion to make a complete protein.

LOAMY SOIL: A loose soil mixture of sand, humus, and silt.

LONGEVITY HERB: A herb that will strengthen the immunity and vitality of an individual to prolong the quality and age of the recipient. Longevity herbs promote fertility as well as creativity.

LONGHOUSES: A multi-dwelling communal log house sheathed with elm bark built by the Iroquois and northeastern woodland Native Americans.

MANO: A handstone used to grind peanuts, maize, and cacao seeds, used by the Mesoamericans with a metate.

MEAD: An alcoholic beverage brewed from honey, malt, yeast, and water.

MEDICATED CLYSTER: Medicated compress.

MEDICINAL: Therapeutic qualities of herbs and plants.

MEDIEVAL PLEASURE GARDEN: Herb gardens and vineyards interplanted with bright, colorful flowers to please the senses.

MERIDIANS: Pathways of energy in the physical body affecting organic and systemic synergy, accessed by acupuncture and acupressure.

METAPHYSICAL: The study of the unseen ultimate nature of various natural laws and aspects of creation.

METATE: A three-legged stone used to grind maize and cacao seeds by the ancient Mesoamericans.

MOONG DAL: Yellow mung beans.

MORDANT: A caustic agent added to brighten the color of a dye, such as alum and cream of tartar. The material is soaked in the mordant before dyeing occurs.

MORTAR: A strong bowl where food or herbs are crushed with a pestle.

MULCH: A protective covering of organic material, such as redwood bark, wheat straw, or black and white newspaper, used to reduce evaporation of water and protect plant roots from heat and cold.

NATURALIZE: A plant that establishes itself in a new area like a native plant. For example, many herbs have naturalized in America from Europe, such as dandelion, yarrow, and thyme.

NEEM: *Azadiracta indica,* a botanical insecticide obtained from the neem tree sap in East India, where it is native. It is used to deter flies and insects during feast days and drunk as a medicinal tonic for malaria fever. It is applied topically in coconut oil to alleviate ringworm.

NIXTAMALIZATION: A Mesoamerican cooking method of soaking ripe maize in water, then cooking it with lime or wood ashes to produce a softer grain.

NOISETTE: A variety of old roses, originating in America. They are a cross of Old Blush and the Musk Rose, *R. moschata,* known for producing clusters of flowers late in the fall as well as spring blooms.

NOSEGAY: A small bouquet of flowers, often worn pinned near the bosom of a young woman.

NYMPH (the one mentioned under mint, not the insect stage): A lesser goddess in ancient mythology represented as a maiden or girl.

NYMPH: An immature insect without wings.

OJIBWA: A Great Lakes tribe also known as the Chippewa, who organized the Grand Medicine Society professing right living and the use of herbal combinations for health and longevity. The Grand Medicine Society is also known as the Midewiwin, including the Winnebego, Omaha, and other Great Lakes and Prairie Tribes.

OLD ROSE: A rose born before 1867. Damask roses can be traced to Babylonian gardens, tea roses to ancient China. They are not descendants of the originals. They are cuttings from the same plants.

OMEN: The sign of a future occurrence.

ORGANIC MATTER: Material containing carbon compounds that decay readily.

ORGANIC: Herbs and foods grown without chemical insecticides or fertilizers.

ORRIS ROOT: The root of the Florentine iris used as a potpourri fixative.

PAGAN: One who celebrates life through nature, the seasons, and lunar and solar cycles.

PANACEA: A remedy that is a cure-all for disease.

PARACHYMOZINE: An enzyme used by medieval monks to curdle milk to make cheese. It was derived from plant material.

PEARLASH: American colonial substitute for yeast made from soda salt obtained from wood ashes.

PENANCE: An act performed to repent sins.

PERENNIAL: A plant that lives throughout each season, or dies down in the winter, like comfrey, and returns with the spring.

PERIMETER (in planning the herb garden): The boundary of an enclosed garden.

PERPETUALS: An everlasting plant, such as an old rose.

PESTLE: Used with a mortar to crush herbs.

PESTS: Insects that eat leaves, stems, and roots of culinary herbs and foods. Pests often have a pointed "nose."

PHARMACOPOEIA: A text describing drug and medicinal preparations.

PHOTOSYNTHESIS: A process of chlorophyll-containing plants producing carbohydrates from water and carbon dioxide in the air.

PINANG KERRIE: The national dish of South Africa.

PINCHING: Removing the top stem growth of herbs to encourage growth. Gardeners pinch the growth off using the thumb and index finger down to the nearest lateral growth of leaves.

PIÑON NUTS: The edible seeds of a variety of low-growing pine in Western North America.

PLANT ROTATION: Alternating crops and plants each year to reduce viral and insect invasion. For example, planting annuals, like chamomile and basil, in different herb beds each year.

POTPOURRI: A mixture of scented, colorful herbs, spices, and flowers used for aromatherapy.

POULTICE: A medicated herbal compound spread on a cloth and applied to a sore or injury.

PRAYER STICK: A ceremonial offering made of eagle down attached to an unpainted wand of a local tree or shrub, such as the willow for the Pima Native Americans, and placed into the dancing ground or in sacred baskets during communal gatherings.

PREDATOR INSECTS: Beneficial as pollinators and predators, such as ladybugs who eat aphids and butterflies who pollinate flowers.

PROPAGATE: To reproduce plants by sowing seeds, rooting cuttings, and starting new plants from dividing one, such as yarrow or irises.

PROPERTIES: Qualities unusual and unique. Example: The property of echinacea root as an antibiotic blood cleanser.

PROTEIN METABOLISM: Changing proteins into simple sugars to build or rebuild the physical body.

PUEBLOS: Village dwellings of large communities that were made from adobe or stone in the desert areas of the Southwest. Underground ceremonial rooms, known as kivas, were built in each village.

PURGATIVE: A strong laxative, such as senna leaves.

PYRETHRIN: The active ingredient in the feverfew pyrethrum plant used as a botanical insecticide. The roots, leaves, and flowers produce pyrethrin. The spray paralyzes insects, who die shortly afterwards. Pyrethrin is toxic to birds and fish.

RADIANT HEALTH: The strengthening of the body and mind, encouraging adaptability and a harmonious synchronization with Nature.

RANUNCULAE: The buttercup family.

RESPIRATION (in plants): The process of oxidation and elimination of gases. Plants take in carbon dioxide and eliminate oxygen.

RHIZOME: A fleshy, rootlike, horizontal, underground plant stem that forms shoots above ground.

ROSARIANS: Specialists who grow and identify roses. They are responsible for propagating new varieties and finding old roses in nature to reintroduce into society.

ROSARY: A circular string of beads representing wholeness and time, endless duration. The rosary was used by many cultures in spiritual invocations.

ROSE HIPS: The ornamental fall fruit of old roses, ranging in color from orange to purple and black. Rose hips are a rich source of vitamin C.

ROTENONE: A botanical insecticide. It is extracted from the Derris plants in Asia and cube plants in South America. It is a slow-acting stomach poison in insects and fish. It is a respiratory irritant to humans. Wear a mask.

SACRISTAN GARDEN: A monastery garden of flowers grown for the altar during church ceremonies.

SALERNO SCHOOL OF MEDICINE: The medieval European school of medicine in Italy.

SAUCEMAKERS: Fourteenth-century professional cooks who created seasonings for fish and variety of foods.

SAUTÉ: To lightly brown in a little oil or fat.

SEA SQUILL: A sea onion that is used for rat poison.

SÉANCE: A meeting to communicate with spirits.

SELF-REALIZATION: Liberation from attitudes restricting our greatest achievements.

SELF-TRUST: The ability to acquire inner guidance and follow it, overcoming any difficulties.

SHAKTI: The nurturing principle of life, referred to as the Divine Mother by the East Indians.

SHAMAN: A Native American priest who uses supernatural powers to cure an ill individual.

SIMPLING: Using one herb to create a therapeutic effect. Example: Mint tea as a digestant.

SIPAPU: A mystical hole in the center of a ceremonial kiva, representing the place of emergence from the Womb of Mother Nature, the power of the feminine.

SOIL pH: A value measuring the acidity or alkalinity of soil, measured from 0 to 14. Below 7.0 is acid, above 7.0 is alkaline. Herbs grow in 7.0 pH, which is considered neutral. Correcting soil pH will assure the proper absorption of nutrients from the soil.

SOPORIFIC: A herb that causes sleep or drowsiness, such as hops or valerian root.

SPECIES: A category of plants that are closely related and may potentially intermix with one another. Example: Mints, basils, and oreganos can cross, losing their flavor.

SPLIT CAKES: A scone-like pancake eaten by American colonists.

STEEP: To allow herbs to set in boiled water, covered and placed away from the heat, to produce an infusion or tea.

STREWING HERBS: Aromatic herbs, such as rosemary and thyme, laid on the floors of medieval banquet halls and homes to dispel odors, which were believed to cause disease. Strewing herbs also repelled insects.

SUPERNATURAL: Phenomenon outside of nature, related to divinity.

Sᴡᴇᴀᴛs (Native American): To use steam and heat in a closed cubicle to draw out toxins from the body.

Sᴡᴇᴇᴛ Bᴀʏs: Bay laurel trees were often referred to as sweet bays; also, an alcove or recessed area.

Sʏɴᴇʀɢʏ: The combination of two separate elements that can achieve together far more than what can be achieved separately.

Sʏɴᴛʜᴇsɪs: The production of a substance by combining two chemically simpler substances.

Sʏʀᴜᴘ: A thickened sugar and water solution, often flavored with herbs or flowers.

T Hᴇʟᴘᴇʀ Cᴇʟʟs: Thymic immune cells which regulate the immune system's response by moderating thymic killer cells and suppressor cells.

T Sᴜᴘᴘʀᴇssᴏʀ Cᴇʟʟs: Immune cells released from the thymus gland that sedate the immune response. These are helpful in autoimmune diseases such as allergic reactions, i.e., hives, hay fever, Crohn's disease.

Tᴀɢɪɴᴇs: A Moroccan slow-cooked meat stew.

Tᴀᴏ: The dynamic flow of nature as an undifferentiated whole.

Tᴀᴘʀᴏᴏᴛ: The main root growing downward of a plant. Examples: Dill, fennel, and comfrey are herbs that have taproots.

Tɪʟʟ: Preparing soil by plowing and turning it several inches into the soil.

Tɪɴᴄᴛᴜʀᴇ: An alcoholic solution of a medicinal herb. Soaking an herb, such as echinacea root, in alcohol for three weeks or more will draw the medicinal properties into the alcohol.

Tᴏɴɪᴄ: An herbal combination blended specifically for certain conditions to nourish, support, and invigorate the body.

Tᴏᴘɪᴀʀʏ: A tree or herb trimmed into a conical shape for decorative purposes.

Tᴏxɪɴ: A substance or byproduct of the metabolism of an organism that is capable of producing antibodies.

TRIDOSHA: The three humor system of fire, water, and air used by the Ayurvedic East Indian healers to balance the body, mind, and spirit.

TUBERS: Underground, fleshy stem, such as a potato plant.

TUSSIE MUSSIE: Victorian nosegay worn by unmarried women and men to exchange messages of love. Each flower and herb had a meaning: rosemary meant remember me; violets vowed innocence; marjoram meant joy; and rose meant success.

UMBELLIFERAE: Carrot and parsley family of herbs with a flower cluster arising near one point of the main stem.

UPANISHADS: Oral and written East Indian doctrines and teachings completed between 700 and 300 B.C., which include ancient stories of mystical revelation.

URAD DAL: Split beans.

VEDAS: The Sanskrit word for "knowledge." The Vedas are books of sacred hymns and rituals originally written for the priests.

VOLATILE OIL: The chemical properties in essential oils and herbs that can change quickly from a liquid to a vapor, releasing aromatic and therapeutic properties.

"WOMEN IN TRAVAIL": Women experiencing labor pains during the birthing process.

Bibliography

Abraham, George and Katy. *Organic Gardening Under Glass*. Emmaus, PA: Rodale Press, Inc., 1975.

Albyn, Carol and Lois Webb. *The Multicultural Cookbook for Students*. Phoenix, AZ: The Oryx Press, 1993.

Barr, Andy, et. al. *Traditional Aboriginal Medicines*. Darwin, Australia: Conservation Commission of the Northern Territory, 1993.

Beales, Peter. *Classic Roses*. NY: Holt, Rineheart, & Winston, 1985.

Beilenson, Evelyn. *Early American Cooking*. NY: Peter Pauper Press Inc., 1985.

Beinfield, H. and E. Korngold. *Between Heaven and Earth*. NY: Ballantine Books, 1991.

Bhumichitr, Vatcharin. *The Taste of Thailand*. NY: Antheum Press, 1988.

Boland, Maureen and Bridges. *Old Wives' Lore for Gardeners*. London: The Bodley Head, Ltd., 1985.

Bugiaali, Juiliano. *The Fine Art of Italian Cooking*. NY: Random House, 1989.

Campbell, Joseph. *Mythologies of the Primitive Planters: The Middle and Southern Americas*. NY: Harper & Row, 1989.

Campbell, Tyrone and Joel Kopp. *Navajo Pictorial Weaving*. NY: Dutton Studio Books, 1991.

Carter, Margaret. *The Little Book of Herbs*. Newark, NJ: Chartwell Books, Inc., 1993.

Chang, W., I. Chang, A. Kutscher, L. Kutscher. *Chinese Dessert Dim Sum, Snack Cookbook*. NY: Sterling Pub. Co., 1986.

Chase, A.W., M.D. *Dr. Chase's Recipe Book and Household Physician*. Detroit: F. B. Dickerson Co., 1899.

Chin, Wu Yeow and Hsuan King. *Chinese Medical Herbs*. Sebastopol, CA: CRCS Publications, 1992.

Christopher, Thomas. *In Search of Lost Roses*. Location: NY: Summit Books, 1989.

Coe, Sophie D. *America's First Cuisines*. Austin, TX: University of Texas Press, 1994.

Cooper, J.C. *An Illustrated Encyclopedia of Traditional Symbols*. London: Thames and Hudson, Ltd., 1978.

Corey, Helen. *Food From Biblical Lands*. Avenel, NJ: Antiochian Orthodox Christian Archdiocese of North America, 1989.

Dehlvi, Hazrat. *Prophetic Medical Sciences*. Delhi: P.M.S. Inc., 1977.

Densmore, Frances. *How Indians Use Wild Plants for Food, Medicine and Crafts*. NY: Dover Publications, Inc, 1974.

DeWitt, Dave and Arthur Pais. *A World of Curries*. NY: Little, Brown and Co., 1994.

Dover Publishing. *The Language of Flowers*. Illustrated by Kate Greenway. Ruston, LA: Dover Publishing, 1965.

Farrington, Doris. *Fireside Cooks and Black Kettle Recipes*. NY: Bobbs-Merrill Co. Inc., 1976.

Fishwick, Marshall. *Thomas Jefferson American Heritage Cookbook*. City: Publisher, 1964.

The Folklore of Plants. Dyer, 1889.

Foster, Steven. "An Aztec Herbal." *The Herb Companion*, Oct./Nov. 1994.

Frawley, David, O.M.D. *Ayurvedic Healing*. Salt Lake City, UT: Passage Press, 1989.

Fussell, Betty. *The Story of Corn*. NY: Alfred Knopf, Inc., 1992.

Griffin, Judy, Ph.D. *Around the World with Herbs.* Fort Worth, TX: Herbal Essence Inc., 1989, 1991, 1992, 1993.

Griffin, Judy, Ph.D. *Healing from the Heart* course (manual and tapes). Fort Worth, TX: Herbal Essence, Inc., 1985, 1986.

Griffin, Judy, Ph.D. *Healing from the Heart.* Ft. Worth, TX: Herbal Essence, Inc., 1985.

Griffin, Judy, Ph.D. *Herbal Aromasignatures.* Fort Worth, TX: Herbal Essence, Inc., 1994.

Griffin, Judy, Ph.D. *Mother Nature's Kitchen.* Fort Worth, TX: Herbal Essence, Inc., 1993.

Griffin, Judy, Ph.D. *Returning to the Source.* Fort Worth, TX: Herbal Essence, Inc., 1983, 1984, 1985, 1988, 1989.

Griffin, Judy, Ph.D. *Romancing the Rose.* Fort Worth, TX: Herbal Essence, Inc., 1995.

Griffin, Judy, Ph.D. *Slice of Life.* Fort Worth, TX: Herbal Essence, Inc., 1986.

Grigson, Jane. *Book of European Cookery.* NY: Antheneum Books, 1983.

Hatfield, Audrey Wynne. *The Weed Herbal.* NY: Sterling Publishing Co., 1983.

Hawkes, Alex. *The Flavors of the Caribbean and Latin America.* NY: Viking Press, 1978.

Health Plants. NY: Crescent Books, 1975.

Hill, Madeline and Gwen Barclay. *Southern Herb Growing.* Fredericksberg, TX: Shearer Publishing, 1987.

Hill, Thomas. *The Gardener's Labyrinth.* Oxford, UK: Oxford University Press, 1985.

Historical Atlas of World Mythology, Vol. II, Part 3. NY: Harper and Row, 1989.

The Inglenook Doctor Book. Elgin, IL: Brethren Publishing House, 1903.

Jones, Evan. *American Food: The Gastronomic Story.* NY: E.P. Dutton & Co. Inc., 1975.

Josephy, Alvin M., ed. *Indians.* NY: Simon and Schuster, Inc., 1961.

Karasch, Barrie. *Native Harvests.* NY: Random House Press, 1977.

Kimball, Yeffe and Jean Anderson. *The Art of American Indian Cooking.* NY: Doubleday and Co., Inc., 1965.

Lad, Vasant. *Ayurveda: The Science of Self Healing.* Santa Fe: Lotus Press, 1984.

Lad, Vassant and David Frawley. *The Yoga of Herbs.* Santa Fe: Lotus Press, 1986.

Lawrence, Martin. *The Country Gardener's Almanac.* NY: Main Street Press, 1990.

Leighton, Ann. *Early American Gardens.* Boston: Houghton Mifflin Co., 1969.

Leonard, Jonathan. *Latin American Cooking.* NY: Time Life Books, 1976.

Mabey, Richard. *The New Age Herbalist.* NY: Macmillan, 1988.

Miller, Gloria. *The Thousand Recipe Chinese Cookbook.* NY: Simon & Schuster, Inc., 1966.

Mitchel, Patricia. *Four Centuries of American Herbs.* Chatham, VA: Sims Mitchell House, 1993.

Mitchell, Patricia. *Cooking in the Young Republic: 1780–1850.* Chatham, VA: Sims Mitchell House, 1992.

Mitchell, Patricia. *Revolutionary Recipes.* Chatham, VA: Sims Mitchell House, 1988, 1991.

Morley, Sylvanus G. *The Ancient Maya.* Stanford, CA: Stanford University Press, 1963.

Murphy, Wendy. *Beds and Borders.* Boston: Houghton Mifflin Co., 1994.

Norman, Jill. *The Complete Book of Spices.* London: Dorling Kindersley Ltd., 1990.

Ortiz, Elizabeth. *The Complete Book of Mexican Cooking.* NY: Ballantine Books, 1965.

Paradissus, Chrissa. *The Best Book of Greek Cookery.* Athens, Greece: Efstathiadis Bros., 1976.

Parkinson, John. *Theatrum Botanicum: The Theator of Plants.* London: Thomas Cotes, 1640.

Peyton, James. *La Cocinera de la Frontera.* Sante Fe: Red Crane Books, 1994.

Prabhavananda, Swami and Frederick Manchester. *The Wisdom of the Hindu Mystics: The Upanishads Breath of the External.* NY: Penguin Books, 1975.

Reader's Digest. *Magic and Medicine of Plants.* NY: The Reader's Digest Association, Inc., 1986, 1989.

Rieske, Bill. *Navajo Hopi Dyes.* Salt Lake City, UT: Indian Publishers, 1940.

Rodale Press, Inc. *The Organic Way to Plant Protection.* Emmaus, PA: Rodale Press, Inc., 1966.

Rodale's Illustrated Encyclopedia of Herbs. Emmaus, PA: Rodale Press, 1987.

Roden, Claudia. *A Book of Middle Eastern Food.* NY: Vintage Books, 1974.

Sahni, Julie. *Classic Indian Vegetarian and Grain Cooking.* NY: William Morrow and Co. Inc., 1985.

Sams, Jaimie and David Carson. *Medicine Cards.* Santa Fe: Bear and Co., 1988.

Seed, Diane. *Favorite Indian Food.* Berkeley, CA: Ten Speed Press, 1990.

Seed, Diane. *The Top One Hundred Italian Dishes.* Berkeley, CA: Ten Speed Press, 1991.

Shaykh Hakim Moinuddin. *The Book of Sufi Healing.* Chisti: Rochester Vt. Inner Traditions International Ltd., 1991.

Starr, Kathy. *The Soul of Southern Cooking.* Jackson: University of Mississippi, 1989.

Stodola, Jiri and Jan Vola. *The Illustrated Books of Herbs*. Edited by Sarah Bunney. NY: Gallery Books, 1984.

Stuart, Malcolm, ed. *The Encyclopedia of Herbs and Herbalism*. NY: Crescent Books, 1979.

Taube, Karl. *Aztec and Maya Myths*. Austin, TX: University of Texas Press, 1993.

Teeguarden, Ron. *Chinese Tonic Herbs*. Tokyo: Japan Publications, Inc., 1984.

The American Heritage Book of Indians. NY: American Heritage Publishing Co., Inc., 1961.

Tierra, Michael. *Planetary Herbology*. Santa Fe: Lotus Press, 1988.

Underhill, Ruth. *Red Man's America*. Chicago: University of Chicago Press, 1953, 1972.

Weiner, Michael. *Earth Medicine Earth Food*. NY: Ballantine Books, 1971.

White, Jon Manchip. *Everyday Life of the North American Indian*. NY: Indian Head Books, 1979.

Yusuf, Ali. *The Meaning of the Illustrious Qur'an*. Lahore, Pakistan: Ashraf Press, 1967.

Acknowledgments

A blessing to the folks who helped make this book happen. Fran Goreham was instrumental in editing, artwork, photography, and friendship. Gail Morris is the fastest typist in the West and Pat Cowan went to great lengths to draw the great landscape designs. Many friends and students offered photos and helped run my business while I wrote: the De Maeres, Judi Martin, Janet Taylor, Leza Wilson, Brenda Spaulding, Harlene Newhart, Peggy Hammel, Denise Stevens, Maxine Briggs, the Hickmans, Lucy Harrell, Shelli Parker and Donna Buie. My children, Vincent, Gina and Jason Ermis, who volunteered to try many of the recipes, complaining that their mom cooked with sticks, and my parents, Howard and Flamina Palombi, who taught me to love gardening. A special thanks to the very friendly and talented staff at Llewellyn, especially Becky Zins, my editor . . . and, of course, Mother Nature, who made this possible for all of us.

Bloom in Peace.

Index

*recipes are in bold print